Surgery for Osteoporotic Fractures

Frankie Leung · Tak Wing Lau
Editors

Surgery for Osteoporotic Fractures

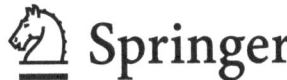 Springer

Editors
Frankie Leung
Department of Orthopaedics and
Traumatology
Queen Mary Hospital
Pokfulam, Hong Kong

Tak Wing Lau
Department of Orthopaedics and
Traumatology
The University of Hong Kong
Pokulam, Hong Kong, Hong Kong

ISBN 978-981-99-9698-8   ISBN 978-981-99-9696-4   (eBook)
https://doi.org/10.1007/978-981-99-9696-4

This Springer imprint is published by the registered company Springer Nature Singapore Pte Ltd.
The registered company address is: 152 Beach Road, #21-01/04 Gateway East, Singapore
189721, Singapore

Paper in this product is recyclable.

Foreword

Osteoporotic fracture is a major cause leading to mortality in the elderly, and this problem is reaching a pandemic level worldwide. Yet, challenges appear at all levels, from fracture healing to fracture fixation, from rehabilitation to secondary prevention, from medical treatment to social care. This requires a team approach involving not only surgeons and therapist but also social workers and policy makers. Further advances will need the collaborative efforts of surgeons, biologists, engineers, sociologists and social advocates.

The authors of this book are all seasoned surgeons who have extensive experience in fracture treatment and also in new designs of implants and method of fixation. They had also won awards for their clinical pathways for osteoporotic fracture treatment. Each chapter is written by authors with personal experience on the topic and illustrated with their own cases. What is most valuable is that the experience comes from one trauma centre. This ensures consistency at all levels. It also sets standards for future works on osteoporotic fractures.

Department of Orthopaedics and Traumatology   Shew-Ping Chow
The University of Hong Kong,
Pokfulam, Hong Kong

Preface

Fracture fixation surgery remains the bread-and-butter job of every orthopaedic surgeon. In the 1990s when we started our residency training, there were only few subspecialized fracture surgeons. Most fracture surgeries were being done by general orthopaedic surgeons and operative results were not always reliable. As surgeons began to focus on improving fracture care, some of them became 'fracture' surgeons. Since the advent of these fracture subspecialists, the knowledge and surgical skills have dramatically improved. New implants such as locking plates were also devised, and we can now successfully treat even the most severe and unstable fractures, including osteoporotic ones.

In the meantime, demographics are changing swiftly throughout the world with life expectancy well above 70 years. Incidence of osteoporotic fractures has been increasing steadily. Moreover, with an active lifestyle of our older patients, there is a huge demand for a prompt and effective treatment and an early return to premorbid level. Our Department at Queen Mary Hospital recognized such need and set up a Division of Orthopaedic Trauma with a designated daily operative list for fracture surgeries. Since then, our practice has evolved and surgeons from various countries are attracted to visit or undergo fellowships at our centre.

The aim of this book is to provide succinct and up-to-date guidance on osteoporotic fracture surgery, based on our philosophy and knowledge gleaned from years of professional practice. We do hope that this book not only covers the vast majority of important issues but also adds to related existing knowledge.

Thanks to all the authors of various chapters who have been 'graduates' from our Orthopaedic Trauma training and are willing to share their knowledge on managing older patients with trauma, along with their personal operative tips and tricks on osteoporotic fractures.

Naturally, our heartiest thanks go to our wives and family members for their unwavering support throughout our careers.

Pokfulam, Hong Kong   Frankie Leung
Pokfulam, Hong Kong   Tak-Wing Lau

Contents

Fracture Healing in Osteoporotic Bone

Janus Siu Him Wong and Frankie Leung

1.1 Introduction

Fracture healing is a delicately choreographed dance between mesenchymal stem cells, osteoblasts, osteoclasts, osteoconductive matrix, osteoinductive mediators, local mechanical environment, vascularity, cellular pathways, local and systemic factors. Ageing, osteoporosis, and drugs used to treat osteoporosis are among risk factors that impact fracture healing. An understanding of physiology, biomechanics, and effects of anti-osteoporotic drugs would be helpful to the orthopaedic surgeon in optimising osteoporotic fracture fixation outcomes and minimising complications.

Despite the common belief that bone healing in the elderly would be slower than younger patients, whether fracture healing is inherently different in elderly patients and the exact mechanism of such remains a conundrum. In general, there are four possible mechanisms in which bone healing can be affected in elderly patients: ageing, osteoporosis, the mechanical environment, and anti-osteoporosis medications.

J. S. H. Wong (✉) · F. Leung
Department of Orthopaedics and Traumatology, Queen Mary Hospital, The University of Hong Kong, Pokfulam, Hong Kong
e-mail: januswong@connect.hku.hk; klleunga@hku.hk

1.2 Fracture Healing in Ageing Bone

The ageing osteoporotic skeleton remodels to maximise strength in face of reduced bone mass. Normal bone continuously remodels through a cycle of osteoclastic bone resorption, coupled with osteoblastic osteoid production which subsequently mineralises to form new bone.

While bone is capable of remodelling in response to normal physiological loads during gait, the skeleton cannot withstand non-habitual loads in twists and falls, which could result in a fracture.

There is strong evidence that fracture healing is delayed in senescence. Aged bone demonstrates impaired response to mechanical stimuli [1], increased stromal and osteoblastic cell-induced osteoclastogenesis [2], decreased bone matrix proteins regulating mineralisation, and decreased collagen cross-linkage [3].

Mesenchymal stem cells (MSC) and colony-forming marrow cells are reduced [4], with diminished proliferation [5] and osteochondrogenic potential [6]. MSC migration [7] and differentiation into osteoblastic lineage [8] are also impaired. In addition to a quantitative defect, there is a qualitative deficiency in subsequent signal transduction [9]. mRNA expression for Indian hedgehog and bone morphogenetic protein-2 in fracture calluses are reduced [10].

Bone vascularisation and angiogenesis [11] are attenuated, with reduced expression of vascular endothelial growth factor [12] contributing to an unfavourable environment for fracture healing. In macrophages, the upregulation of M1/proinflammatory genes and dysregulation of immune-related genes [13] have been reported. Coupled with increased oxidative stress and reduced anti-inflammatory M2 macrophages, these factors contribute to attenuated responses to adverse stimuli [14] and diminished bone callus revascularisation [15].

Reductions in cell differentiation, osteoblast function, and endochondral ossification are well described in animal models. In early stages of fracture healing, collagen II expression from chondrocytes and osteocalcin expression from osteoblasts are reduced, with subsequent delays in collagen X expression and vascular invasion [16]. This culminates in longer time for callus maturation in terms of callus bridging, microstructure, and mineralisation [17], and temporal delays in regaining mechanical strength [18].

Despite similar compositional and nanostructural characterisations [19], inferior callus mechanical properties have been reported [20], with lower rigidity, breaking load in 3-point bending, and callus mineral accretion [21].

1.3 Fracture Healing in Osteoporotic Bone

The effects of osteoporosis on fracture healing are less clear (Fig. 1.1). In early stages, bone turnover markers are reduced [22], with large volume of unmineralised tissue in osteoporotic fracture callus and impaired bone remodelling [23]. Late stages of fracture healing are also affected—histomorphologically, there is delayed endochondral bone formation, increased trabecular osteoclasts, and loose irregular arrangement of new bone trabeculae [24]. Callus cross-sectional area is smaller [25] with delayed callus mineral accretion [26]. Consistently reduced bone mineral density at all time points has been observed, with reduced total and bony callus, newly formed bone, and total connectivity. This amounts to 17% less failure load, 15% less bending stiffness, 20% less bending stress, and 28% less energy to failure [27].

However, the clinical evidence of osteoporosis affecting fracture healing remains nebulous. Despite earlier reports of delayed fracture healing in nailed femoral shaft fractures in osteoporotic patients [28], subsequent studies did not confirm such association. Osteoporosis was not

Ageing
↓mesenchymal stem cells
↓mechanoresponse
↓angiogenesis
↓osteochondrogenic potential

Mechanical environment
↓cortical bone thickness
↓cortical bone stiffness and strength
↓screw pull-out strength
↑risk of fixation failure

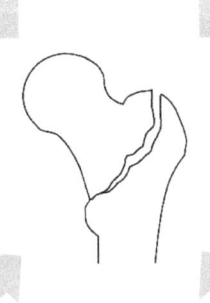
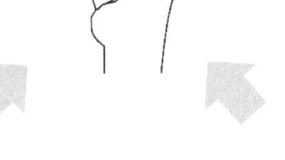

Osteoporosis
↓bone turnover markers
↓callus size
↓mechanical properties

Anti-osteoporosis medication
Bisphosphonates ↓osteoclastic resorption
Parathyroid hormone as anabolic agent

Fig. 1.1 Elements affecting osteoporotic fracture healing

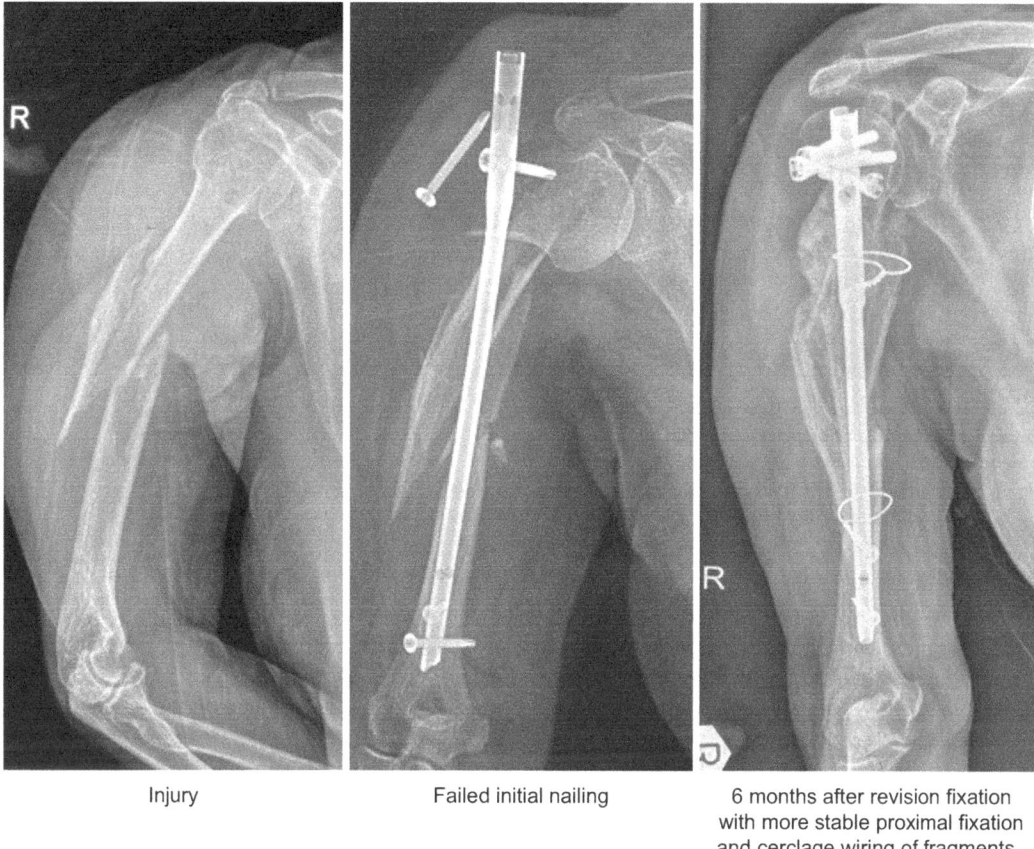

| Injury | Failed initial nailing | 6 months after revision fixation with more stable proximal fixation and cerclage wiring of fragments |

Fig. 1.2 Abundant callus formation after stable fixation in an osteoporotic humeral shaft fracture after failed intramedullary nailing

an independent risk factor for non-union in a large database case-control study [29]. No radiological difference in fracture healing was observed between osteoporotic patients and controls with plated distal radius fractures [30]. Osteoporosis was not associated with an increased risk of delayed or non-union of distal radius and proximal humerus fractures in a retrospective cohort study [31]. Figure 1.2 illustrates the point that good fracture healing and callus formation is still possible in an appropriately fixed osteoporotic humeral fracture. Paucity of data in fracture healing of young osteoporotic patients in the absence of skeletal dysplasia or metabolic bone diseases pose practical limitations in appreciating the effects of osteoporosis in isolation from senescence and postmenopausal changes.

1.4   Mechanical Environment After Fixation

An effective fracture fixation provides a stable mechanical environment for normal fracture healing to take place (Fig. 1.3). Even if the biological environment is favourable for healing to occur, an unstable situation may destroy early callus and lead to excessive bone resorption.

Bone is the weak point where construct failure occurs, with osteoporotic bone exhibiting altered cortical and trabecular bone structural and material properties [32]. Cortical bone thickness is crucial to stability of fixation implants [33]. As cortical stiffness and strength deteriorates through age [34], implant anchorage and ingrowth is compromised [35]. Bone mineral density corresponds linearly with screw holding power [36].

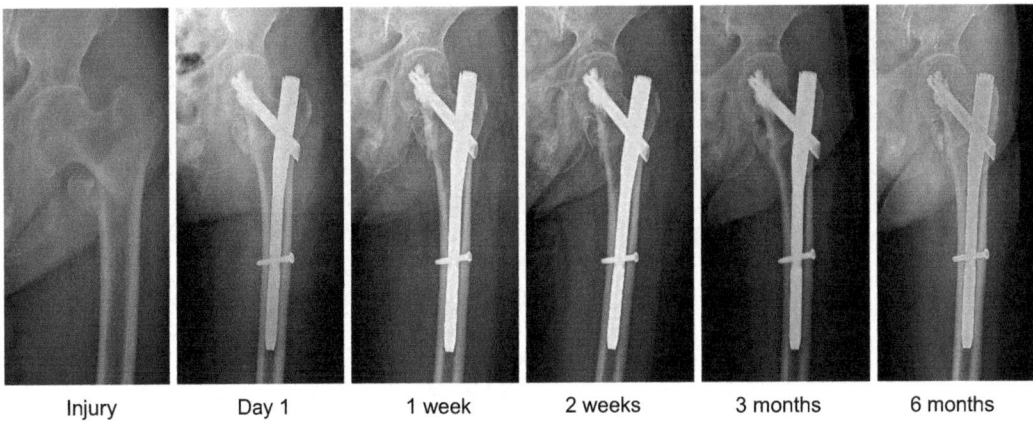

| Injury | Day 1 | 1 week | 2 weeks | 3 months | 6 months |

Caption: Fracture healing occurs rapidly after effective fixation.

Fig. 1.3 Healing of an osteoporotic trochanteric hip fracture treated with closed reduction and proximal femoral nailing with cement augmentation. Fracture healing occurs rapidly after effective fixation

Torque production at the screw thread-bone interface is reduced, with the advantage of cancellous screw geometry nullified when bone mineral density falls below $0.4g/cm^3$ [37]. When strain tolerance falls below load transmitted at the bone-implant interface, microfracture, bone resorption, and implant loosening can occur [38].

In clinical studies, fixation in osteoporotic bone has been associated with higher failure rates of 10–25% [39]. In trochanteric hip fracture fixation, there are increased risks of varus collapse and mechanical failure (including femoral head perforation, nail migration, and plate loosening) in patients with osteoporosis [40]. Higher risk of compression hip screw cut-out in osteoporotic bone [41] has been reported. In femoral neck fracture fixation, there is a higher risk for revision surgery in patients with osteoporosis [42].

A number of strategies are employed to reduce the chance of fixation failure. Locking plates improve fatigue strength and ultimate failure loads [43], reduce tensile strain in bone around screws [44], and screw loosening [45]. Fixation augmentation with polymethylmethacrylate cement enhances purchase and increases pull-out force [46]. Other augmentation options include allograft such as fibula [47], as well as bone substitutes such as demineralised bone matrix and calcium phosphate [48]. Hydroxyapatite coating has been shown to improve fixation of external fixator pins [49] and reduce lag screw cut-out in

trochanteric fracture fixation [50]. Screws coated with bisphosphonate have been reported to be associated with increased pull-out force [51].

Biomechanics of osteoporotic fracture fixation are covered in detail in the next chapter.

1.5 Effect of Anti-osteoporotic Drugs on Fracture Healing

1.5.1 Bisphosphonates

Bisphosphonate acts by inhibiting osteoclastic bone resorption and is the most commonly used osteoporosis drug. It has a long half-life, conferring a protective effect against fractures even after drug cessation [52]. However, there are concerns that disrupting the osteoblast-osteoclast balance harbours complications such as atypical femoral fractures, with the potential of derailing fracture healing mechanisms. Primary bone healing achieved via fracture compression and rigid fixation involves bone resorption in the initial stage. In cortical bone, remodelling proceeds in tunnels with osteoclasts forming "cutting cones" removing damaged bone followed by refilling by osteoblasts in the "closing cone" occurring behind the osteoclasts. However, primary bone healing via cortical remodelling is hard to achieve in osteoporotic bone. Secondary healing via callus formation is often the main form of bone union.

Animal studies show that early stages of fracture healing are not impaired by bisphosphonate use [53]. Bisphosphonates are associated with increased callus size [53–56], predominantly cartilage-like undifferentiated mesenchymal tissue at post fracture 6 weeks [57], and reduced bone turnover [58]. Subsequent endochondral ossification [54] and remodelling [55, 59, 60] are delayed, with retention of trabecular cancellous woven bone [59, 60] and postponed remodelling to lamellar bone [54, 61]. Biomechanical reports on callus strength are varied [53–55, 57, 61]. On the whole, delay in bone healing for rigidly and non-rigidly fixed fractures have been observed with continuous bisphosphonate usage [62].

In clinical studies, there is yet to be conclusive evidence against bisphosphonates with regard to fracture healing. Bisphosphonate use is not associated with delayed forearm fracture healing in a prospective randomised controlled study [63]. Similar findings are observed in distal radius fractures managed conservatively [64] or treated with volar locking plates [65].

At the shoulder, despite earlier reports of increased risk of non-union in humerus fracture, a subsequent study reported similar radiographic and clinical outcomes in proximal humerus fracture patients treated with locking plate fixation regardless of bisphosphonate use [66].

At the hip, prior exposure to bisphosphonates before trochanteric femoral fracture is associated with increased risk of delayed union at three months [67]. However, no increased risk of non-union in trochanteric hip fracture was observed in patients receiving zoledronate [68].

At the spine, bisphosphonate use is associated with radiological findings of intervertebral clefts in spinal fracture patients, albeit with similar clinical outcomes [69].

The timing for starting bisphosphonate therapy after fracture is another area of contention. Current studies do not show any effect on fracture healing. No delay in trochanteric hip fracture healing is observed among patients receiving bisphosphonate [70, 71]. Similarly, no difference in fracture union was observed in operatively treated distal radius fracture patients who started alendronate a few days or four months after surgery. Clinical outcomes of qDASH, grip strength, wrist ROM, and tenderness were similar at 6 months [72].

To summarise, bisphosphonates do not appear to impede fracture healing in clinical settings. It is generally safe to start bisphosphonates after fracture fixation.

1.5.2 Denosumab

Denosumab is an antibody against the receptor activator of nuclear factor-kappa B ligand (RANKL). Through osteoclast inhibition and decreasing bone resorption, denosumab has been shown to reduce the risk of hip, non-vertebral, and vertebral fractures [73]. In a randomised controlled trial, denosumab was not associated with delayed union or non-union in non-vertebral fractures [74].

1.5.3 Teriparatide

Teriparatide (recombinant parathyroid hormone 1–34) is an anabolic agent that promotes new bone formation. Parathyroid hormone converts quiescent lining cell to active osteoblasts [75], with a potential increase in osteoblastogenesis and decrease in adipocytogenesis [76]. Parathyroid hormone increases the number of osteoblasts in trabecular bone, while reducing sclerostin-positive osteocytes in cortical bone [77]. Chondrocyte recruitment and differentiation are enhanced [78], influencing cartilaginous and mineralised callus formation [79]. Callus mineralisation [80] and consolidation [81] are promoted, with a sustained anabolic effect extending to the remodelling phase [82]. Bone mineral content, density, and cartilage volume are enhanced, with superior mechanical properties [83] in terms of improved callus torsional strength and stiffness [82].

Clinical studies have generally demonstrated favourable effects on fracture healing. In a multicentre randomised controlled trial, teriparatide usage was associated with shorter time to healing in non-operatively treated distal radius fractures [84]. At the pelvis, parathyroid hormone (1–84) treatment was associated with faster healing of pubic fractures [85] and sacral insufficiency fractures [86]. Teriparatide was associated with quicker union for trochanteric hip fractures, with better quality of life [87, 88].

1.5.4 Oestrogen and Raloxifene

Oestrogen enhances endosteal bone formation [89], while raloxifene induces total callus formation [89]. Both oestrogen and raloxifene are associated with calluses with larger chondrocyte areas, greater mineralisation, with thicker trabeculae and neocortices [90, 91]. Although callus remodelling in endochondral ossification was impaired in an animal study, fracture repair was not impeded [92].

1.5.5 Strontium Ranelate

In rodent studies, strontium ranelate is associated with increased bone formation, bone mineral density, biomechanical strength, total bone volume of callus, osteogenesis, and more mature

and tightly arranged woven and lamellar bone [93]. Despite initial optimism on enhanced fracture healing [94], a subsequent RCT did not show accelerated fracture healing with strontium in conservatively treated distal radius fractures [95].

1.5.6 Calcitonin

In a double-blinded randomised controlled trial, calcitonin was associated with better radiographic healing in hip fracture patients [96]. However, calcitonin is rarely used for treatment of osteoporosis in view of concerns for carcinogenicity.

1.5.7 Antisclerostin Antibody

Romosozumab, an antibody against sclerostin, increases bone formation and decreases bone resorption through its effect on the Wnt pathway. Antisclerostin monoclonal antibody was associated with increased callus size and higher load to failure in an animal study [97]. Its effects on fracture healing await further elucidation from future human clinical trials.

The effects of anti-osteoporotic drugs on fracture healing are summarised in Table 1.1.

Table 1.1 Summary on effects of anti-osteoporotic drugs on fracture healing

	Effect	Strength of evidence	Type of study
Bisphosphonates [52–72]	Equivocal; impaired fracture healing in animal studies, but equivocal effect in clinical studies	++	Clinical and animal
Denosumab [73, 74]	No association with delayed or non-union	+	Clinical
Teriparatide [75–88]	Promote fracture healing	++	Clinical and animal
Oestrogen and raloxifene [89–92]	Promote fracture healing	+	Animal
Strontium ranelate [93–95]	Promote fracture healing	+	Clinical and animal
Calcitonin [96]	Promote fracture healing	+	Clinical
Romosozumab [97]	Promote fracture healing	+	Animal

1.6 Conclusion

Ageing and osteoporosis present challenges in fracture healing and fixation. Bone healing can be affected by ageing bone, osteoporosis, mechanical environment after fixation and anti-osteoporosis drugs. How these factors interplay to affect bone healing is complex and the cause for delayed union is often multifactorial. As for osteoporosis drugs, bisphosphonates are not associated with delays in fracture healing in systematic reviews, while teriparatide may expedite fracture healing.

References

1. Borgiani E, Figge C, Kruck B, Willie BM, Duda GN, Checa S. Age-related changes in the mechanical regulation of bone healing are explained by altered cellular mechanoresponse. J Bone Miner Res. 2019;34(10):1923–37. https://doi.org/10.1002/jbmr.3801.
2. Cao JJ, Wronski TJ, Iwaniec U, Phleger L, Kurimoto P, Boudignon B, et al. Aging increases stromal/osteoblastic cell-induced osteoclastogenesis and alters the osteoclast precursor pool in the mouse. J Bone Miner Res. 2005;20(9):1659–68. https://doi.org/10.1359/JBMR.050503.
3. Nyman JS, Roy A, Acuna RL, Gayle HJ, Reyes MJ, Tyler JH, et al. Age-related effect on the concentration of collagen crosslinks in human osteonal and interstitial bone tissue. Bone. 2006;39(6):1210–7. https://doi.org/10.1016/j.bone.2006.06.026.
4. Ahmed AS, Sheng MH, Wasnik S, Baylink DJ, Lau KW. Effect of aging on stem cells. World J Exp Med. 2017;7(1):1–10. https://doi.org/10.5493/wjem.v7.i1.1.
5. Lopas LA, Belkin NS, Mutyaba PL, Gray CF, Hankenson KD, Ahn J. Fractures in geriatric mice show decreased callus expansion and bone volume. Clin Orthop Relat Res. 2014;472(11):3523–32. https://doi.org/10.1007/s11999-014-3829-x.
6. Ambrosi TH, Goodnough LH, Steininger HM, Hoover MY, Kim E, Koepke LS, et al. Geriatric fragility fractures are associated with a human skeletal stem cell defect. Aging Cell. 2020;19(7):e13164. https://doi.org/10.1111/acel.13164.
7. Sanghani-Kerai A, Coathup M, Samazideh S, Kalia P, Silvio LD, Idowu B, et al. Osteoporosis and ageing affects the migration of stem cells and this is ameliorated by transfection with CXCR4. Bone Joint Res. 2017;6(6):358–65. https://doi.org/10.1302/2046-3758.66.BJR-2016-0259.R1.
8. Tang Z, Wei J, Yu Y, Zhang J, Liu L, Tang W, et al. gamma-Secretase inhibitor reverts the Notch signaling attenuation of osteogenic differentiation in aged bone marrow mesenchymal stem cells. Cell Biol Int. 2016;40(4):439–47. https://doi.org/10.1002/cbin.10583.
9. Prall WC, Haasters F, Heggebo J, Polzer H, Schwarz C, Gassner C, et al. Mesenchymal stem cells from osteoporotic patients feature impaired signal transduction but sustained osteoinduction in response to BMP-2 stimulation. Biochem Biophys Res Commun. 2013;440(4):617–22. https://doi.org/10.1016/j.bbrc.2013.09.114.
10. Meyer RA Jr, Meyer MH, Tenholder M, Wondracek S, Wasserman R, Garges P. Gene expression in older rats with delayed union of femoral fractures. J Bone Joint Surg Am. 2003;85(7):1243–54. https://doi.org/10.2106/00004623-200307000-00010.
11. Lu C, Hansen E, Sapozhnikova A, Hu D, Miclau T, Marcucio RS. Effect of age on vascularization during fracture repair. J Orthop Res. 2008;26(10):1384–9. https://doi.org/10.1002/jor.20667.
12. Rivard A, Berthou-Soulie L, Principe N, Kearney M, Curry C, Branellec D, et al. Age-dependent defect in vascular endothelial growth factor expression is associated with reduced hypoxia-inducible factor 1 activity. J Biol Chem. 2000;275(38):29643–7. https://doi.org/10.1074/jbc.M001029200.
13. Clark D, Brazina S, Yang F, Hu D, Hsieh CL, Niemi EC, et al. Age-related changes to macrophages are detrimental to fracture healing in mice. Aging Cell. 2020;19(3):e13112. https://doi.org/10.1111/acel.13112.
14. Gibon E, Loi F, Cordova LA, Pajarinen J, Lin T, Lu L, et al. Aging affects bone marrow macrophage polarization: relevance to bone healing. Regen Eng Transl Med. 2016;2(2):98–104. https://doi.org/10.1007/s40883-016-0016-5.
15. Loffler J, Sass FA, Filter S, Rose A, Ellinghaus A, Duda GN, et al. Compromised bone healing in aged rats is associated with impaired M2 macrophage function. Front Immunol. 2019;10:2443. https://doi.org/10.3389/fimmu.2019.02443.
16. Lu C, Miclau T, Hu D, Hansen E, Tsui K, Puttlitz C, et al. Cellular basis for age-related changes in fracture repair. J Orthop Res. 2005;23(6):1300–7. https://doi.org/10.1016/j.orthres.2005.04.003.1100230610.
17. Mehta M, Strube P, Peters A, Perka C, Hutmacher D, Fratzl P, et al. Influences of age and mechanical stability on volume, microstructure, and mineralization of the fracture callus during bone healing: is osteoclast activity the key to age-related impaired healing? Bone. 2010;47(2):219–28. https://doi.org/10.1016/j.bone.2010.05.029.
18. Bak B, Andreassen TT. The effect of aging on fracture healing in the rat. Calcif Tissue Int. 1989;45(5):292–7. https://doi.org/10.1007/BF02556022.

19. Mathavan N, Turunen MJ, Guizar-Sicairos M, Bech M, Schaff F, Tagil M, et al. The compositional and nano-structural basis of fracture healing in healthy and osteoporotic bone. Sci Rep. 2018;8(1):1591. https://doi.org/10.1038/s41598-018-19296-z.

20. Strube P, Sentuerk U, Riha T, Kaspar K, Mueller M, Kasper G, et al. Influence of age and mechanical stability on bone defect healing: age reverses mechanical effects. Bone. 2008;42(4):758–64. https://doi.org/10.1016/j.bone.2007.12.223.

21. Meyer RA Jr, Tsahakis PJ, Martin DF, Banks DM, Harrow ME, Kiebzak GM. Age and ovariectomy impair both the normalization of mechanical properties and the accretion of mineral by the fracture callus in rats. J Orthop Res. 2001;19(3):428–35. https://doi.org/10.1016/S0736-0266(00)90034-2.

22. Kolios L, Hitzler M, Moghaddam A, Takur C, Schmidt-Gayk H, Honer B, et al. Characteristics of bone metabolism markers during the healing of osteoporotic versus nonosteoporotic metaphyseal long bone fractures: a matched pair analysis. Eur J Trauma Emerg Surg. 2012;38(4):457–62. https://doi.org/10.1007/s00068-012-0190-1.

23. Thormann U, El Khawassna T, Ray S, Duerselen L, Kampschulte M, Lips K, et al. Differences of bone healing in metaphyseal defect fractures between osteoporotic and physiological bone in rats. Injury. 2014;45(3):487–93. https://doi.org/10.1016/j.injury.2013.10.033.

24. Wang JW, Li W, Xu SW, Yang DS, Wang Y, Lin M, et al. Osteoporosis influences the middle and late periods of fracture healing in a rat osteoporotic model. Chin J Traumatol. 2005;8(2):111–6.

25. Kubo T, Shiga T, Hashimoto J, Yoshioka M, Honjo H, Urabe M, et al. Osteoporosis influences the late period of fracture healing in a rat model prepared by ovariectomy and low calcium diet. J Steroid Biochem Mol Biol. 1999;68(5-6):197–202. https://doi.org/10.1016/s0960-0760(99)00032-1.

26. Lill CA, Hesseln J, Schlegel U, Eckhardt C, Goldhahn J, Schneider E. Biomechanical evaluation of healing in a non-critical defect in a large animal model of osteoporosis. J Orthop Res. 2003;21(5):836–42. https://doi.org/10.1016/S0736-0266(02)00266-8.

27. Hao YJ, Zhang G, Wang YS, Qin L, Hung WY, Leung K, et al. Changes of microstructure and mineralized tissue in the middle and late phase of osteoporotic fracture healing in rats. Bone. 2007;41(4):631–8. https://doi.org/10.1016/j.bone.2007.06.006.

28. Nikolaou VS, Efstathopoulos N, Kontakis G, Kanakaris NK, Giannoudis PV. The influence of osteoporosis in femoral fracture healing time. Injury. 2009;40(6):663–8. https://doi.org/10.1016/j.injury.2008.10.035.

29. van Wunnik BP, Weijers PH, van Helden SH, Brink PR, Poeze M. Osteoporosis is not a risk factor for the development of nonunion: a cohort nested case-control study. Injury. 2011;42(12):1491–4. https://doi.org/10.1016/j.injury.2011.08.019.

30. Buyukkurt CD, Bulbul M, Ayanoglu S, Esenyel CZ, Ozturk K, Gurbuz H. The effects of osteoporosis on functional outcome in patients with distal radius fracture treated with plate osteosynthesis. Acta Orthop Traumatol Turc. 2012;46(2):89–95. https://doi.org/10.3944/AOTT.2012.2440.

31. Gorter EA, Gerretsen BM, Krijnen P, Appelman-Dijkstra NM, Schipper IB. Does osteoporosis affect the healing of subcapital humerus and distal radius fractures? J Orthop. 2020;22:237–41. https://doi.org/10.1016/j.jor.2020.05.004.

32. Chao EY, Inoue N, Koo TK, Kim YH. Biomechanical considerations of fracture treatment and bone quality maintenance in elderly patients and patients with osteoporosis. Clin Orthop Relat Res. 2004;425:12–25. https://doi.org/10.1097/01.blo.0000132263.14046.0c.

33. Seebeck J, Goldhahn J, Morlock MM, Schneider E. Mechanical behavior of screws in normal and osteoporotic bone. Osteoporos Int. 2005;16(Suppl 2):S107–11. https://doi.org/10.1007/s00198-004-1777-0.

34. Burstein AH, Reilly DT, Martens M. Aging of bone tissue: mechanical properties. J Bone Joint Surg Am. 1976;58(1):82–6.

35. Giannoudis P, Tzioupis C, Almalki T, Buckley R. Fracture healing in osteoporotic fractures: is it really different? A basic science perspective. Injury. 2007;38(Suppl 1):S90–9. https://doi.org/10.1016/j.injury.2007.02.014.

36. Perren SM. Backgrounds of the technology of internal fixators. Injury. 2003;34(Suppl 2):B1–3. https://doi.org/10.1016/j.injury.2003.09.018.

37. Turner IG, Rice GN. Comparison of bone screw holding strength in healthy bovine and osteoporotic human cancellous bone. Clin Mater. 1992;9(2):105–7. https://doi.org/10.1016/0267-6605(92)90054-w.

38. Koval KJ, Meek R, Schemitsch E, Liporace F, Strauss E, Zuckerman JD. An AOA critical issue. Geriatric trauma: young ideas. J Bone Joint Surg Am. 2003;85(7):1380–8.

39. Cornell CN. Internal fracture fixation in patients with osteoporosis. J Am Acad Orthop Surg. 2003;11(2):109–19. https://doi.org/10.5435/00124635-200303000-00005.

40. Barrios C, Broström LA, Stark A, Walheim G. Healing complications after internal fixation of trochanteric hip fractures: the prognostic value of osteoporosis. J Orthop Trauma. 1993;7(5):438–42. https://doi.org/10.1097/00005131-199310000-00006.

41. Yoshimine F, Latta LL, Milne EL. Sliding characteristics of compression hip screws in the intertrochanteric fracture: a clinical study. J Orthop Trauma. 1993;7(4):348–53. https://doi.org/10.1097/00005131-199308000-00011.

42. Spangler L, Cummings P, Tencer AF, Mueller BA, Mock C. Biomechanical factors and failure of trans-

cervical hip fracture repair. Injury. 2001;32(3):223–8. https://doi.org/10.1016/s0020-1383(00)00186-8.

43. Seide K, Triebe J, Faschingbauer M, Schulz AP, Püschel K, Mehrtens G, et al. Locked vs. unlocked plate osteosynthesis of the proximal humerus - a biomechanical study Clinical Biomechanics 2007;22(2):176-182. doi: https://doi.org/10.1016/j.clinbiomech.2006.08.009.

44. MacLeod AR, Pankaj P, Simpson AH. Does screw-bone interface modelling matter in finite element analyses? J Biomech. 2012;45(9):1712–6. https://doi.org/10.1016/j.jbiomech.2012.04.008.

45. Bottlang M, Doornink J, Byrd GD, Fitzpatrick DC, Madey SM. A nonlocking end screw can decrease fracture risk caused by locked plating in the osteoporotic diaphysis. J Bone Joint Surg Am. 2009;91(3):620–7. https://doi.org/10.2106/jbjs.H.00408.

46. McKoy BE, An YH. An injectable cementing screw for fixation in osteoporotic bone. J Biomed Mater Res. 2000;53(3):216–20. https://doi.org/10.1002/(sici)1097-4636(2000)53:3<216::aid-jbm5>3.0.co;2-o.

47. Bae JH, Oh JK, Chon CS, Oh CW, Hwang JH, Yoon YC. The biomechanical performance of locking plate fixation with intramedullary fibular strut graft augmentation in the treatment of unstable fractures of the proximal humerus. J Bone Joint Surg Br. 2011;93(7):937–41. https://doi.org/10.1302/0301-620x.93b7.26125.

48. Kammerlander C, Neuerburg C, Verlaan JJ, Schmoelz W, Miclau T, Larsson S. The use of augmentation techniques in osteoporotic fracture fixation. Injury. 2016;47(Suppl 2):S36–43. https://doi.org/10.1016/s0020-1383(16)47007-5.

49. Moroni A, Faldini C, Marchetti S, Manca M, Consoli V, Giannini S. Improvement of the bone-pin interface strength in osteoporotic bone with use of hydroxyapatite-coated tapered external-fixation pins. A prospective, randomized clinical study of wrist fractures. J Bone Joint Surg Am. 2001;83(5):717–21. https://doi.org/10.2106/00004623-200105000-00010.

50. Moroni A, Faldini C, Pegreffi F, Giannini S. HA-coated screws decrease the incidence of fixation failure in osteoporotic trochanteric fractures. Clin Orthop Relat Res. 2004;425:87–92. https://doi.org/10.1097/01.blo.0000132405.30139.bb.

51. Tengvall P, Skoglund B, Askendal A, Aspenberg P. Surface immobilized bisphosphonate improves stainless-steel screw fixation in rats. Biomaterials. 2004;25(11):2133–8. https://doi.org/10.1016/j.biomaterials.2003.08.049.

52. Black DM, Schwartz AV, Ensrud KE, Cauley JA, Levis S, Quandt SA, et al. Effects of continuing or stopping alendronate after 5 years of treatment: the Fracture Intervention Trial Long-term Extension (FLEX): a randomized trial. JAMA. 2006;296(24):2927–38. https://doi.org/10.1001/jama.296.24.2927.

53. Hao Y, Wang X, Wang L, Lu Y, Mao Z, Ge S, et al. Zoledronic acid suppresses callus remodeling but enhances callus strength in an osteoporotic rat model of fracture healing. Bone. 2015;81:702–11. https://doi.org/10.1016/j.bone.2015.09.018.

54. Fu LJ, Tang TT, Hao YQ, Dai KR. Long-term effects of alendronate on fracture healing and bone remodeling of femoral shaft in ovariectomized rats. Acta Pharmacol Sin. 2013;34(3):387–92. https://doi.org/10.1038/aps.2012.170.

55. Peter CP, Cook WO, Nunamaker DM, Provost MT, Seedor JG, Rodan GA. Effect of alendronate on fracture healing and bone remodeling in dogs. J Orthop Res. 1996;14(1):74–9. https://doi.org/10.1002/jor.1100140113.

56. Menzdorf L, Weuster M, Klüter T, Brüggemann S, Behrendt P, Fitchen-Oestern S, et al. Local pamidronate influences fracture healing in a rodent femur fracture model: an experimental study. BMC Musculoskelet Disord. 2016;17:255. https://doi.org/10.1186/s12891-016-1113-9.

57. Savaridas T, Wallace RJ, Salter DM, Simpson AH. Do bisphosphonates inhibit direct fracture healing? A laboratory investigation using an animal model. Bone Joint J. 2013;95(9):1263–8. https://doi.org/10.1302/0301-620X.95B9.31562.

58. Morse A, McDonald MM, Mikulec K, Schindeler A, Munns CF, Little DG. Pretreatment with pamidronate decreases bone formation but increases callus bone volume in a rat closed fracture model. Calcif Tissue Int. 2020;106(2):172–9. https://doi.org/10.1007/s00223-019-00615-z.

59. Amanat N, McDonald M, Godfrey C, Bilston L, Little D. Optimal timing of a single dose of zoledronic acid to increase strength in rat fracture repair. J Bone Miner Res. 2007;22(6):867–76. https://doi.org/10.1359/jbmr.070318.

60. Matos MA, Tannuri U, Guarniero R. The effect of zoledronate during bone healing. J Orthop Traumatol. 2010;11(1):7–12. https://doi.org/10.1007/s10195-010-0083-1.

61. Li J, Mori S, Kaji Y, Mashiba T, Kawanishi J, Norimatsu H. Effect of bisphosphonate (incadronate) on fracture healing of long bones in rats. J Bone Miner Res. 1999;14(6):969–79. https://doi.org/10.1359/jbmr.1999.14.6.969.

62. Hauser M, Siegrist M, Keller I, Hofstetter W. Healing of fractures in osteoporotic bones in mice treated with bisphosphonates - a transcriptome analysis. Bone. 2018;112:107–19. https://doi.org/10.1016/j.bone.2018.04.017.

63. van der Poest CE, Patka P, Vandormael K, Haarman H, Lips P. The effect of alendronate on bone mass after distal forearm fracture. J Bone Miner Res. 2000;15(3):586–93. https://doi.org/10.1359/jbmr.2000.15.3.586.

64. Shoji KE, Earp BE, Rozental TD. The effect of bisphosphonates on the clinical and radiographic outcomes of distal radius fractures in women. J Hand Surg Am. 2018;43(2):115–22. https://doi.org/10.1016/j.jhsa.2017.09.006.

65. Gong HS, Song CH, Lee YH, Rhee SH, Lee HJ, Baek GH. Early initiation of bisphosphonate does not affect healing and outcomes of volar plate fixation of osteoporotic distal radial fractures. J Bone Joint Surg Am. 2012;94(19):1729–36. https://doi.org/10.2106/JBJS.K.01434.

66. Seo JB, Yoo JS, Ryu JW, Yu KW. Influence of early bisphosphonate administration for fracture healing in patients with osteoporotic proximal humerus fractures. Clin Orthop Surg. 2016;8(4):437–43. https://doi.org/10.4055/cios.2016.8.4.437.

67. Lim EJ, Kim JT, Kim CH, Kim JW, Chang JS, Yoon PW. Effect of preoperative bisphosphonate treatment on fracture healing after internal fixation treatment of intertrochanteric femoral fractures. Hip Pelvis. 2019;31(2):75–81. https://doi.org/10.5371/hp.2019.31.2.75.

68. Lyles KW, Colon-Emeric CS, Magaziner JS, Adachi JD, Pieper CF, Mautalen C, et al. Zoledronic acid and clinical fractures and mortality after hip fracture. N Engl J Med. 2007;357(18):1799–809. https://doi.org/10.1056/NEJMoa074941.

69. Ha KY, Park KS, Kim SI, Kim YH. Does bisphosphonate-based anti-osteoporosis medication affect osteoporotic spinal fracture healing? Osteoporos Int. 2016;27(2):483–8. https://doi.org/10.1007/s00198-015-3243-6.

70. Kim TY, Ha YC, Kang BJ, Lee YK, Koo KH. Does early administration of bisphosphonate affect fracture healing in patients with intertrochanteric fractures? J Bone Joint Surg Br. 2012;94(7):956–60. https://doi.org/10.1302/0301-620X.94B7.29079.

71. Cho YJ, Chun YS, Rhyu KH, Kang JS, Jung GY, Lee JH. Does the time of postoperative bisphosphonate administration affect the bone union in osteoporotic intertrochanteric fracture of femur? Hip Pelvis. 2015;27(4):258–64. https://doi.org/10.5371/hp.2015.27.4.258.

72. Uchiyama S, Itsubo T, Nakamura K, Fujinaga Y, Sato N, Imaeda T, et al. Effect of early administration of alendronate after surgery for distal radial fragility fracture on radiological fracture healing time. Bone Joint J. 2013;95(11):1544–50. https://doi.org/10.1302/0301-620X.95B11.31652.

73. Cummings SR, San Martin J, McClung MR, Siris ES, Eastell R, Reid IR, et al. Denosumab for prevention of fractures in postmenopausal women with osteoporosis. N Engl J Med. 2009;361(8):756–65. https://doi.org/10.1056/NEJMoa0809493.

74. Adami S, Libanati C, Boonen S, Cummings SR, Ho PR, Wang A, et al. Denosumab treatment in postmenopausal women with osteoporosis does not interfere with fracture-healing: results from the FREEDOM trial. J Bone Joint Surg Am. 2012;94(23):2113–9. https://doi.org/10.2106/jbjs.K.00774.

75. Kim SW, Pajevic PD, Selig M, Barry KJ, Yang JY, Shin CS, et al. Intermittent parathyroid hormone administration converts quiescent lining cells to active osteoblasts. J Bone Miner Res. 2012;27(10):2075–84. https://doi.org/10.1002/jbmr.1665.

76. Fan Y, Hanai JI, Le PT, Bi R, Maridas D, DeMambro V, et al. Parathyroid hormone directs bone marrow mesenchymal cell fate. Cell Metab. 2017;25(3):661–72. https://doi.org/10.1016/j.cmet.2017.01.001.

77. Ogura K, Iimura T, Makino Y, Sugie-Oya A, Takakura A, Takao-Kawabata R, et al. Short-term intermittent administration of parathyroid hormone facilitates osteogenesis by different mechanisms in cancellous and cortical bone. Bone Rep. 2016;5:7–14. https://doi.org/10.1016/j.bonr.2016.01.002.

78. Kakar S, Einhorn TA, Vora S, Miara LJ, Hon G, Wigner NA, et al. Enhanced chondrogenesis and Wnt signaling in PTH-treated fractures. J Bone Miner Res. 2007;22(12):1903–12. https://doi.org/10.1359/jbmr.070724.

79. Nakazawa T, Nakajima A, Shiomi K, Moriya H, Einhorn TA, Yamazaki M. Effects of low-dose, intermittent treatment with recombinant human parathyroid hormone (1-34) on chondrogenesis in a model of experimental fracture healing. Bone. 2005;37(5):711–9. https://doi.org/10.1016/j.bone.2005.06.013.

80. Manabe T, Mori S, Mashiba T, Kaji Y, Iwata K, Komatsubara S, et al. Human parathyroid hormone (1-34) accelerates natural fracture healing process in the femoral osteotomy model of cynomolgus monkeys. Bone. 2007;40(6):1475–82. https://doi.org/10.1016/j.bone.2007.01.015.

81. Mognetti B, Marino S, Barberis A, Martin AS, Bala Y, Di Carlo F, et al. Experimental stimulation of bone healing with teriparatide: histomorphometric and microhardness analysis in a mouse model of closed fracture. Calcif Tissue Int. 2011;89(2):163–71. https://doi.org/10.1007/s00223-011-9503-3.

82. Alkhiary YM, Gerstenfeld LC, Krall E, Westmore M, Sato M, Mitlak BH, et al. Enhancement of experimental fracture-healing by systemic administration of recombinant human parathyroid hormone (PTH 1-34). J Bone Joint Surg Am. 2005;87(4):731–41. https://doi.org/10.2106/JBJS.D.02115.

83. Andreassen TT, Ejersted C, Oxlund H. Intermittent parathyroid hormone (1-34) treatment increases callus formation and mechanical strength of healing rat fractures. J Bone Miner Res. 1999;14(6):960–8. https://doi.org/10.1359/jbmr.1999.14.6.960.

84. Aspenberg P, Johansson T. Teriparatide improves early callus formation in distal radial fractures. Acta Orthop. 2010;81(2):234–6. https://doi.org/10.3109/17453671003761946.

85. Peichl P, Holzer LA, Maier R, Holzer G. Parathyroid hormone 1-84 accelerates fracture-healing in pubic

bones of elderly osteoporotic women. J Bone Joint Surg Am. 2011;93(17):1583–7. https://doi.org/10.2106/JBJS.J.01379.

86. Yoo JI, Ha YC, Ryu HJ, Chang GW, Lee YK, Yoo MJ, et al. Teriparatide treatment in elderly patients with sacral insufficiency fracture. J Clin Endocrinol Metab. 2017;102(2):560–5. https://doi.org/10.1210/jc.2016-3582.

87. Huang TW, Chuang PY, Lin SJ, Lee CY, Huang KC, Shih HN, et al. Teriparatide improves fracture healing and early functional recovery in treatment of osteoporotic intertrochanteric fractures. Medicine. 2016;95(19):e3626. https://doi.org/10.1097/MD.0000000000003626.

88. Huang TW, Yang TY, Huang KC, Peng KT, Lee MS, Hsu RW. Effect of teriparatide on unstable pertrochanteric fractures. Biomed Res Int. 2015;2015:568390. https://doi.org/10.1155/2015/568390.

89. Stuermer EK, Sehmisch S, Rack T, Wenda E, Seidlova-Wuttke D, Tezval M, et al. Estrogen and raloxifene improve metaphyseal fracture healing in the early phase of osteoporosis. A new fracture-healing model at the tibia in rat. Langenbeck's Arch Surg. 2010;395(2):163–72. https://doi.org/10.1007/s00423-008-0436-x.

90. Beil FT, Barvencik F, Gebauer M, Seitz S, Rueger JM, Ignatius A, et al. Effects of estrogen on fracture healing in mice. J Trauma. 2010;69(5):1259–65. https://doi.org/10.1097/TA.0b013e3181c4544d.

91. Spiro AS, Khadem S, Jeschke A, Marshall RP, Pogoda P, Ignatius A, et al. The SERM raloxifene improves diaphyseal fracture healing in mice. J Bone Miner Metab. 2013;31(6):629–36. https://doi.org/10.1007/s00774-013-0461-x.

92. Cao Y, Mori S, Mashiba T, Westmore MS, Ma L, Sato M, et al. Raloxifene, estrogen, and alendronate affect the processes of fracture repair differently in ovariectomized rats. J Bone Miner Res. 2002;17(12):2237–46. https://doi.org/10.1359/jbmr.2002.17.12.2237.

93. Li YF, Luo E, Feng G, Zhu SS, Li JH, Hu J. Systemic treatment with strontium ranelate promotes tibial fracture healing in ovariectomized rats. Osteoporos Int. 2010;21(11):1889–97. https://doi.org/10.1007/s00198-009-1140-6.

94. Tarantino U, Celi M, Saturnino L, Scialdoni A, Cerocchi I. Strontium ranelate and bone healing: report of two cases. Clin Cases Miner Bone Metab. 2010;7(1):65–8.

95. Scaglione M, Fabbri L, Casella F, Guido G. Strontium ranelate as an adjuvant for fracture healing: clinical, radiological, and ultrasound findings in a randomized controlled study on wrist fractures. Osteoporos Int. 2016;27(1):211–8. https://doi.org/10.1007/s00198-015-3266-z.

96. Huusko TM, Karppi P, Kautiainen H, Suominen H, Avikainen V, Sulkava R. Randomized, double-blind, clinically controlled trial of intranasal calcitonin treatment in patients with hip fracture. Calcif Tissue Int. 2002;71(6):478–84. https://doi.org/10.1007/s00223-001-2111-x.

97. Ominsky MS, Li C, Li X, Tan HL, Lee E, Barrero M, et al. Inhibition of sclerostin by monoclonal antibody enhances bone healing and improves bone density and strength of nonfractured bones. J Bone Miner Res. 2011;26(5):1012–21. https://doi.org/10.1002/jbmr.307.

Biomechanics of Osteoporotic Fracture Fixation

2

Xiaoreng Feng, Frankie Leung, Sloan Kulper, and Erica Ueda

2.1 Introduction

Bone mass usually peaks at around 25–30 years of age and remains relatively stable in healthy individuals until it begins to decline at around 45 years of age. Age-related bone loss is most acute in post-menopausal women due to estrogen deficiency. Approximately half of all women and one-fifth of men experience osteoporosis by the time they reach 80 years of age.

Osteoporosis exposes individuals to a higher risk of fragility fractures and increases the difficulty of subsequent fracture repair. Fracture healing is regarded as a race between bony union and fixation failure. Surgeons may lessen the risk of complications if they have a thorough understanding of how osteoporotic fractures occur, why implants fail after surgery, and what practical strategies may be adopted to enhance fixation strength.

X. Feng (✉)
Department of Orthopaedics and Traumatology, Queen Mary Hospital, The University of Hong Kong, Pokfulam, Hong Kong

Department of Orthopaedics and Traumatology, Yangjiang People's Hospital, Yangjiang, China

F. Leung
Department of Orthopaedics and Traumatology, Queen Mary Hospital, The University of Hong Kong, Pokfulam, Hong Kong
e-mail: klleunga@hku.hk

S. Kulper · E. Ueda
Lifespans, Ltd., Wong Chuk Hang, Hong Kong
e-mail: sloan@lifespans.net; erica@lifespans.net

2.2 Strength and Morphology Changes in Osteoporotic Bone

While osteoporosis is a systemic disease that affects the strength of bone tissue throughout the body, it increases the likelihood of fractures most acutely in select anatomic locations. Typically, osteoporotic fractures occur in the spine, the distal radius, the proximal humerus, and the proximal femur.

Osteoporosis changes bone strength in several ways:

Firstly, osteoporosis causes bone tissue to become more brittle. Bone tissue in healthy young adults is a viscoelastic material that is flexible under normal loading conditions and stiff during rapid impact [1–5]. The reversible, rate-dependent stiffening of bone tissue is an emergent property of its composite structure, which consists of flexible collagen fibers adorned with crystals of comparably rigid hydroxyapatite formed from calcium dissolved in the blood serum. Viscoelasticity protects bone tissue from injury by varying its mechanical properties to suit the loading conditions at any moment in time. Healthy bone tissue remains elastic during normal ambulation, preventing fatigue injuries such as the formation and growth of cracks caused by repetitive cycles of low-magnitude stress (Fig. 2.1). The elasticity of bone tissue under slowly-applied, low-magnitude stress allows it to safely store and release a large quantity of mechanical energy by increasing its ability to reversibly deform (i.e., by taking advan-

© The Author(s), under exclusive license to Springer Nature Singapore Pte Ltd. 2024
F. Leung, T. W. Lau (eds.), *Surgery for Osteoporotic Fractures*,
https://doi.org/10.1007/978-981-99-9696-4_2

Fig. 2.1 Schematic stress-strain diagrams illustrating the viscoelastic behavior of (**a**) healthy adult bone tissue, and (**b**) osteoporotic bone tissue, showing the sum effect of reduced viscoelasticity, elastic modulus (the slope of the elastic region), and strength (stress at failure)

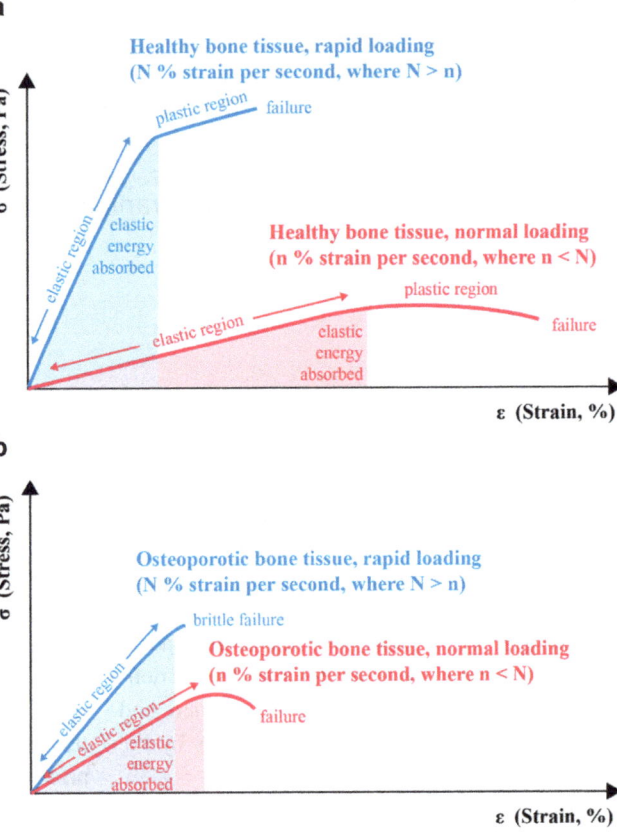

tage of the ability of collagen to behave like a spring). Bone tissue initially behaves elastically under impact and then quickly stiffens, protecting it from rapidly-applied, high magnitude loads by resisting deformation more vigorously (i.e., by taking advantage of the rigidity of the hydroxyapatite mineral). This prevents material damage such as crushing and large-scale cracks caused by excessive deformation. In individuals with osteoporosis, bone becomes more brittle, increasing its stiffness but reducing its ability to undergo as much reversible elastic strain. As a result, the benefits of the viscoelastic phenomenon observed in healthy bone tissue are greatly diminished.

Secondly, both bone strength and elastic modulus increase as bone mineralizes and evolves from childhood through adulthood, then gradually decreases during middle age [6, 7]. These values are directly correlated to the amount of energy that bone is able to absorb during loading (Fig. 2.1) [8]. The modulus of bone is highly sensitive to density, being proportional to its third power [1, 9–12], while bone strength is propor-

tional to bone mineral density squared [13]. For example, it may be reasonably assumed that osteoporotic bone tissue with half the normal bone mineral density will be one-eighth as stiff, and half as strong, as healthy bone tissue.

Thirdly, osteoporosis influences the geometry of the diaphysis and metaphysis of long bones in different ways. In the diaphysis, osteoporosis changes its cross-sectional shape by increasing both the endosteal diameter and periosteal diameter. The increase in endosteal diameter is more than the increase in periosteal diameter, thereby decreasing the thickness of the cortex (Fig. 2.2a). The geometry of bone affects its moment of inertia, thus influencing its overall response to loading. Calculating the moment of inertia can help to assess how the material is distributed in the cross section of the object relative to the applied load. It indicates that if the material is farther away from the beam's center, its stiffness is greater. With the femur as an example, the cortical outer diameter is increased while the cortical thickness is reduced approximately the same rate. The effect of these

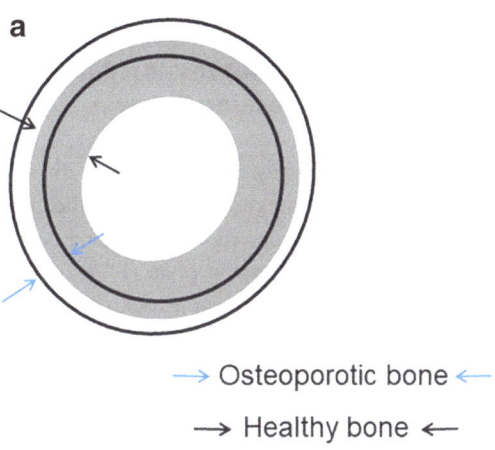

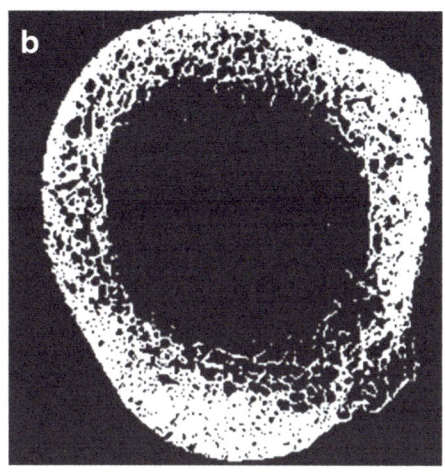

→ Osteoporotic bone ←

→ Healthy bone ←

Fig. 2.2 Geometry change in the diaphysis cross-sectional shape because of osteoporosis. (**a**) Both the endosteal diameter and periosteal diameter increase in osteoporotic bone in comparison with healthy bone. The increase in endosteal diameter is more than the increase in periosteal diameter, and therefore thickness of the cortex decreases. (**b**) The inner surface of the cortex becomes more irregular and porous in osteoporotic bone

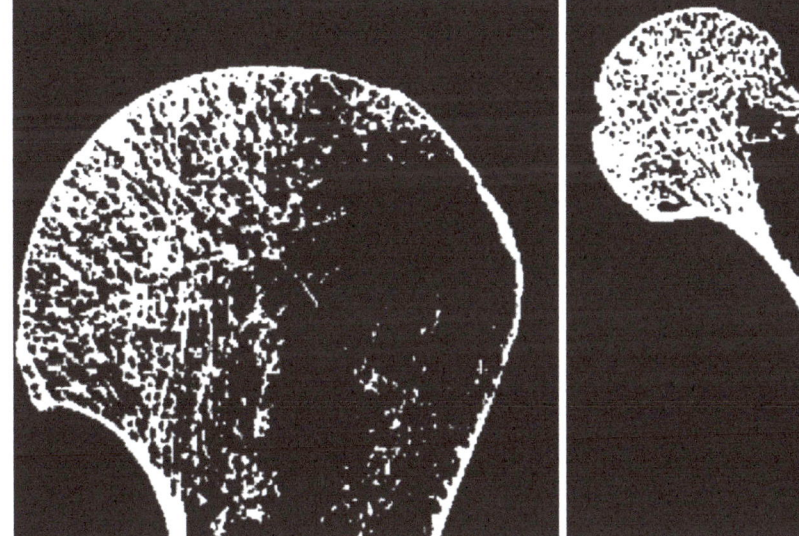

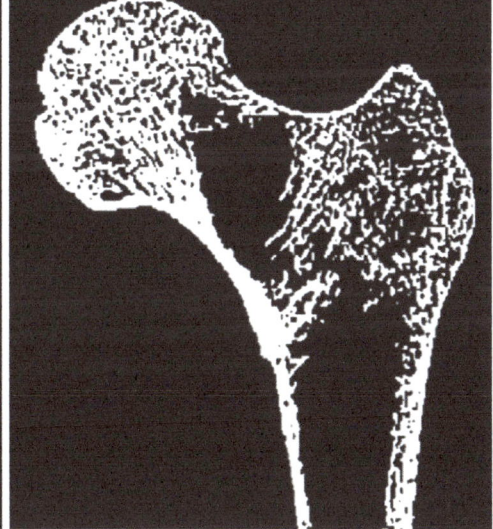

Fig. 2.3 Change in geometry of the metaphysis because of osteoporosis. Osteoporosis causes reduction in bone mass and density of the metaphysis, especially in the center part of this region

changes is to increase the moment of inertia, and thereby the overall strength, of the femoral shaft. As an analogy to daily life, small-diameter tubing with a relatively thick wall may be replaced with thin-walled large-diameter tubing in order to save weight without sacrificing strength (i.e., within the limitations of the material used). In general, such similar geometric changes to the diaphysis of long bones are beneficial to bone strength, and may be regarded as a self-protective mechanism of aging bone. Not all changes to bone geometry are beneficial, however: in the osteoporotic femur, the inner surface of the cortex also becomes more irregular and porous, eventually reducing the overall material strength (Fig. 2.2b).

In the metaphysis that is largely trabecular bone, osteoporosis mainly lowers the bone mass and density, especially the center part of this region (Fig. 2.3). Therefore, in the proximal humerus and the proximal femur of a patient with osteoporosis, the central region lacks bone tissue or only has scarce trabecular bone. However, some amount of trabecular bone tissue exists at the periphery beneath the cortex and the subchondral bone. With the understanding of this change, surgeons should insert screws as close to the subchondral bone as possible (usually within 10 mm of the joint) to obtain enough bone purchase for enhancement of the screw holding power.

2.3   Biomechanical Principles of Commonly Used Implants

The density of local bone around an implant directly determines the strength of fixation to bone. Since osteoporotic bone has very low density, fixation of osteoporotic fractures using implants is challenging. Understanding the biomechanical principles and concepts of commonly used fracture fixation devices will help to maximize the fixation stability of osteoporotic fractures.

2.4   Plates

2.4.1   Dynamic Compression Plate and Non-locking Screw

Fracture fixation plates can be adopted for several different functions, depending on the plate design and how it is applied. One common design is the dynamic compression plate (DCP), which is attached to bone by non-locking screws. Stability is achieved by bringing the fracture fragments together and attaining compression across the fracture site. This offers rigid stability and allows for the healing of primary bone with minimum callus.

Dynamic compression plates are compressed against the bone fragments by the screws and the friction between the bone and plate maintains the stability of the fracture fixation construct (Fig. 2.4a). As long as the frictional force at the bone–plate interface is greater than the load, the fracture fixation construct remains stable. If the frictional force is less than the load, the construct becomes unstable and screw fixation failure

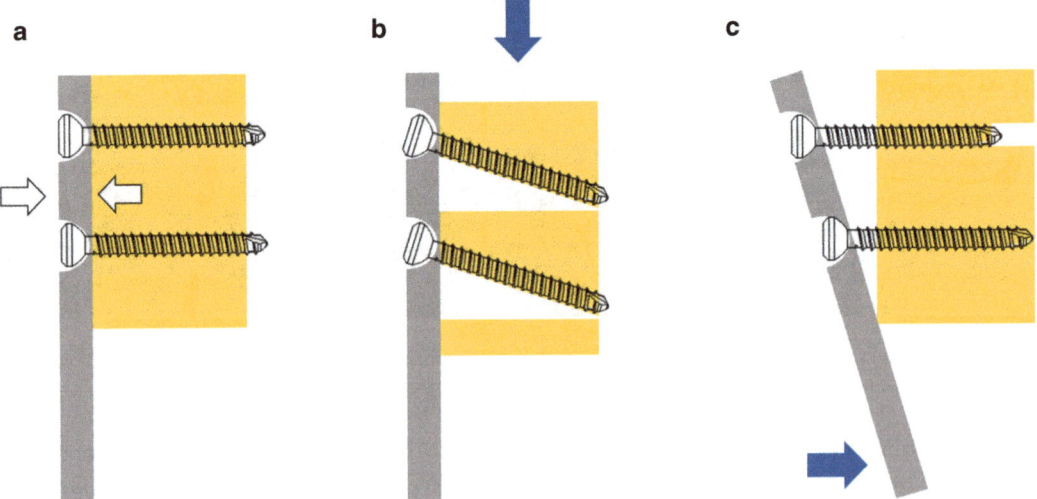

Fig. 2.4 (**a**) The friction between the bone and plate maintains the stability of the fracture fixation construct; (**b**) When the frictional force generated is less than the load applied, the construct becomes unstable and screw fixation failure occurs; (**c**) When DCP constructs fail, the screws are sequentially pulled out from the bone due to loss of bony purchase

occurs (Fig. 2.4b). In addition, when DCP and non-locking screw constructs fail, the screws usually sequentially pullout due to the loss of bony purchase (Fig. 2.4c). Conventional non-locking screws require good bony purchase to create sufficient compression in order to secure the construct.

2.4.2 Locking Plate and Locking Screw

Locking plates work using a different biomechanical principle as compared to non-locking compression plates. Locking plates are effective for treating fractures, especially in the presence of poor bone quality. Locking screws have threaded screw heads, which can be inserted into the threaded screw hole of the locking plate, thereby locking to the plate. The resultant fixation is a fixed angle device acting as a single construct (Fig. 2.5). The anti-pullout ability of the locking screw is not as critical as its resistance to bending forces. Thus, the locking screw is designed with a larger core diameter and a finer thread to best fit the loading conditions (Fig. 2.5).

Locking screws are rigidly connected to the locking plate, creating a device that is like an external fixator [14]. Every screw acts as a fixed implant and does not depend on the bone quality to compress the plate to the bone (Fig. 2.5). Instead, the locking screw relies on the plate–screw interface, the screw's shear strength, as well as the bone's compression strength for attaining stability of the construct. The biomechanical loading share principle of the locking plate construct and the special locking screw design make it especially suitable for patients with poor quality bone. It is important to note that the construction of a locking plate and locking screws is unable to create compression at the place of fracture, so fixation relies on the overall mechanical stability of the rigid construct. Locking plates offer more stability in cases of comminuted fractures and in osteoporotic bone, where it is hard to attain cortical apposition and compression [15].

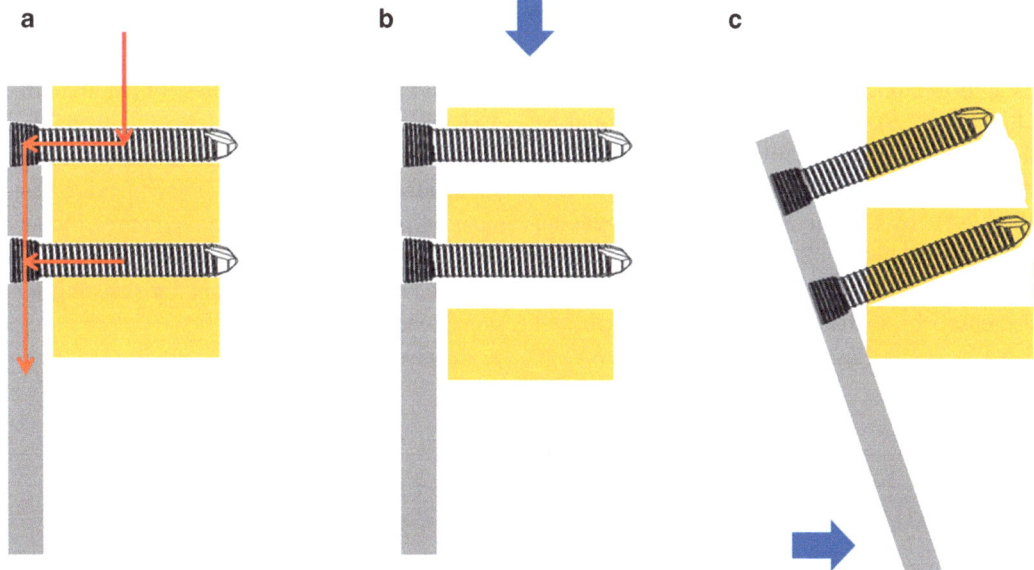

Fig. 2.5 (**a**) Locking screws have threaded screw heads, which lock into the threaded screw holes of the locking plate, thus forming a rigid, fixed angle device. Forces applied on the bone transfer from the screws to the plate directly and does not depend on friction between the plate and bone; (**b, c**) Because all of the screws are locked to the plate, fixation of the screws all fail at the same time when fixation of the entire construct ultimately fails. The locking screws fail mainly due to lateral migration through the bone tissue rather than by pullout

Locking plate constructs have a different failure mode than non-locking plate constructs (Fig. 2.5). In contrast to the sequential pullout of the non-locking screws, the locking screws should undergo fixation failure at the same time as fixation of the whole rigid construct finally fails after compressive failure of the bone. The locking screws fail mainly due to lateral migration through the bone tissue, thus there is less reliance on the screw pullout strength to maintain stability.

Another advantage of locking plates over non-locking plates is that the construct does not rely on compression of the locking plate directly against the bone, so the blood supply of the periosteum is preserved and there is less interference with the biologic process of fracture healing.

For bridge plating techniques to fix a comminuted fracture where it is difficult to compress the fracture, a gap is left at the fracture site. The fracture site can turn into a fulcrum, around which the plate bends and fails under compressive and bending loads. The working length of the plate, the total length of the plate, as well as the number and position of the screws are very important in reducing the strain of the plate and the screws. The distance between the two screws nearest to the fracture site (working length) should be long enough to reduce the strain concentration in the plate (Fig. 2.6). In addition, the plate should be long enough to increase the moment arm of the distal screws to reduce the force applied to them (Fig. 2.7) [16]. The fixation construct's bending and torsional fixation strength can then be enhanced. Also the plate strain can be greatly decreased by increasing the overall length and

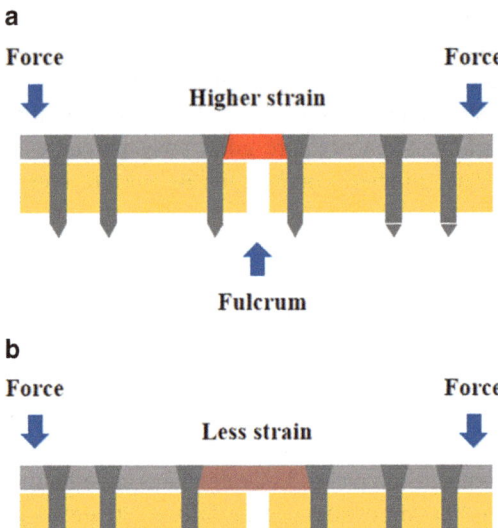

Fig. 2.6 Working length is the distance between the two screws nearest to the fracture site. Increasing the working length can reduce the strain in the plate, thus reducing the risk of breakage of the plate

working length of the plate [17]. To a certain extent, the plate stiffness will be strengthened by increasing the number of cortex fixation points. However, not all plate holes need to have screws inserted to offer similar stiffness of fixation [18]. A plate screw density which is smaller than 0.5 is enough to maintain the fixation stability. It is recommended that six cortices at each feature fragment be present to resist axial compression and bending forces. Meanwhile, eight cortices at each fracture fragment is sufficient for resisting torsional loading.

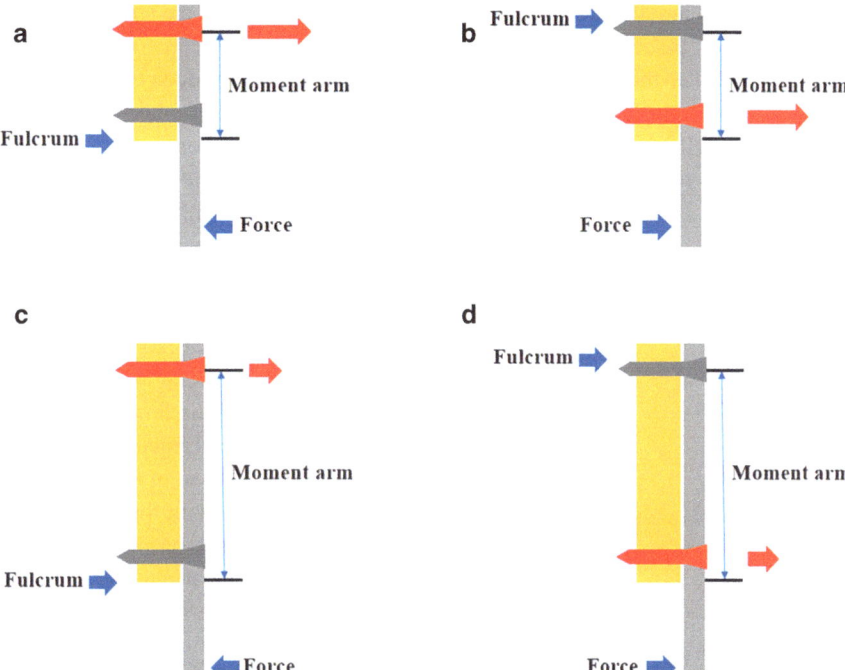

Fig. 2.7 Enhancing the whole length of the plate increases the moment arm of the most distal screw, thus lowering the force acting on it and increasing the stability of the fixation construct. Red arrows represent the forces acting on the red screws. The longer the arrow, the greater the force

2.5   Intramedullary Nail

An intramedullary nail (IM nail) with interlocking screws is the standard treatment choice for diaphysis fracture of the long bones. It is also used commonly in treating proximal femur and proximal humerus fractures. The friction between the nail and the inner surface of the medullary canal as well as the holding power of the interlocking screws in bone are the main source of stability. IM nails provide relative stability for the fracture, and thus the fracture will have secondary bone healing with callus formation. In contrast to eccentric fixation provided by a plate, an IM nail provides central fixation, thus possessing a natural biomechanical advantage in fracture fixation over plating. Additionally, a cylindrical implant has the structural advantage compared with a flat implant in resisting bending and torsional forces. In contrast to most plating techniques, an IM nail is inserted in a minimally invasive way without exposing the fracture site. The soft tissue envelop and the periosteal blood

supply of the bone are preserved, leading to faster fracture healing.

Failure of the interlocking screws occurs occasionally during healing in the form of either screw breakage or screw cutout from the bone. In comminuted fractures, no load is being borne by the bone cortices at the fracture site, and stresses on the interlocking screws are obviously increased. In younger or denser bone, screw bending and breakage can occur. However, in patients with osteoporosis or poor bone quality, bone damage around the screw (i.e., screw cutout) usually happens before screw breakage.

Additionally, the location of the interlocking screw also affects the stress on the screw. For distal screws, the screw is supported mainly by the cortices when the distal screws are positioned into bone that has comparatively low bone density. The distal end of the femur widens suddenly, and thus the unsupported length (the span) of the screw between the cortices varies (Fig. 2.8). The stiffness and strength of a screw under a bending force reduces with the third power of its span for screws with the same diameter and material. If the span of one screw is twice as long as that of another, it is assumed that the deformation will be eight times greater under the same load. Therefore, a more distally located interlocking screw will increase the risk of screw breakage.

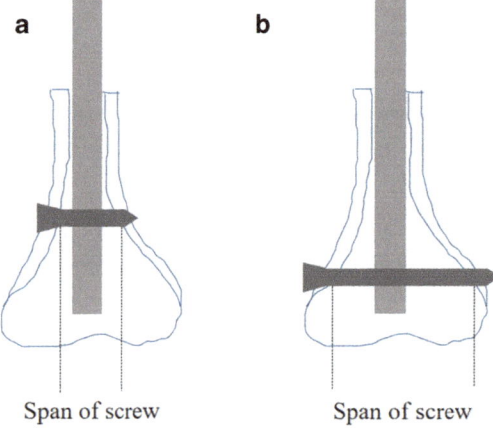

Span of screw   Span of screw

Fig. 2.8 The distal end of the long bones, such as femur and tibia, flares rapidly, thus the length of the locking screw required to lock the rod can be quite variable. The bending strength decreases with the third power of its length between cortices (the span of screw). If the screw length doubles, the deformation of the screw under the same load enhances by a factor of eight. However, increasing the span of the screw can be regarded as an increase in moment arm of the screw, which will decrease the stress acting on the screw-bone interface, thus reducing the risk of the screw migrating or cutting out from the bone

However, increasing the span of the screw can be regarded as an increase in moment arm of the screw, which will reduce the stress acting on the screw–bone interface, thus reducing the risk of the screw migrating or cutting out from the bone. The fatigue life of the distal locking screws is in direct association with the inner diameter of the screw and the resulting moment of inertia, and thus it is better to reduce the depth of the threads to increase the inner diameter of the screw, thus increasing its fatigue life [19].

The other demanding mechanical situation for IM nail fixation of the femur or tibia takes place with extremely distal fractures. In distal fractures where no cortical bone of the distal fracture fragment is associated with the nail to share the off-axial forces, stresses on the interlocking screws are significantly enhanced (Fig. 2.9). For fracture at the isthmus of the shaft, one or two interlocking screws in the same plane are enough to maintain the stability. However, for distal fractures, at least three interlocking screws at different planes should be applied to resist the off-axial forces. In addition, poller or blocking screws can also be used in some cases to increase the fixation stability.

For the fixation of proximal femur fractures, cephalomedullary nails with a helical blade design has been widely used [20]. The blade has a larger transverse diameter as compared to a

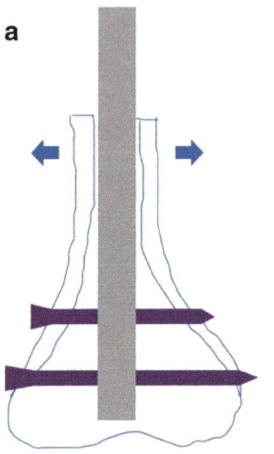

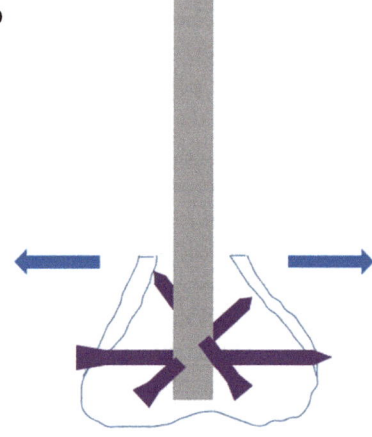

Fig. 2.9 (**a**) For fracture at the isthmus of the shaft, where nail–bone contact can prevent lateral fragment displacement, less stress will be transferred to the interlocking screws. (**b**) For distal fractures, where no nail–bone contact at the distal bone is available to share the off-axial forces, much higher stress is borne by the interlocking screws. At least three interlocking screws in different planes should be applied to resist the off-axial forces

large lag screw, thus offering greater resistance to lateral migration. Its insertion also involves use of a smaller drill and thus removes less bone. The blade is inserted by impaction of surrounding trabecular bone undergoing volumetric compression. The result is enhanced anchorage and rotational stability within the femoral head.

2.6   Future Direction

Since bone quality of the patient cannot be changed by the surgeon, development of novel bone screws with increasing holding power in the osteoporotic bone is a feasible and promising way to reduce the fixation failure rate. Since screw thread is the determinant component that governs the initial screw fixation stability, choosing the right thread profile for the bone screw is extremely important. However, the currently widely used buttress thread in bone screw design is derived from the industrial screw, [21] which has been proven cannot adequately resist multiaxial forces and is prone to stripping at the bone–screw interface, therefore having inferior fixation stability in osteoporotic bone [22]. The optimal

bone screw thread design for osteoporotic bone remains unclear.

The authors of this chapter have conducted a series of researches in this topic. Our clinical and biomechanical studies revealed that apart from the axial pullout strength, lateral migration resistance should also be used to evaluate the bone screw fixation stability and guide the bone screw thread design [23, 24]. Our biomechanical study found that the barb thread design has the worst pullout strength, while the reverse buttress thread has the best pullout strength as compared with standard buttress thread, which indicates that a proximal flank angle of larger than 90°can improve the pullout strength of bone screws (Fig. 2.10) [25]. Bone screw thread with a flat crest and undercut feature has been proven to have superior lateral migration resistance [26, 27]. Novel thread designs with an undercut structure have been proposed and initially validated in osteoporotic synthetic bone, showing better fixation stability than the traditional buttress thread [26, 27]. Our bone screw-related research indicated that bone screw thread design is a promising direction that is helpful to reduce the bone screw failure rate in osteoporotic bone.

a   b

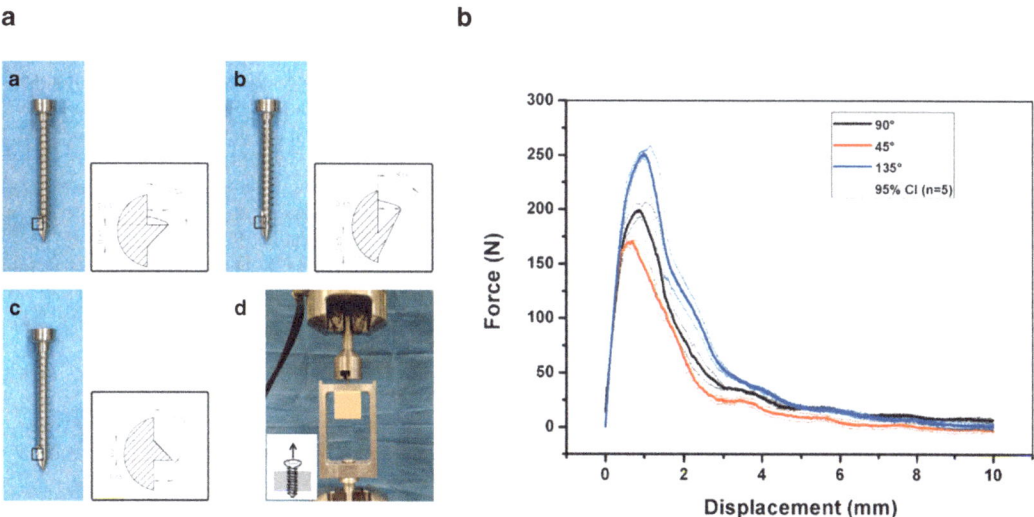

Fig. 2.10 (**a**) Bone screws with typical buttress thread ((**a**)with a proximal flank angle of 90°), barb thread ((**b**) with a proximal flank angle of 45°), and reverse buttress thread ((**c**) with a proximal flank angle of 135°) were tested by pullout in a synthetic cancellous bone (**c**). (**b**) The force-displacement curve showed that the barb thread

is the worst, while the reverse buttress thread is the best in pullout strength among the three thread types. (Figures from: Feng X, Qi W, Fang CX, et al. 2021. Can barb thread design improve the pullout strength of bone screws? A biomechanical study and finite element analysis. Bone Joint Res 10: 105–112)

2.7   Summary

Effective fixation of fragility fractures requires a biomechanical appreciation of the change in bone geometry and structure due to osteoporosis and the fundamental mechanisms of where these loads are transferred when using commonly applied fixation devices. Correctly fixing the implant devices according to their biomechanical principles to maximize the fixation stability is very important for surgical treatment of fragility fractures.

References

1. Burstein AH, Reilly DT, Martens M. Aging of bone tissue: mechanical properties. J Bone Joint Surg Am. 1976;58(1):82–6.
2. Crowninshield RD, Pope MH. The response of compact bone in tension at various strain rates. Ann Biomed Eng. 1974;2(2):217–25.
3. Currey JD. The effects of strain rate, reconstruction and mineral content on some mechanical properties of bovine bone. J Biomech. 1975;8(1):81–6.
4. McElhaney JH. Dynamic response of bone and muscle tissue. J Appl Physiol. 1966;21(4):1231–6.
5. Merk BR, Stern SH, Cordes S, Lautenschlager EP. A fatigue life analysis of small fragment screws. J Orthop Trauma. 2001;15(7):494–9.
6. Currey JD, Butler G. The mechanical properties of bone tissue in children. J Bone Joint Surg Am. 1975;57(6):810–4.
7. Weaver JK, Chalmers J. Cancellous bone: its strength and changes with aging and an evaluation of some methods for measuring its mineral content: I. Age changes in cancellous bone. JBJS. 1966;48(2):289–99.
8. Currey JD. Changes in the impact energy absorption of bone with age. J Biomech. 1979;12(6):459–69.
9. Bartley MH Jr, Arnold JS, Haslam RK, Jee WSS. The relationship of bone strength and bone quantity in health, disease and aging 12. J Gerontol. 1966;21(4):517–21.
10. Bell GH, Dunbar O, Beck JS, Gibb A. Variations in strength of vertebrae with age and their relation to osteoporosis. Calcif Tissue Res. 1967;1(1):75–86.
11. Cody DD, Goldstein SA, Flynn MJ, Brown EB. Correlations between vertebral regional bone mineral density (rBMD) and whole bone fracture load. Spine. 1991;16(2):146–54.
12. Galante J, Rostoker W, Ray RD. Physical properties of trabecular bone. Calcif Tissue Res. 1970;5(1):236–46.
13. Carter DR, Hayes WC. The compressive behavior of bone as a two-phase porous structure. J Bone Joint Surg Am. 1977;59(7):954–62.
14. Frigg R, Appenzeller A, Christensen R, Frenk A, Gilbert S, Schavan R. The development of the distal femur less invasive stabilization system (LISS). Injury. 2001;32:24–31.
15. Egol KA, Kubiak EN, Fulkerson E, Kummer FJ, Koval KJ. Biomechanics of locked plates and screws. J Orthop Trauma. 2004;18(8):488–93.
16. Ellis T, Bourgeault CA, Kyle RF. Screw position affects dynamic compression plate strain in an in vitro fracture model. J Orthop Trauma. 2001;15(5):333–7.
17. Sanders R, Haidukewych GJ, Milne T, Dennis J, Latta LL. Minimal versus maximal plate fixation techniques of the ulna: the biomechanical effect of number of screws and plate length. J Orthop Trauma. 2002;16(3):166–71.
18. ElMaraghy AW, ElMaraghy MW, Nousiainen M, Richards RR, Schemitsch EH. Influence of the number of cortices on the stiffness of plate fixation of diaphyseal fractures. J Orthop Trauma. 2001;15(3):186–91.
19. Hou S-M, Wang J-L, Lin J. Mechanical strength, fatigue life, and failure analysis of two prototypes and five conventional tibial locking screws. J Orthop Trauma. 2002;16(10):701–8.
20. Yee DKH, Lau W, Tiu KL, Leung F, Fang E, Pineda JPS, et al. Cementation: for better or worse? Interim results of a multi-centre cohort study using a fenestrated spiral blade cephalomedullary device for pertrochanteric fractures in the elderly. Arch Orthop Trauma Surg. 2020;140(12):1957–64.
21. Roberts TT, Prummer CM, Papaliodis DN, Uhl RL, Wagner TA. History of the orthopedic screw. Orthopedics. 2013;36:12–4.
22. Stahel PF, Alfonso NA, Henderson C, Baldini T. Introducing the "bone-screw-fastener" for improved screw fixation in orthopedic surgery: a revolutionary paradigm shift? Patient Saf Surg. 2017;11:6.
23. Feng X, Lin G, Fang CX, et al. Bone resorption triggered by high radial stress: the mechanism of screw loosening in plate fixation of long bone fractures. J Orthop Res. 2019;37:1498–507.
24. Feng X, Qi W, Zhang T, et al. Lateral migration resistance of screw is essential in evaluating bone screw stability of plate fixation. Sci Rep. 2021;11:12510.
25. Feng X, Qi W, Fang CX, et al. Can barb thread design improve the pullout strength of bone screws? A biomechanical study and finite element analysis. Bone Joint Res. 2021;10:105–12.
26. Feng X, Zhang S, Liang H, Chen B, Leung F. Development and initial validation of a novel undercut thread design for locking screws. Injury. 2022;53(7):2533–40. https://doi.org/10.1016/j.injury.2022.02.048.
27. Feng X, Zhang S, Luo Z, Liang H, Chen B, Leung F. Development and initial validation of a novel thread design for non-locking cancellous screws. J Orthop Res. 2022;40(12):2813–21. https://doi.org/10.1002/jor.25305.

Tak Wing Lau

3.1 Introduction

In geriatric patients, fixing the osteoporotic and comminuted fractures are challenging. However, before we are actually fixing the fracture on the operative table, preparing the geriatric patients for operation is even more challenging. This is particularly obvious when the geriatric patients are under the care of orthopaedic surgeons, whom are not professionally trained to deal with the pre-existing medical conditions, polypharmacy and/or borderline cardiac and pulmonary functions. It can be challenging to proceed to a quick and safe operation. As hip fracture is the commonest reason for geriatric patients admitted, and the best management for hip fracture is to operate early, we could not avoid dealing with the "unfamiliar" medical aspects ourselves. To make the situation worse, the average age of the hip fracture patients is increasing yearly with increase in number of comorbidities [1], the difficulty in pre-operative management can only be getting more difficult and complicated.

There is good evidence that accelerated surgery does not harm patients but could reduce post-operative delirium and length of hospital stay [2]. Although age is frequently described as a predictor of perioperative risk, it is more likely that age is a proxy for a number of underlying vulnerabilities to decompensation during or after surgery. The following chapter is a general guide for orthopaedic surgeons to deal with the commonest pre-operative issues in geriatric patients. This could help us to better understand and prepare the geriatric patients for surgery. However, this could never replace the efficiency and benefit of a well-organized multidisciplinary orthogeriatric comanaged team [3].

3.2 Pre-operative Assessment

From British orthopaedic Association on "The Care of Patients with Fragility Fracture" [4], the followings should be completed as a pre-operative assessment and preparation:

- Diagnosis established
- Pressure relieving mattress used
- Patient assessed for other injuries and medical conditions
- Pain relief
- Routine bloods
- Electrocardiogram (ECG)
- Pre-operative chest X-ray
- Immediate fluid resuscitation with intravenous saline.

Pre-operative assessment in geriatric patients is particularly challenging for all the parties

T. W. Lau (✉)
Department of Orthopaedics and Traumatology, The
University of Hong Kong, Pokfulam, Hong Kong

involved, namely orthopaedic surgeons, anaesthetists, geriatricians, and physicians. One of the most common fractures in geriatric patients, hip fracture, is considered probably the most difficult group of patients. First, the average age is relatively high, which is around 85 [5]. Second, these patients has multiple comorbidities involving cardiovascular, pulmonary, and central nervous systems [5]. Third, although hip fracture surgery is not considered as an emergency, it should preferably be done within 48 hours after admission [4, 6].

Even though they have high anaesthetic and surgical risks, we know that early surgical treatment is the best form of analgesia and it also minimizes the rate of complications due to immobilization. Yet, delay in surgery is very common in these patients mostly because of medical reasons. This is especially frustrating when the operation is cancelled in the last minute before going into the operating theatre. Often this is related to the fact that surgeons are not familiar with the risk assessments. We are not sure which patients are actually not fit for surgery and need to be optimized. The balance between the risks of anaesthesia and surgical trauma versus the benefits of early surgery become an art of practice which should be based on both evidence and experience.

The most important aim of pre-operative assessment is to identify those patients that are likely to develop life-threatening events during or after surgery. Most of the time, the post-operative period is more risky than intra-operative period. In essence, the capacity of the patient to withstand the acute physiological perturbations resulting from the entire operative period extends into the recovery phase. If the patient can meet the increased oxygen demand due to the acute stress response to surgery, he/she should be ready to be operated.

In general, the pre-operative management of the geriatric fracture patients involves the following areas:

- Pain control
- Thromboprophylaxis
- Cardiac function assessment
- Pulmonary function assessment
- Central nervous system assessment.

3.3   Pain Control

The best pain control for the hip fracture patients is immediate surgical management. However, no matter how efficiently we could operate on these patients, there are still some patients that require some time for optimization. During this window period, pain control becomes very important. Good pain management can also help to decrease post-operative delirium and complications in frail geriatric patients [7, 8].

Pain management should be started immediately after admission to emergency department when hip fracture is suspected [9]. Many geriatric patients, especially when they have pre-existing cognitive impairment, are not good at expressing their pain [7, 8]. From our data, half of our hip fracture patients has dementia [5]. It becomes very important to give appropriate, adequate and not excessive analgesics in pre-operative period even many of our hip fracture patients may not be able to express their pain level.

The first choice is paracetamol and, if it is insufficient, an opioid can be added [9]. Non-steroidal anti-inflammatory drugs (NSAID) are not recommended because of gastrointestinal, cardiovascular, and renal side effects with possibility of other drug interactions [9, 10]. Nerve blocks are very useful in pre-operative pain control and also in patients where operation could not be performed in a considerable time [6, 11]. The nerve block could be given in the emergency department or in the admission ward. Femoral nerve block or fascia iliaca block are both quick and effective for hip fracture patients. Pre-operative skeletal or skin traction is not effective [6, 12]. They do not result in any significant pain relief.

3.4   Thromboprophylaxis

Venous thromboembolism can lead to perioperative mortality in geriatric fracture patients. Therefore, thromboprophylaxis should be a standard pre-operative management for all these patients.

Early mobilization is effective in lowering the risk of clinical thrombosis [4]. There is good evidence to support the use of venus thromboemolism prophylaxis in hip fracture patients [6]. Several medications are commonly used; intravenous unfractionated heparin, subcutaneous low molecular weight heparin or even oral aspirin have been reported with good evidences to support [6, 13]. Currently, low molecular weight heparin is a common choice for thromboprophylaxis. It has been shown to reduce the risk of symptomatic venous thromboembolic events in hip and knee arthroplasties by about three-fifths [14].

For patients that are not on any pre-existing anticoagulants or antiplatelet agents, the administration of thromboprophylaxis depends on timing of surgery (Fig. 3.1) [15]. If the operation can be done immediately, no pre-operative thromboprophylaxis is required. By 12–24 hours after surgery, subcutaneous enoxaparin should be started. If the surgery is planned in 6–24 hours, the shorter half-life intravenous unfractionated heparin is recommended because of the better controllability. It should be stopped 4–6 hours prior to surgery. If the surgery is done after 24 hours, a standard prophylactic dose of subcutaneous low molecular weight heparin is given with the last dose administered up to 12 hours pre-operatively [13, 15–17]. All prophylaxis should be continued until the patient is fully ambulatory and if the patient has increased risk of thromboembolism, up to 35 days post-operatively [13, 15].

Fig. 3.1 Flow chart for thromboprophylaxis

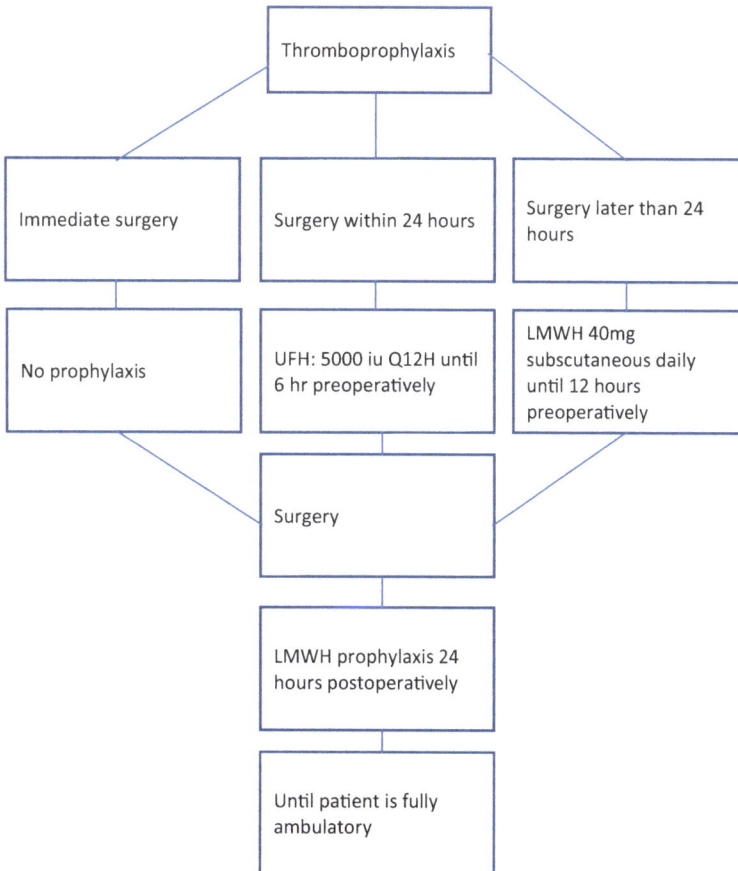

3.5 Cardiac Function Assessment

The purpose of pre-operative evaluation is not to give medical clearance but to perform an evaluation of the patient's current medical status. It should help with the evaluation, management, and risk of cardiac problems. No test should be performed unless it is likely to affect the choice of treatment. In order to avoid delay, ECG should be best performed in the emergency department [4] or in the admission ward [5]. Some conditions that need a cardiac consultation for a more detailed cardiac assessment [18]:

Pre-operative urgent cardiac specialist consultation	Conditions
	• Unstable coronary syndromes, such as unstable or severe angina or a recent myocardial infarction (7 days to 1 month)
	• Decompensated heart failure
	• Significant arrhythmias (including supraventricular arrhythmias with ventricular rate above 100, high-grade atrioventricular heart blocks)
	• Severe valvular disease

The goal of a cardiac consultation is the optimal care of the patient [19]. The purpose is to confirm diagnosis, delineate the severity of the disease and whether there is any room for improvement with medical treatment in the context of a surgery that should be done as early as possible.

3.6 Systolic Heart Murmurs and Echocardiogram

The presence of systolic heart murmurs during pre-operative assessment is common and often "silent" until they are discovered during the routine pre-operative assessment. This systolic murmur could be a benign one or represent a significant aortic stenosis. The latter is significant as this is a relative contra-indication to spinal anaesthesia. Echocardiography would help to make a definitive diagnosis and a quantitative assessment of the condition. However, the treatment of any valvular disease is unlikely to precede surgery. Therefore, the results of echocardiography will not change in the anaesthetic management of these patients [20]. The absence of the echocardiography should not lead to delay [4]. Management should involve carefully administered and monitored general or spinal anaesthesia. The aim is to maintain coronary and cerebral perfusion pressures during surgeries. One can also consider short-term admission to a higher-level care unit postoperatively [20].

3.7 Warfarin and Direct Oral Anticoagulant Drugs

For hip fracture patients that are already on warfarin, the management includes witholding the drug or bridging therapy [15, 20].

```
┌─────────────────────────────┐
│      Patient on warfarin     │
└─────────────────────────────┘
```

```
┌─────────────────────────┐        ┌─────────────────────────┐
│  Patient with AF/ DVT/ PE │        │  Patient with mechanical │
│                           │        │        heart valve       │
└─────────────────────────┘        └─────────────────────────┘
```

```
        ┌──────────────┐              ┌──────────┐   ┌──────────┐
        │ Stop Warfarin │              │ Low risk  │   │ High risk │
        └──────────────┘              └──────────┘   └──────────┘
```

```
┌──────────┐   ┌──────────┐                      ┌──────────────────┐
│ INR ≤ 1.5 │   │ INR > 1.5 │                      │ Bridging therapy  │
└──────────┘   └──────────┘                      └──────────────────┘
```

```
              ┌──────────────────┐              ┌──────────────────────┐
              │ Give intravenous  │              │ Heparin intravenous   │
              │    Vit K 5mg      │              │    infusion or Low     │
              └──────────────────┘              │   Molecular weight     │
                                                 │       heparin          │
                                                 └──────────────────────┘
```

```
              ┌──────────────────┐
              │  Recheck INR 4-6  │
              │   hours later      │
              └──────────────────┘
```

```
┌────────────────────────────────────────────────────────────────┐
│              Normal thromboprophylaxis,                          │
│            Consider spinal anaesthesia,                          │
│                 Proceed to surgery                               │
│        Resume Warfarin when hemostasis achieved                  │
└────────────────────────────────────────────────────────────────┘
```

The direct oral anticoagulant drugs (apixaban, edoxaban, rivaroxaban, dabigatran) pose a different challenge to warfarin, especially in terms of prompt time to theatre. These drugs are eliminated by the kidneys. Reversal agents could be given for life-threatening situations. In general, waiting out two half-lives (approximate residual anticoagulant effect of around 25%) between the last dose and surgery provides an appropriate balance between bleeding risk and benefit of early surgeries [20]. The half-lives of these drugs are generally within 15 h, thus stopping them for 1.5 days should be enough for a relative safe surgery if the patient has an estimated eGFR ≥60 ml/min/1.73 m² [20]. Since the thrombin time is very sensitive to the dabigatran blood level, if the TT is normal, anaesthesia and surgery should be safe.

3.8 Anti-platelet Therapy

Another common issue in patients having cardiovascular diseases is the use of aspirin or dual anti-platelet agents. Aspirin works by blockade of the formation of thromboxane and the effect lasts for 7–10 days [21]. In general, if aspirin is used for only prophylaxis without specific cardiovascular risk, it should be stopped and surgery can be performed as soon as possible. On the other hand, if patient has higher cardiovascular risk, aspirin could be continued during the surgery without witholding it [6, 15]. Spinal anaesthesia is possible in both scenarios [22]. Standard thromboprophylaxis should be started 6–24 hours post-operatively. Aspirin should be resumed when haemostasis is achieved [15, 22].

It becomes more challenging when patient is on dual anti-platelet agents. This is getting commoner because of recent advances and popularity of percutaneous coronary angioplasty with or without stenting. Drug such as clopidogrel (Plavix®) is commonly used together with aspirin. Normal platelet function returns after stopping clopidogrel for 7–10 days, and hence withholding the drug for 1 week is practiced for elective orthopaedic surgeries [23]. If a hip fracture patient is taking clopidogrel due to a previous cardiovascular or cerebrovascular event, it should be stopped upon admission. The surgery should not be delayed once patient is stabilized [6, 15]. Spinal anaesthesia is generally not recommended [15] and one should proceed to general anaesthesia if there are no contra-indications [20]. In patients having dual antiplatelet agents for coronary artery stent, the situation is much more complex. In general, if a bare metal stent has been placed within 6 weeks or a drug-eluting stent has been placed within 6 months, both aspirin and clopidogrel should be continued [15, 22]. On the other hand, if the stent is placed not within this period, stopping the clopidogrel while continuing aspirin is possible. In both circumstances, the cardiovascular status should be assessed and optimized by physician and anaesthetist pre-operatively [4]. There is no advantage of delaying the surgery if the patient is stable [6, 20].

3.9 Pulmonary Function

The reason for pre-operative pulmonary assessment is to prevent post-operative pulmonary complications. Patients at risk of developing pneumonia include [18, 24]:

- Advanced age
- American Society of Anaesthesiologists (ASA) class 2 or higher
- Functional dependence
- Chronic obstructive pulmonary disease
- Congestive heart failure
- Emergency surgery
- General anaesthesia
- Prolonged surgery

- Serum albumin level less than 30g/L.

Pre-operative chest radiograph should be done as a standard in the emergency department as the investigation is not costly and can improve efficiency in case the patient requires surgical treatment [4]. Other tests such as repeated chest radiograph, spirometry, or arterial blood gas should not be ordered as a routine [25].

Oxygen saturation below 90% with room air represents an important finding, as from this point a small decrement of partial pressure will lead to a large decrease in saturation. Those with low haemoglobin will have a reduced oxygen carrying capacity. Several factors can result in respiratory failure in post-operative period. The systemic inflammatory response could simply elevate the oxygen consumption. Occult sepsis can also increase oxygen demand and carbon dioxide production. If patient has undergone general or spinal anaesthesia, the chance of atelectasis increases [26]. Some opioids analgesia can depress respiration and the urge to cough together with impaired mucociliary clearance mechanism of the respiratory epithelium [27]. All these factors can predispose the frail hip fracture geriatric patients to develop chest complications in post-operative phase.

One common dilemma in pre-operative period is concomitant chest infection. Generally speaking, the acute chest infection without sepsis or decompensation can be safely managed simultaneously with the hip fracture surgery. Delay of the hip fracture surgery, expecting the chest infection could be managed with antibiotics alone, with an immobilized painful hip fracture, results in more harm than good [28]. Besides, unlike abdominal or thoracic surgery, the operative site is well away from the respiratory muscles and by itself is unlikely to interfere with breathing in the post-operative period.

Chronic obstructive pulmonary disease, asthma, and obstructive sleep apnoea are also common pulmonary conditions in geriatric patients. A detailed history taking and a good clinical examination are usually enough for pre-operative assessment [25]. Asymptomatic patients or those with mild symptoms do not require any specific optimization before surgery. In case of severe symptoms, steroids and bronchodilators may be required.

3.10 Central Nervous System

Delirium is common in hospitalized patients [29] and is common in those with pre-existing cognitive impairment [30]. Development of acute delirium before surgery in hip fracture patients could be up to 16% [11]. Post-operative delirium is associated with increased morbidity, mortality and prolonged length of stay [31, 32]. Moreover, this condition is often underdiagnosed due to the subtle clinical presentation [33]. From our experience, about half of hip fracture patients could not pass the mental test and considered as dementia [5]. Early diagnosis of pre-operative delirium is important and can be achieved by use of validated tools such as short Confusion Assessment Method (CAM) and modified Barthel index [11].

Once delirium is suspected, major organic conditions should be ruled out. These include hypoxia, hypoglycaemia, fluid and electrolytes imbalances, sepsis or organic disorders of the central nervous system. Reversible conditions such as electrolyte disturbances should be treated promptly. Multi-component Care Bundle has been shown to effectively reduce post-operative delirium [11]. It involves multiple measures at various levels involving hospital and the orthopaedic or geriatric ward, as follows.

1. A specially designed cubicle for geriatric patients with adequate lighting and space
2. Education and empower caretaker visits and involvement in patients' training
3. Longer visiting hours for caretakers
4. Enhanced analgesic protocol with the use of Fascia Iliaca block on top of oral analgesics

3.11 Conclusion

There is very strong evidence that delaying the surgery in general will increase in morbidity and mortality in hip fracture patients. Goal of preoperative optimisation is to allow the patients to be operated safely and quickly. However, in some situations, some more time is required to optimise the patients better.

Acceptable reasons for delaying surgeries of hip fracture of patients [20, 28]
Haemoglobin <80 g/L
Plasma sodium concentration <120 or >150/mmol
Potassium concentration <2.8 or >6.0/mmol
Uncontrolled diabetes
Uncontrolled or acute onset left ventricular failure
Correctable cardiac arrhythmia with a ventricular rate >120/min
Chest infection with sepsis
Reversible coagulopathy

Afterall, an efficient and well organized multidisciplinary team involving orthopaedic surgeons, geriatricians, and anaesthetists is important for treating this group of patients. All team members should work closely to optimize the patients for surgery as soon as possible to give the best clinical outcomes for the geriatric fracture patients [1, 3–5, 9].

Problem	Recommendation
Timing of surgery	Early (<24–48 h) to decrease complications
Fluid management	Restore fluid status
Cardiovascular high risk	Cardiology consultation, most need beta-blockers
Aortic stenosis	Cardiac testing only if advised by medical
Pulmonary conditions	Optimize medical treatment pre-operatively
Delirium	Avoidance is best, treat contributing conditions
Diabetes	Maintain glucose levels between 100 and 180 mg/dL
Anaemia	Correct haemoglobin to ≥8 g/dL
Clopidogrel (Plavix) use	Proceed with early surgery
Warfarin use	Correct INR to ≤1.5

References

1. Lau TW, Fang C, Leung F. The effectiveness of a geriatric hip fracture clinical pathway in reducing hospital and rehabilitation length of stay and improving short-term mortality rates. Geriatr Orthop Surg Rehabil. 2013;4(1):3–9.
2. HIP Attack Investigators. Accelerated surgery versus standard care in hip fracture (HIP ATTACK): an international, randomised, controlled trial. Lancet. 2020;395:698–708.
3. Friedman SM, Mendelson DA, Kates SL, McCann RM. Geriatric co-management of proximal femur fractures: total quality management and protocol-driven care result in better outcomes for a frail patient population. J Am Geriatr Soc. 2008;56(7):1349–56.
4. British Orthopaedic Association. The care of patients with fragility fracture. London: British Orthopaedic Association; 2007.
5. Lau TW, et al. Geriatric hip fracture clinical pathway: the Hong Kong experience. Osteoporos Int. 2010;21(Suppl 4):S627–36.
6. Roberts KC, Timothy Brox W, Jevsevar DS, Sevarino K. Management of hip fractures in the elderly. J Am Acad Orthop Surg. 2015;23(2):131–7.
7. Feast AR, White N, Lord K, Kupeli N, Vickerstaff V, Sampson EL. Pain and delirium in people with dementia in the acute general hospital setting. Age Ageing. 2018;47:841–6.
8. Feldt KS, Ryden MB, Miles S. Treatment of pain in cognitively impaired compared with cognitively intact older patients with hip fracture. J Am Geriatr Soc. 1998;46:1079–85.
9. NICE. The management of hip fractures in adults. 2017. https://www.nice.org.uk/guidance/cg124.
10. Wongrakpanich S, Wongrakpanich A, Melhado K, Rangaswami J. A comprehensive review of non-steroidal anti-inflammatory drug use in the elderly. Aging Dis. 2018;9:143–50.
11. Lam DMH, Wang C, Lee AKH, Chung YF, Lau TW, Fang C, Leung F, Chan TCW. Multi-component care bundle in geriatric fracture hip for reducing post-operative delirium. Geri Orthop Surh Rehab. 2021;12:21514593211004530.
12. Handoll HH, Queally JM, Parker MJ. Pre-operative traction for hip fracture in adults. Cochrane Database Syst Rev. 2011;12:CD000168.
13. Falck-Ytter Y, et al. Prevention of VTE in orthopedic surgery patients: antithrombotic therapy and prevention of thrombosis, 9th ed: American College of Chest Physicians evidence-based clinical practice guidelines. Chest. 2012;141:e278S–325S.
14. Eikelboom JWJ, Quinlan DJD, Douketis JDJ. Extended-duration prophylaxis against venous thromboembolism after total hip or knee replacement: a meta-analysis of the randomised trials. Lancet. 2001;358:7.
15. Wendl-Soeldner MA, Moll CW, Kammerlander C, Gosch M, Roth T. Algorithm for anticoagulation management in geriatric hip fracture patients – surgeons save blood. Z Gerontol Geriat. 2014;47:95–104.
16. Bucking B, Bliemel C, Waschnick L, et al. Anticoagulation medication for proximal femoral fractures: prospective validation study of new institutional guidelines. Unfallchirurg. 2013;116:909–15.
17. Chassot PG, Delabays A, Spahn DR. Perioperative antiplatelet therapy: the case for continuing therapy in patients at risk of myocardial infarction. Br J Anaesth. 2007;99:316–28.
18. Wong GTC, Sun NCH. Providing perioperative care for patients with hip fractures. Osteoporos Int. 2010;21(suppl 4):S547–53.
19. Fleisher LA, Beckman JA, Brown KA, Calkins H, Chaikof EL, Fleischmann KE, Freeman WK, Froehlich JB, Kasper EK, Kersten JR, Riegel B, Robb JF. ACCF/AHA focused update on perioperative beta blockade incorporated into the ACC/AHA 2007 guidelines on perioperative cardiovascular evaluation and care for noncardiac surgery: a report of the American College of Cardiology Foundation/American Heart Association task force on practice guidelines. Circulation. 2009;120:e169–276.
20. Griffiths R, et al. Guideline for the management of hip fractures 2020: guideline by the Association of Anaesthetists. Anaesthesia. 2021;76(2):225–37.
21. Tohgi H, Konno S, Tamura K, et al. Effects of low-to-high doses of aspirin on platelet aggregability and metabolites of thromboxane A2 and prostacyclin. Stroke. 1992;23:1400–3.
22. Douketis JD, et al. Perioperative management of antithrombotic therapy: antithrombotic therapy and prevention of thrombosis, 9th ed: American College of Chest Physicians evidence-based clinical practice guidelines. Chest. 2012;141:e326S–50S.
23. Li CC, Hirsh JJ, Xie CC, et al. Reversal of the antiplatelet effects of aspirin and clopidogrel. J Thromb Haemost. 2012;10:521–8.
24. Smetana GW, Lawrence VA, Cornell JE, American College of Physicians. Preoperative pulmonary risk stratification for noncardiothoracic surgery: systematic review for the American college of physicians. Ann Intern Med. 2006;144:581–95.
25. Lo I, Siu CW, Tse HF, Lau TW, Leung F, Wong M. Preoperative pulmonary assessment for patients with hip fracture. Osteoporos Int. 2010;21:579–86.
26. Magnusson L, Spahn DR. New concepts of atelectasis during general anaesthesia. Br J Anaesth. 2003;91:61–72.
27. Gamsu G, Singer MM, Vincent HH, Berry S, Nadel JA. Postoperative impairment of mucous transport in the lung. Am Rev Respir Dis. 1976;114:673–9.
28. Griffiths R, Alper J, Beckingsale A, Goldhill D, Heyburn G, et al. Association of Anaesthetists of Great Britain and Ireland Management of proximal femoral fractures 2011: association of anaesthetists of Great Britain and Ireland. Anaesthesia. 2012;67:85–98.
29. Trzepacz PT. Delirium. Advances in diagnosis, pathophysiology, and treatment. Psychiatr Clin North Am. 1996;19:429–48.

30. American Psychiatric Association. Practice guideline for the treatment of patients with delirium. Am J Psychiatry. 1999;156:20–9.
31. Mullen JO, Mullen NL. A prospective, multifactorial study to predict and minimize death risk. Hip fracture mortality. Clin Orthop Relat Res. 1992;280:214–22.
32. Nightingale S, Holmes J, Mason J, House A. Psychiatric illness and mortality after hip fracture. Lancet. 2001;357:1264–126531.
33. Inouye SK. The dilemma of delirium: clinical and research controversies regarding diagnosis and evaluation of delirium in hospitalized elderly medical patients. Am J Med. 1994;97:278–88.

Choice of Management and Techniques of Proximal Humeral Fixation

4

Dennis King Hang Yee, Tak Man Wong, and Christian Fang

4.1 Introduction

Proximal humeral fractures account for 4–6% of all fractures [1] and are the third most common fracture in patients with osteoporosis [2]. More than 80% of patients are older adults. Most of such fractures can be treated non-operatively, with the more complicated cases requiring surgical intervention [3, 4]. The advantages of surgical intervention are anatomical reduction, rigid fixation, and early mobilization. However, it is still a challenge to manage proximal humerus fractures surgically due to poor bone quality and therefore poor anchorage [5, 6]. According to literature, implant loosening is not uncommon and is reported in a range between 14% and 22% [7]. Besides, the rate of reoperation is reported to be up to 29% [8]. To prevent such complications, it is important to know in detail the bone density of the proximal humerus to maximize screw purchase.

4.2 Bone Density Around the Proximal Humerus

Several studies have been performed for bone density and strength measurement of the proximal humerus. Barvencil et al. showed that proximal humerus bone density is highest over the superior and medial region [9]. Hep et al. found the posterior and medial parts of the proximal humerus have higher bone density compared with the other regions, while proximal and lessor tuberosities had the lowest bone density [10]. Other studies also showed that the highest bone density was over the posterior, superior, and medial parts of the proximal humerus [11–13]. Therefore, the trajectory of screws should be superior, posterior, and medial, to allow for stronger screws.

Clinically, two methods have been proposed to predict the bone density of the proximal humerus and the likelihood of screw cutout by measuring the cortical bone thickness of the shaft of the humerus (Fig. 4.1), namely the Tingart measurement [14] and the deltoid tuberosity index (Table 4.1) [15].

D. K. H. Yee (✉) · T. M. Wong · C. Fang
Department of Orthopaedics and Traumatology,
Queen Mary Hospital, The University of Hong Kong,
Pokfulam, Hong Kong
e-mail: yeedns@ortho.hku.hk; wongtm@hku.hk

© The Author(s), under exclusive license to Springer Nature Singapore Pte Ltd. 2024
F. Leung, T. W. Lau (eds.), *Surgery for Osteoporotic Fractures*,
https://doi.org/10.1007/978-981-99-9696-4_4

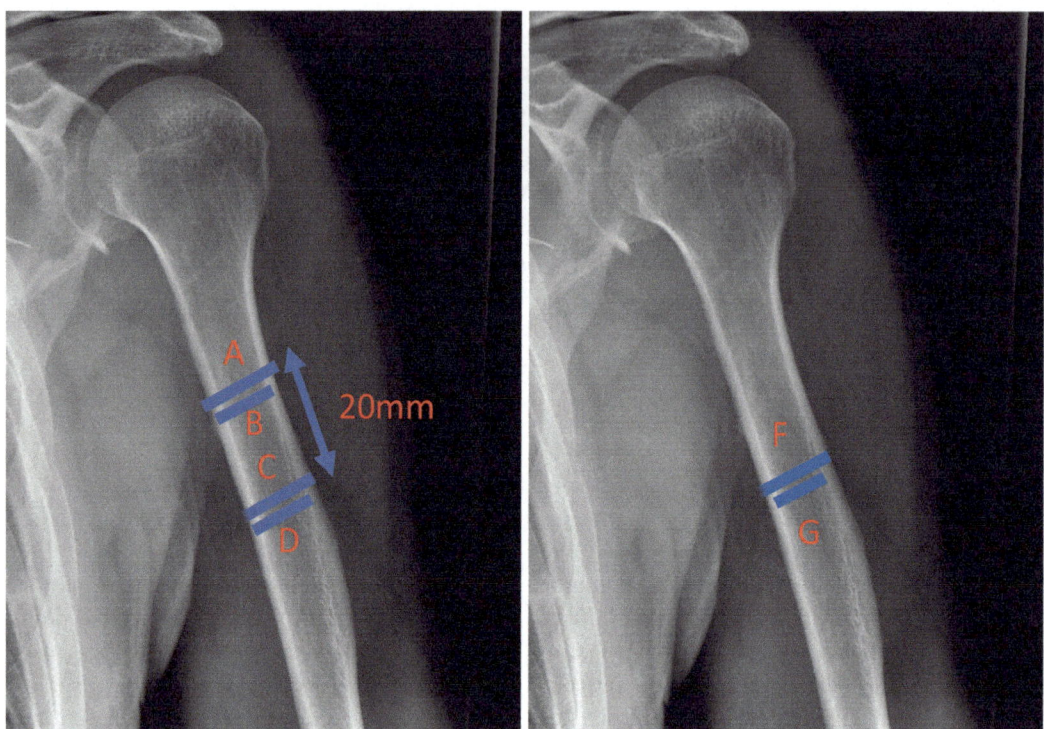

Fig. 4.1 Demonstration of how to estimate the bone density based on Tingart measurement and deltoid tuberosity index

Table 4.1 Tingart measurement and deltoid tuberosity index for predicting the local bone density of the proximal humerus. Tingart measurement <6 or deltoid tuberosity index <1.4 correlated with low local bone mineral density

	X-ray view	Measurements	Formula	Cut-off value	Accuracy
Tingart measurement	Anteroposterior	Two levels: proximal and distal, 20 mm apart	(A + B + C − D)/2	<6	93% sensitive 52% specific
Deltoid tuberosity index	Anteroposterior with shoulder internal rotated	One level proximal to deltoid tuberosity	F/G	<1.4	88% sensitive 80% specific

4.3 Classification

The two most common systems are the Neer classification and the AO/OTA classification. In Neer Classification, 2-part, 3-part, and 4-part fractures are based on whether the greater tuberosity, lesser tuberosity, surgical or anatomical necks of the humerus are involved. A displaced fragment is defined as either 1cm separation or 45-degree angulation.

The AO/OTA classification categorizes proximal humerus fractures into types, groups, and subgroups with reference to Neer Classification. AO/OTA classification 11A, 11B, and 11C represents 2-part, 3-part, and 4-part fractures, respectively (Fig. 4.2).

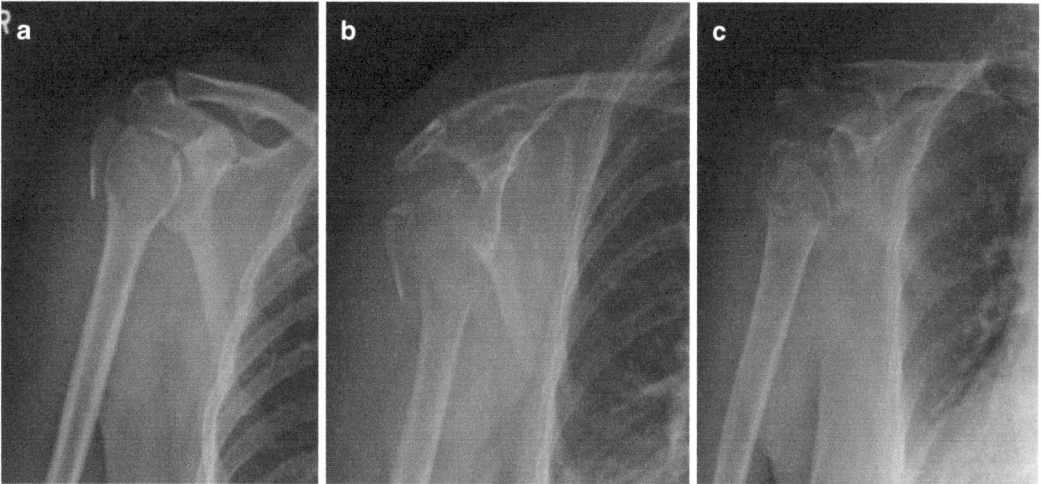

Fig. 4.2 Examples of AO/OTA classification 11A, 11B and 11C (left to right)

4.4 Management

The treatment of proximal humerus fractures remains controversial. The PROFHER trial is the largest multicentred randomized controlled trial on the management of proximal humerus fractures. It concluded that there was no significance between the conservative and operative groups in terms of functional outcome [16]. A 2015 Cochrane review also found that there was no evidence that surgical treatment achieved a better result compared with the non-operative treatment. Low-demand patients, poor surgical candidates, or patients with very osteoporotic bones are not suitable for surgical fixation. Operative fixation is indicated in significantly displaced fractures and high demand patients with acceptable bone quality, head-splitting fractures, pathological fractures or fracture dislocation, as the results of non-operative treatment are generally poor. The most commonly used implants for proximal humerus fractures are locking plate, intramedullary nail, and shoulder arthroplasty. In this chapter, we propose an algorithm to decide on the management approach of proximal humerus fracture (Fig. 4.3) combining concepts from O'Donnell and Gage [17] and Kralinger [18] with our own. Please note that associated neurovascular injury, glenohumeral joint dislocation not reducible with closed means,

open fracture, multiple injuries, and pathological fractures are additional indications for operative treatment.

The incidence of avascular necrosis of the head of the humerus after proximal humerus fracture is between 3 and 68% [19, 20]. The main blood supply of the proximal humerus is by both anterior and posterior humeral circumflex arteries (Fig. 4.4). The anterior humeral circumflex artery supplies 36% of the blood supply to the humeral head overall, while the posterior humeral circumflex artery provides 64%. The posterior humeral circumflex artery also provides significantly more of the blood supply in three of the four quadrants of the humeral head [21]. The most relevant predictors of ischemia are the length of the dorsomedial metaphyseal extension, the integrity of the medial hinge, and the basic fracture type determined with the binary description system [22]. A combination of anatomical neck, short calcar, and disrupted hinge predicts positive values of fracture induced humeral head ischemia of up to 97% [22]. Particularly in elderly patients, shoulder arthroplasty should be considered if such risk factors are present (Fig. 4.5).

Locking intramedullary nails compared with locking plates
1. Biomechanical studies have been conducted comparing fixation of proximal humerus frac-

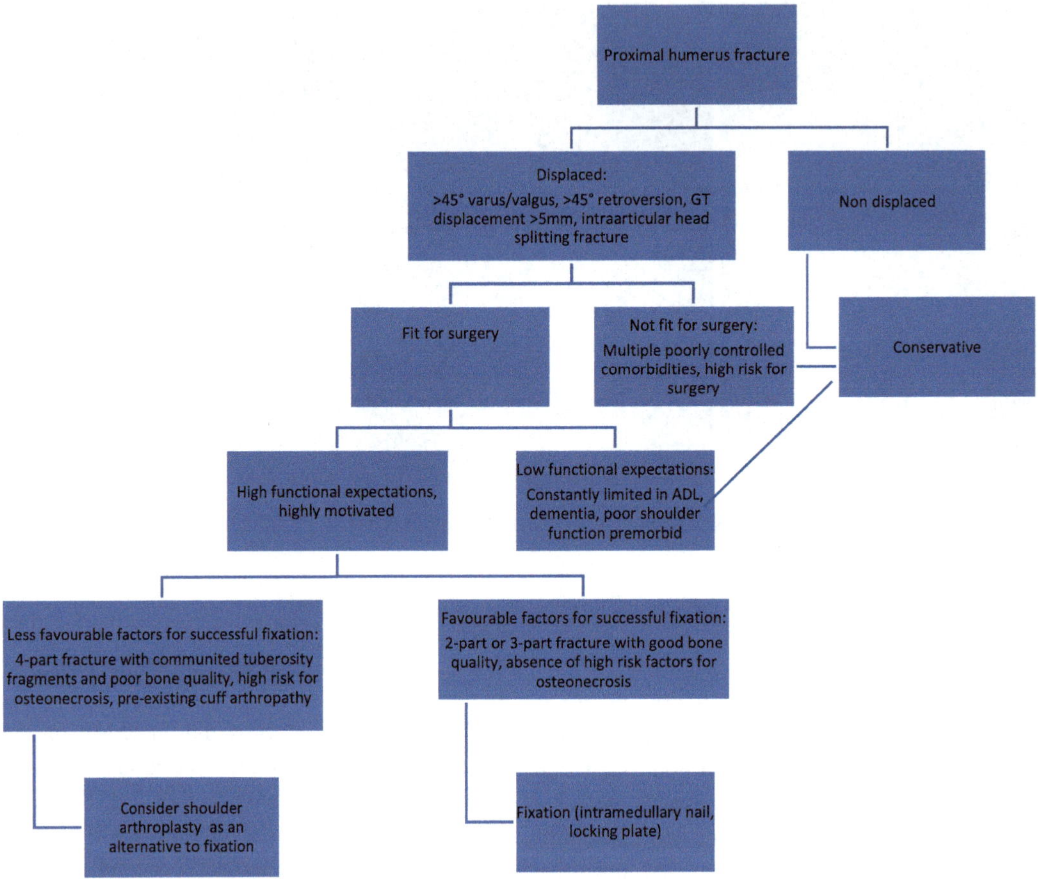

Proximal humerus fracture
Displaced:
>45° varus/valgus, >45° retroversion, GT displacement >5mm, intraarticular head splitting fracture
Non displaced
Fit for surgery
Not fit for surgery:
Multiple poorly controlled comorbidities, high risk for surgery
Conservative
High functional expectations, highly motivated
Low functional expectations:
Constantly limited in ADL, dementia, poor shoulder function premorbid
Less favourable factors for successful fixation:
4-part fracture with communited tuberosity fragments and poor bone quality, high risk for osteonecrosis, pre-existing cuff arthropathy
Favourable factors for successful fixation:
2-part or 3-part fracture with good bone quality, absence of high risk factors for osteonecrosis
Consider shoulder arthroplasty as an alternative to fixation
Fixation (intramedullary nail, locking plate)

Fig. 4.3 Algorithm for management approach of proximal humerus fracture

Anterior circumflex humeral artery
Axillary artery
Posterior circumflex humeral artery

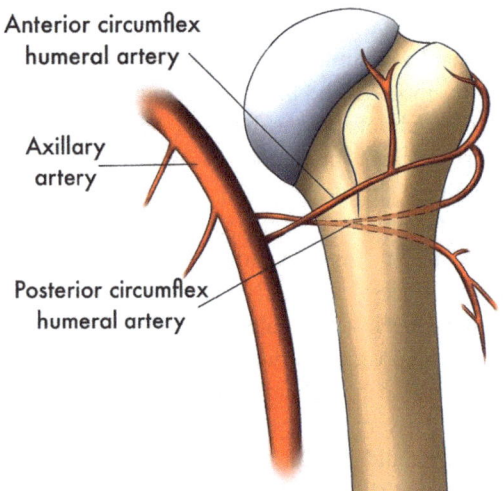

Fig. 4.4 Blood supply of proximal humerus

ture with locking intramedullary nails and locking plates. Table 4.2 summarizes key principles from ex vivo studies. Intramedullary nail fixation has superior biomechanical stability in 2-part proximal humerus fractures.

2. There are three randomized controlled trials with a total of 204 patients comparing the use of locking intramedullary nails and locking plates in fixation of proximal humerus fracture (Table 4.3). The results are inconsistent with regard to functional outcomes at 1 year, and complication rates. Gracitelli et al. [26] showed no significant differences for all parameters except higher total complication rate (P = 0.002) and reoperation rate (P = 0.041) in the nail group. Contrarily, Plath et al. [27] showed the locking blade nail group

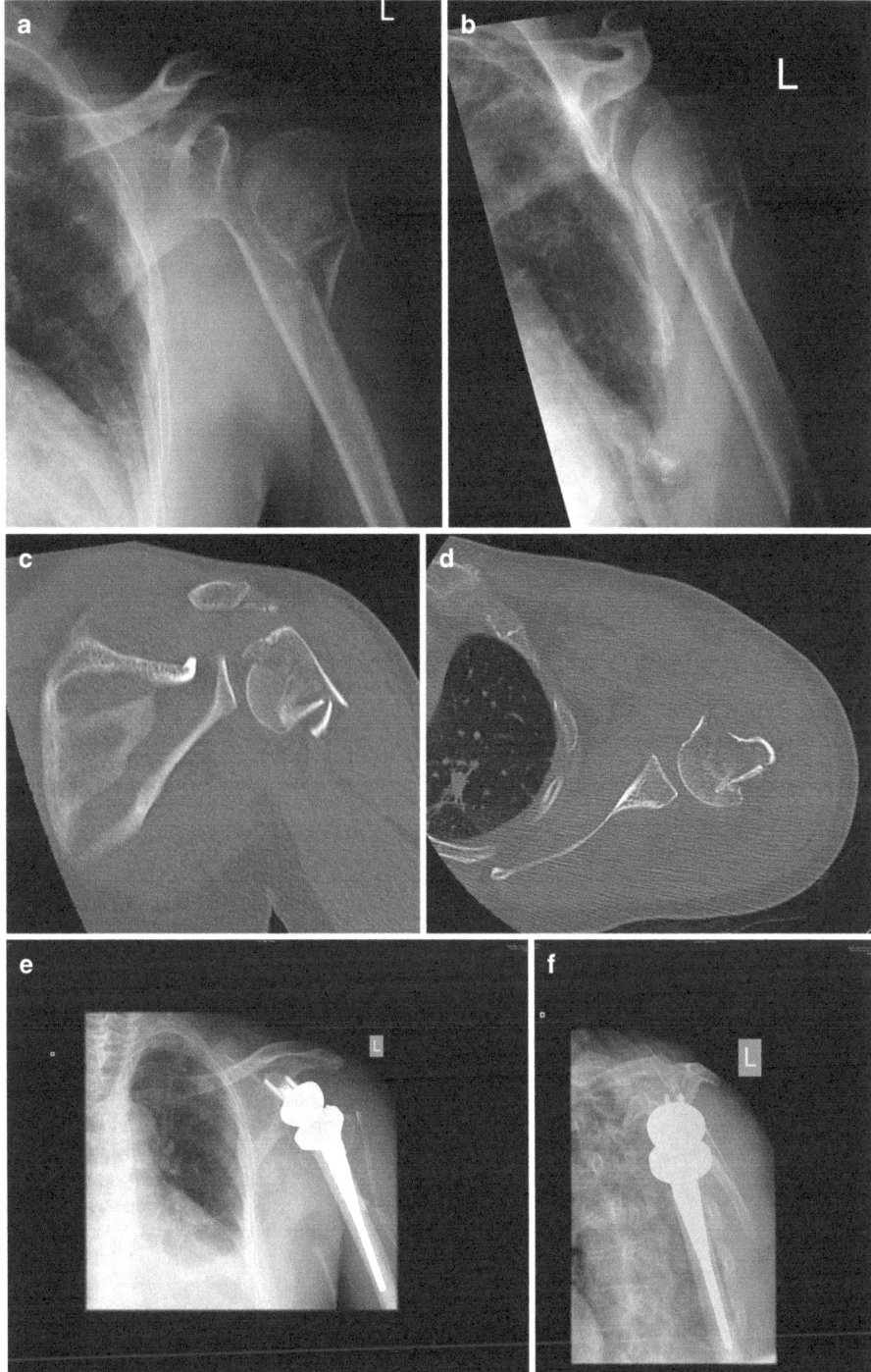

Fig. 4.5 (**a–d**) 76/F suffered from 4-part proximal humerus fracture after falling from three steps of stairs. X-ray showed fractures involving the anatomical head, with short calcar fragment, and breakage of the medial hinge. (**e, f**) Reverse shoulder arthroplasty was performed in view of high risk of avascular necrosis and other complications associated with fracture fixation

Table 4.2 Biomechanical studies that compared fixation of proximal humerus fracture with locking intramedullary nails and locking plates

Study	N	Comparisons	Outcome measured	Key findings
Strasser et al. [23]	Twelve fresh frozen humeri with 2-part fracture model	(a) The Expert Humerus Nail with the angular stable locking system (b) PHILOS stainless steel locking plate	The varus impaction, varus per cycle motion, tilt, and tilt per cycle were analysed	The plate group showed a significantly higher median varus impaction
Füchtmeier et al. [24]	12 matched pairs of human cadaver humeri	(a) Humerus nail (Sirus) (b) Proximal humeral nail with spiral blade (c) PHILOS stainless steel locking plate (d) 4.5 mm AO T-plate	Bending and torsional stiffness	Intramedullary nails were biomechanically superior when compared to plating systems
Yoon et al. [25]	Sixteen match-paired (32 total) fresh frozen, cadaveric specimens following creation of an AO/OTA Type 11A3 (2-part) proximal humerus fractures	(a) 3.5 mm fixed angle plate (3.5-FAP) (b) 4.5 mm fixed angle plate (4.5-FAP) (c) Humeral intramedullary nail (IMN) (d) Humeral intramedullary nail with a fixed angle blade (IMN-FAB)	Constructs were tested for stiffness and ultimate load to failure	Biomechanical testing of modern fixation options for 2-part proximal humerus fracture exhibited that the stiffest and highest load to failure construct was the IMN-FAB followed by the IMN, 3.5-FAP and then the 4.5-FAP constructs

Table 4.3 Randomized controlled studies that compared fixation of proximal humerus fracture with locking intramedullary nails and locking plates

Study	N	Comparisons	Outcome measured	Key findings
Gracitelli et al. [26]	72 patients with 2- or 3-part proximal humerus fracture	(a) Centronail intramedullary nail with three proximal locking screws (b) PHILOS stainless steel locking plate	12-month Constant-Murley score, DASH, the VAS pain score, the shoulder passive range of motion, the neck shaft angle, and complication rates.	There were no significant differences for all parameters except the nail group experienced higher total complication rates ($P = 0.002$) and reoperation rates ($P = 0.041$)
Plath et al. [27]	81 patients >60 years old with proximal humerus fracture	(a) Locking Blade Nail (b) PHILOS stainless steel locking plate	Constant score, age and gender adjusted Constant score, DASH score, VAS for pain, subjective overall condition of the shoulder (1–6) and active shoulder range of motion in flexion and abduction	The LBN group showed improved DASH scores as compared to PHILOS at 12 months ($p = 0.042$) with fewer incidences of secondary loss of reduction and screw cutout ($p = 0.039$)

Table 4.3 (continued)

Study	N	Comparisons	Outcome measured	Key findings
Zhu et al. [28]	Fifty-one consecutive patients with a fresh 2-part surgical neck fracture were randomized to be treated with a locking intramedullary nail (*n* = 25) or a locking plate (*n* = 26)	(a) Locking intramedullary nail (b) Locking plate	Clinical and radiographic assessments were conducted at 1 year and 3 years after the surgery. A visual analogue scale (VAS) was used to assess shoulder pain. The American Shoulder and Elbow Surgeons (ASES) scores and Constant-Murley scores were recorded to evaluate shoulder function	Satisfactory results can be achieved with either implant in the treatment of 2-part proximal humeral surgical neck fractures. There was no difference regarding the ASES scores between these two implants at the time of the final, 3-year follow-up. The complication rate was lower in the locking intramedullary nail group, while fixation with a locking plate had the advantage of a better 1-year outcome

had improved DASH scores ($p = 0.042$) with few incidences of secondary loss of reduction and screw cutout ($p = 0.039$). Zhu et al. [28] was the only study with 3 years follow-up and showed there was no difference in ASES scores among the two implants.

3. Nevertheless, locking plate fixation of displaced surgical neck fracture is still favoured by most surgeons [29]. Iatrogenic rotator cuff injury from nail introduction is one of the main reasons surgeons reject antegrade humeral intramedullary nails [30].

4. Modern straight humeral nails enter the intramedullary canal through the rotator cuff muscle. This minimizes damage to the rotator cuff insertion, which is identified as a possible cause of shoulder pain in older generation curvilinear humeral nails [31].

5. Authors' preference:
   (a) For 2-part fracture or 3-part fracture with varus displacement, especially with poor bone quality (as measured by on Tingart measurement and Deltoid tuberosity index), nail fixation is preferred due to its biomechanical superiority.
   (b) For valgus 3-part fracture or 4-part fracture, secure tuberosity fixation is the main focus and plate fixation may help accomplish this goal easier in authors' hands.

4.5 Setup for Proximal Humerus Fixation

1. The setup and positioning of the patients for both proximal humerus nailing and plating are similar (Fig. 4.6). The author prefers supine position on a radiolucent table, with the torso positioned on the edge of the table so the shoulder can be hyperextended if necessary. A small rolled towel bump is placed under the ipsilateral scapula. The C-arm approaches the patient from the contralateral side. Lateral view is obtained with internal rotation of the shoulder coupled with "external rotation" of the C-arm. Some surgeons advocate beach chair position, however, it is more difficult to obtain true AP view of the humeral head especially with the shoulder extended. Dynamic fluoroscopy is useful to assess optimal screw depth and should optimally be perpendicular to the plane of the screw.

Open reduction and internal fixation of proximal humerus fracture with locking plate

1. The author prefers split deltoid approach for the majority of fracture patterns (Fig. 4.7). A lateral incision is made from the anterolateral edge of acromion, and the wound is extended distally to 5 cm to avoid injury to the axillary nerve (Fig. 4.8). Subacromial space is devel-

Fig. 4.6 Typical set up for proximal humeral fracture fixation. One assistant sits on the right side of the surgeon (for right sided fracture) and controls the limb position

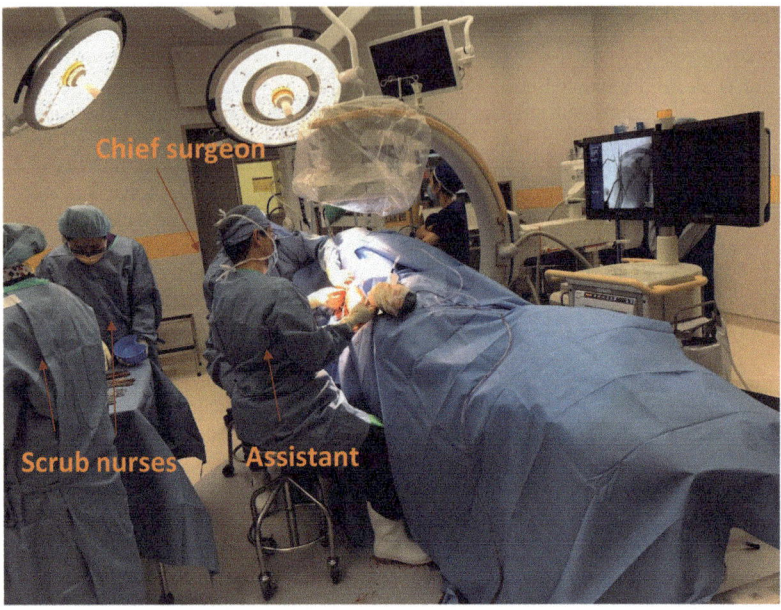

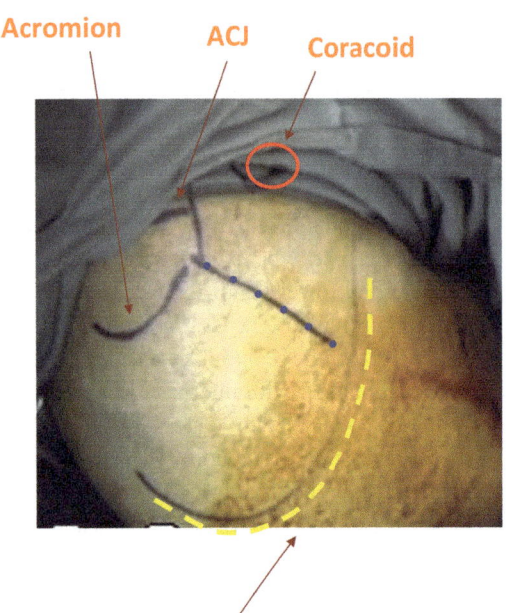

Course of Axillary Nerve

Fig. 4.7 Split deltoid approach with the proximal incision limited to the anticipated course of the axillary nerve. Proximal extension of the incision with partial deltoid detachment from the acromion allows improved visualization of the lesser tuberosity fragment

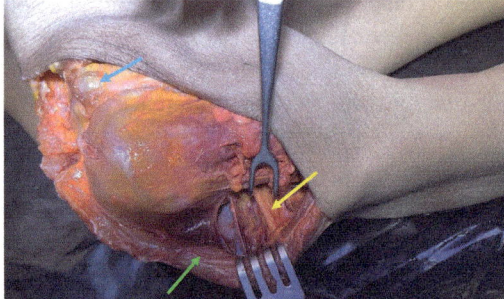

Fig. 4.8 Anterior deltoid is detached from the acromion and clavicle, and it is retracted posteriorly. Yellow arrow: axillary nerve. Green arrow: deltoid muscle. Blue arrow: coracoid process

oped by sweeping finger after deltoid is split. Axillary nerve may be identified by palpation under the deltoid muscle but this is often not necessary.

2. For fracture dislocation which has failed closed reduction and for head-splitting fracture, deltopectoral approach is preferred. An anterior incision is made, starting from the coracoid process and extended distally 10–15 cm towards the shaft of the humerus.

An interval between pectoralis major and deltoid is developed, and cephalic vein is retracted laterally. After incision of clavipectoral fascia, a Hofmann retractor is placed laterally to retract the deltoid. Medial retraction should be avoided because of musculocutaneous nerve which enters coracobrachialis 2.5 cm distal to coracoid process. If humeral head or glenoid is involved, division of subscapularis attachment is needed for better exposure with later repair.

3. *Step 1: Suture fixation of rotator cuff*

Supraspinatus and infraspinatus tendons are identified and anchored with strong non-absorbable sutures. These sutures can help pull the head out of varus and will be anchored to the plate as a supplementary fixation. The sutures placed at tendon-bone junction are better in resisting cut through particularly in elderly patients [32].

4. *Step 2: Reduction of head fragment*

Firstly, the humeral head fragment is reduced to the shaft. Retroversion of the head is corrected using 2.0 K wire as a joystick, inserted from anterior to posterior. Elevation of the shaft with towels under the elbow help to reduce posterior angulation of the fracture which is commonly seen. Residual varus deformity is corrected using a similar technique with the K wire inserted from lateral to medial. An axial K wire is inserted through the humeral head to intramedullary canal to temporarily hold this reduction. Alternatively, K wire aiming from anterolateral shaft to humeral head proximally may be used (Fig. 4.9).

5. *Step 3: Reduction of the tuberosity fragments*

The greater tuberosity is frequently displaced cephalic and posterior. One to two 1.6 mm K wire can be used to reduce the tuberosity fragment using Kapendji technique (Fig. 4.10). After reduction of the greater tuberosity, transosseous suture between the greater tuberosity and the head fragment are tightened to close the gap anterior to the greater tuberosity.

6. *Step 4: Plate assisted reduction of the medial translation of shaft*

The pull of the pectoralis major muscle often causes medial translation of the humeral shaft. The plate is slid extraperiosteally underneath the deltoid and the axillary nerve to 5mm distal to the top of greater tuberosity and 2–4 mm posterior to the bicipital groove to minimize subacromial impingement and compression of ascending branch of anterior circumflex respectively. The shaft is pulled laterally with a 3.5 mm cortical screw introduced to the proximal combi hole of the locking plate (Fig. 4.11). Full tightening of the cortical screw may result in loss of medial neck cortical support and should be avoided.

7. *Step 5: Optimize fixation*

To avoid intraarticular drill bit penetration especially in osteoporotic bones, woodpecker drilling technique is used. The surgeon advances the drill bit only for a short distance each time until the hard subchondral bone is felt. For soft bone, only the near cortex is drilled, followed by pushing the depth gauge to reach the subchondral region. However, in these situations, the surgeon must always be very mindful about the screw trajectory—it is very easy for the screw to false tract and fail to lock with the fixed angle locking plate. At least five proximal locking screws should be placed into the head of humerus to provide sufficient stability (Fig. 4.12). Calcar screw is required for fractures with deficient medial support [33, 34]. Finally, screw positions must be scrutinized on multiple radiographic views to look for any intraarticular violation.

8. Rehabilitation

Immediate passive mobilization and assisted active mobilization is advised for most patients after surgical fixation for the first 6 weeks. This is in line with current evidence that emphasizes placing controlled stresses throughout the fracture site at an early stage [35]. Active mobilization and gentle strengthening exercises are started after 6 weeks post-operation.

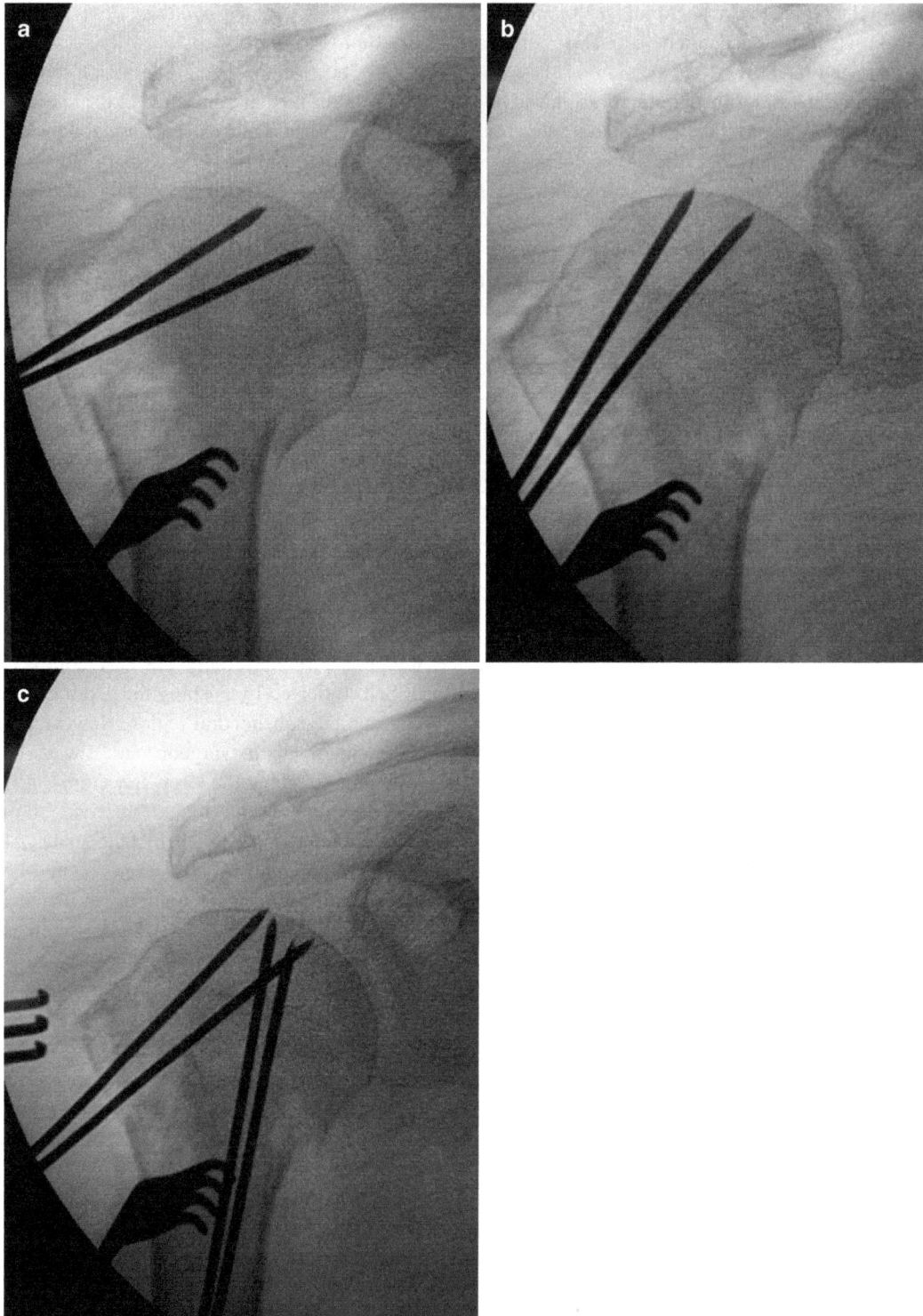

Fig. 4.9 (**a–c**) Lateral to medial joystick K wire to correct the residual varus deformity. This is temporarily held with 2 K wires from anterolateral shaft to humeral head

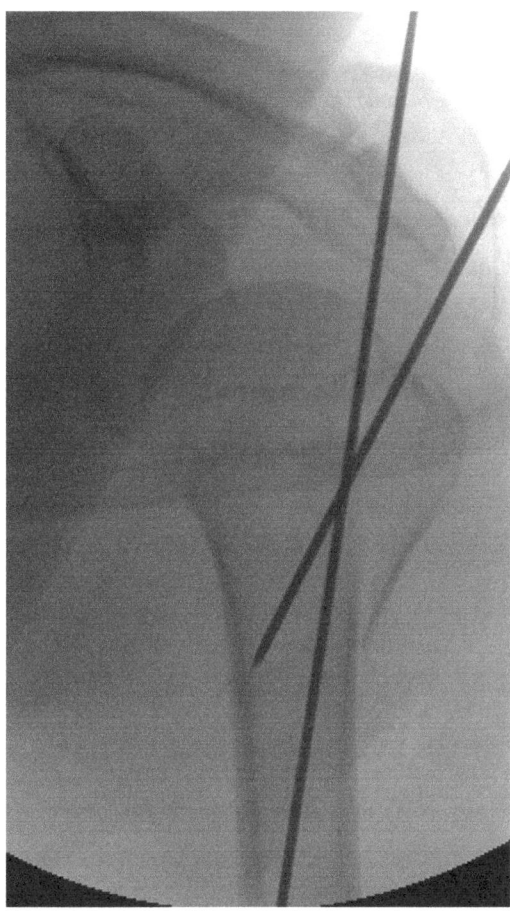

Fig. 4.10 Two 1.6 mm K wire inserted as Kapendji technique to control the cephalic and posterior translation of the greater tuberosity fragment, respectively

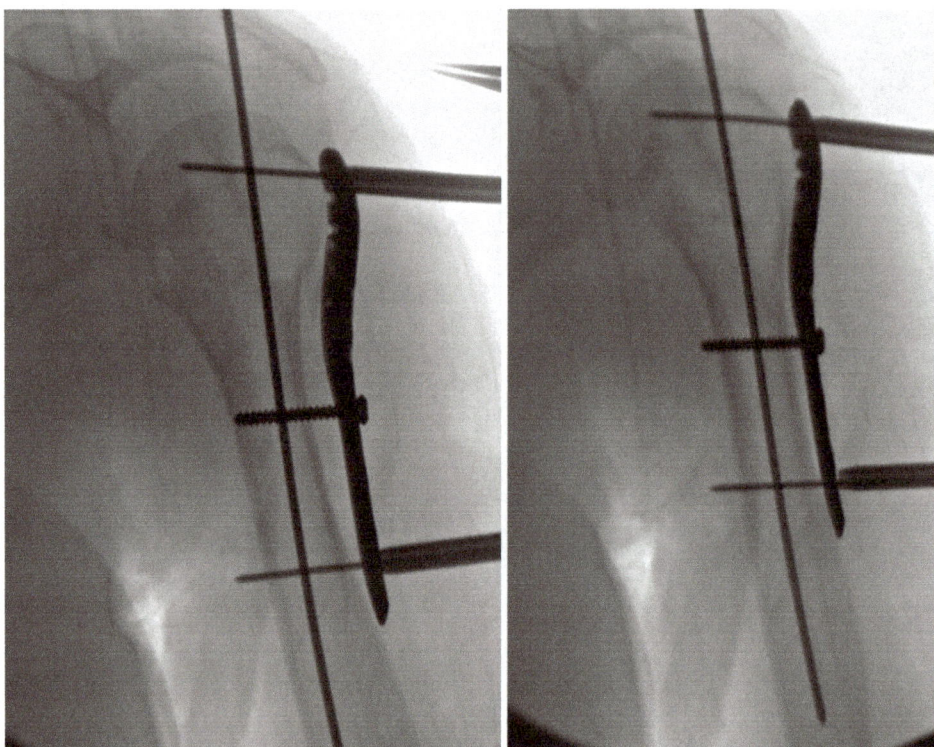

Fig. 4.11 Medial translation of the humeral shaft corrected with cortical screw introduction through the locking plate

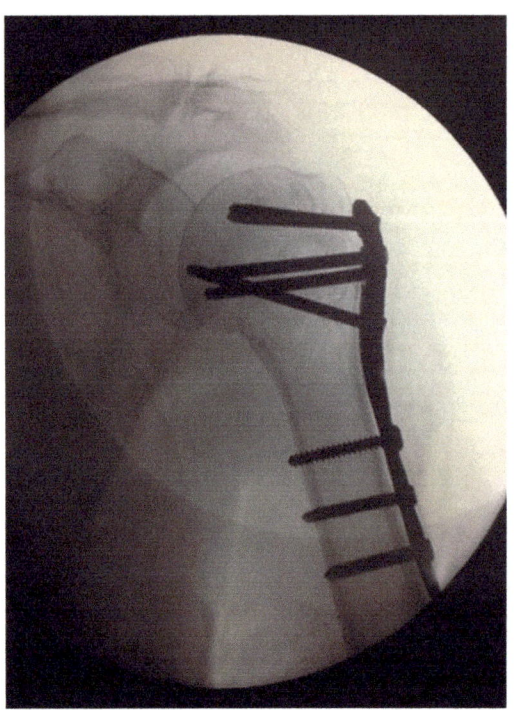

Fig. 4.12 At least five proximal screws should be placed to achieve maximal stability

4.6   Augmentation of Osteosynthesis in Proximal Humerus Plating

The most common techniques for augmentation of plate osteosyntheses included fibula bone graft, to enhance medial support, metaphyseal void filler with either synthetic bone substitute or bone graft, and screw tip augmentation with cement. A systematic review by Biermann et al included 15 biomechanical studies and 30 clinical studies and concluded any kind of augmentation positively enhances mechanical stability, reduces the rate of secondary dislocation, and improves patients' clinical outcome with no additional associated complications [36].

4.7 Surgical Techniques in Fixation of Two-Part Fractures Involving the Greater Tuberosity

Displaced greater tuberosity fractures benefit from surgery to prevent subacromial impingement and loss of range of motion. The indication of surgery is controversial and ranges from 3 to 10 mm of displacement of the greater tuberosity [36]. Surgical options for isolated greater tuberosity fracture include open reduction internal fixation or arthroscopic fixation. Depending on the size and the amount of comminution, either isolated screw fixation (non-comminuted large fragment), buttress plate fixation (large fragment with questionable bone quality) or tension band suture (small fragment) may be utilized (Fig. 4.13a, b).

For small to medium sized greater tuberosity fractures (<3 cm in length), double row tension band suture via open or arthroscopic approach is possible [37]. After debridement and clearing of the fracture haematoma, two suture anchors are inserted into the articular edge of the humeral head through the rotator cuff (Fig. 4.14a, b). The medial row is tightened using "double pulley suture bridges technique" (Fig. 4.14c). The frag-

Fig. 4.13 (a, b) Fracture of greater tuberosity fixed with two lag screws and tension band sutures

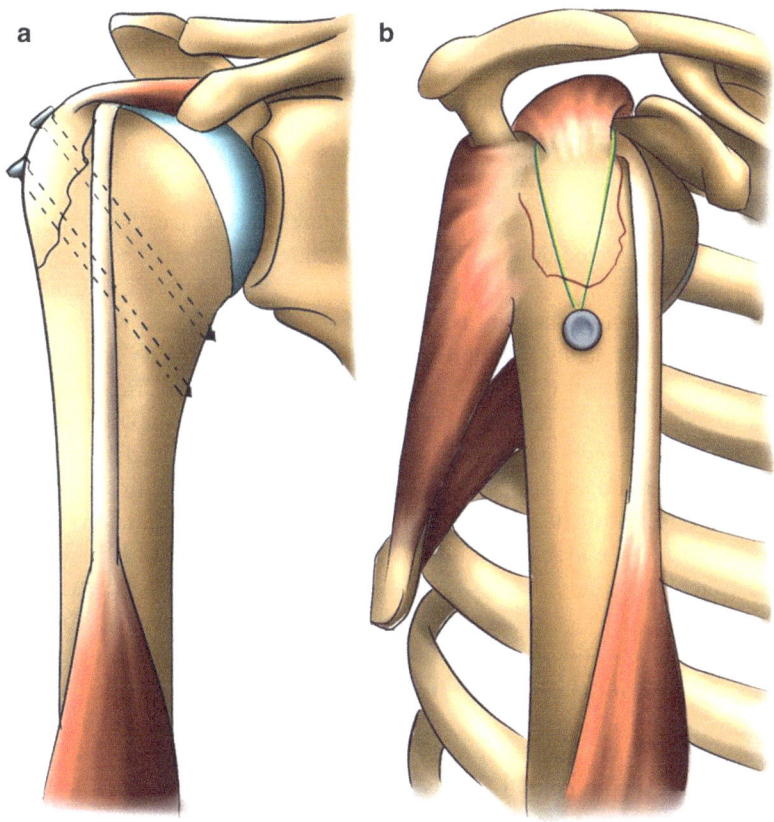

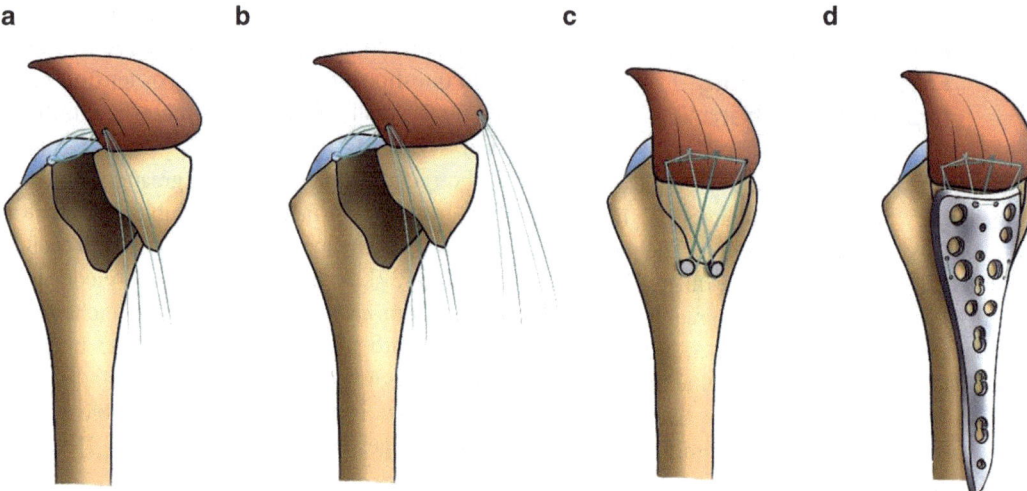

Fig. 4.14 Arthroscopic fixation of greater tuberosity fracture. (**a, b**) Two medial row suture anchors are inserted into the articular edge of the humeral head through rotator cuff. (**c**) The medial row is tightened using "double pulley suture bridges technique". The fragment is reduced by pulling sutures, which are then fixed by knotless suture anchors. (**d**) If fragments are multiple and large, an additional plating is added and sutures are tied to the available holes of the plate

ment is then reduced by pulling the sutures, which are then fixed by knotless suture anchors (Fig. 4.14c)

A rehabilitation plan similar to usual proximal humeral fracture fixation can be implemented, except with small greater tuberosity fractures which are analogous to rotator cuff repair, in which a more conservative mobilization plan should be adopted. This involves 6 weeks of pendulum exercise followed by 6 weeks of passive mobilization before allowing active mobilization.

4.8 Proximal humeral nail

1. For Neer 3-part and 4-part proximal humerus fracture, a split deltoid approach is used for tuberosity reduction. For Neer 2-part proximal humerus fracture, joystick percutaneous fixation is the preferred method. Neer 3-part and 4-part fractures should be converted to 2-part fracture first, by fixation of the tuberosities to the head fragment with sutures, before fixing the neck of humerus.

2. *Step 1: K wire joystick reduction*

   Two 2.5 mm K wires are inserted to the head fragment by percutaneous technique as joysticks. The anterior–posterior K wire is inserted from proximal anterior to distal posterior to correct the posterior angulation and retroversion deformity, and the lateral-medial K wire is inserted from proximal lateral to distal medial to control the varus deformity. They are at 90° to each other to allow good control of humeral head fragment in all planes of motion (Fig. 4.15). K wires thinner than 2.5 mm will yield easily and fail to correct the deformity. These K wires should avoid the path of the nail entry. Both K wires are pivoted distally to affect the reduction. The aim is to uncover the entry site of the nail from acromioclavicular joint and lateral clavicle.

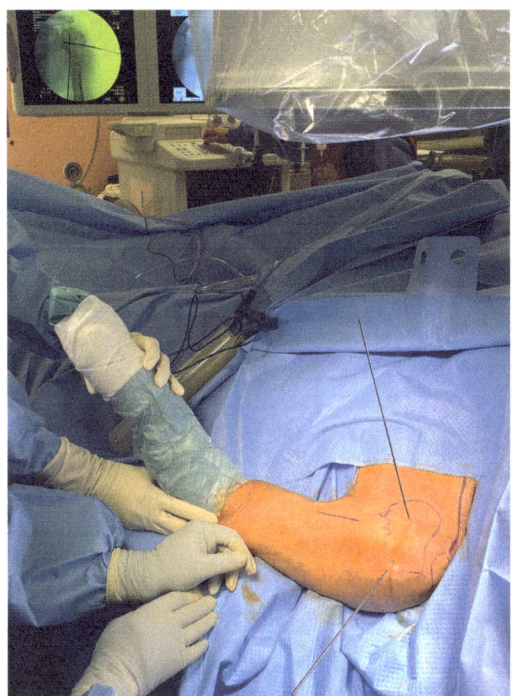

Fig. 4.15 Two 2.5 mm K wires used as joysticks: anterior to posterior K wire controls the posterior angulation and retroversion of the head fragment while the lateral to medial K wire controls the varus deformity. See the C-arm monitor at the left upper corner for the K wire position in the humeral head

3. *Step 2: Nail entry site preparation*

The apex of the humeral head is identified on both anteroposterior and lateral radiograph. A 2.5 mm K wire is inserted percutaneously, through the apex of the humeral head to the humeral shaft. This is usually just anterior to the acromioclavicular joint. The entry site must be scrutinized meticulously on fluoroscopy as lateral and anterior entry site will result in varus and retroversion deformity, respectively. The 2 joystick K wires allow rotation of the head fragment under fluoroscopic screening (Fig. 4.16a, b), and the entry site K wire should appear to be centred on the apex the head on all views. A 2 cm incision is made over the entry site K wire. Deltoid muscle is split bluntly.

4. *Step 3: Nail instrumentation*

A cannulated awl is preferred over a trephine reamer for entry hole creation, as the awl tends to split the rotator cuff muscle instead of removal of a circular cuff of muscle. A long guide rod is inserted from the entry site across the fracture, and the humeral nail is railroaded through the guide rod. If any K wire joystick blocks the passage of the nail, it can be removed at this stage. Passage of the nail should be gentle to avoid injury to the bone cuff around the entry site. The nail should be flush with the subchondral bone, and excessive countersinking of the nail more than 5 mm below the subchondral bone should be avoided [38], as this places the proximal bolts in suboptimal position, decreasing the stability of the "fifth anchoring point" which is the proximal end of the nail.

5. *Step 4: Adjust rotation and manual compression of the fracture*

The proximal locking bolts are inserted with percutaneous stab incisions. Specifically for the MultiLoc nail (Depuy Synthes), "screw-in-screw" option with 3.5 mm locking screw improves stability and purchase of the head fragment [39]. Prior to distal locking bolt placement, correct rotation of the fracture should be checked. This is accomplished by fluoroscopic examination, comparing the width and cortical diameter, and also by examining the range of rotation of the shoulder when the forearm and the jig of the nail are moved together. Axial loading of the fracture by manual compression between the elbow and the jig of the nail allows fracture compression prior to distal locking.

6. *Step 5: Tuberosities stabilization*

For 3-part and 4-part proximal humerus fracture, an extended split deltoid approach is used in which part of the anterior deltoid is released from the acromion. The head shaft relationship is restored first and insertion of the nail will stabilize the reduction.

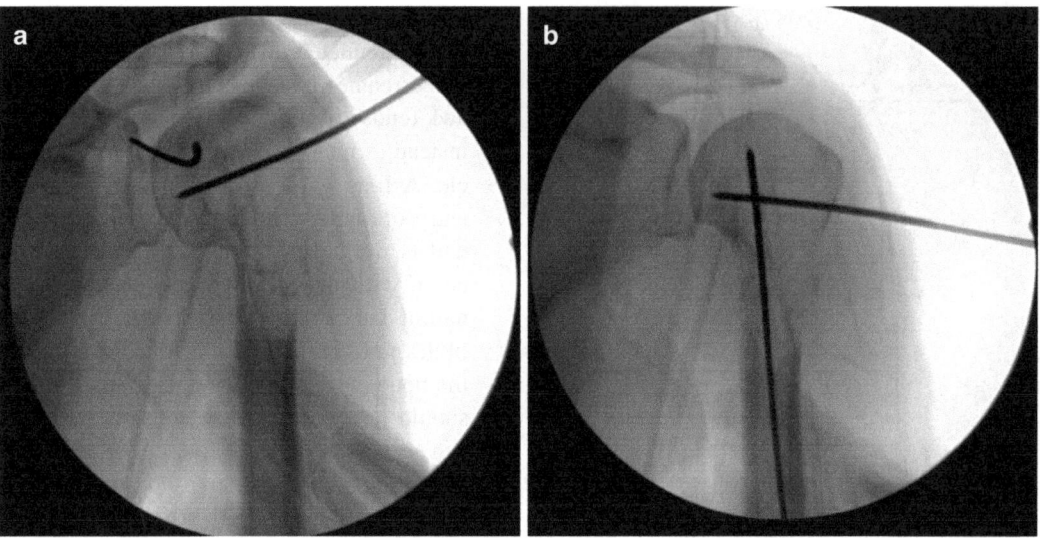

Fig. 4.16 (**a**, **b**) Varus malalignment and retroversion corrected to anatomical alignment with K wire joystick manipulation

Tuberosities are tied to each other with strong non-absorbable sutures, before the insertion of locking bolt. Sutures anchored on rotator cuff are tied onto the head of the locking bolt to neutralize their deforming force (Fig. 4.17a–f).

7. *Rehabilitation*

Passive mobilization by therapist and assisted active forward flexion, with the help of the contralateral upper limb, are started on the first day after operation. From the seventh week after surgery, patients begin active shoulder mobilization and strengthening exercises.

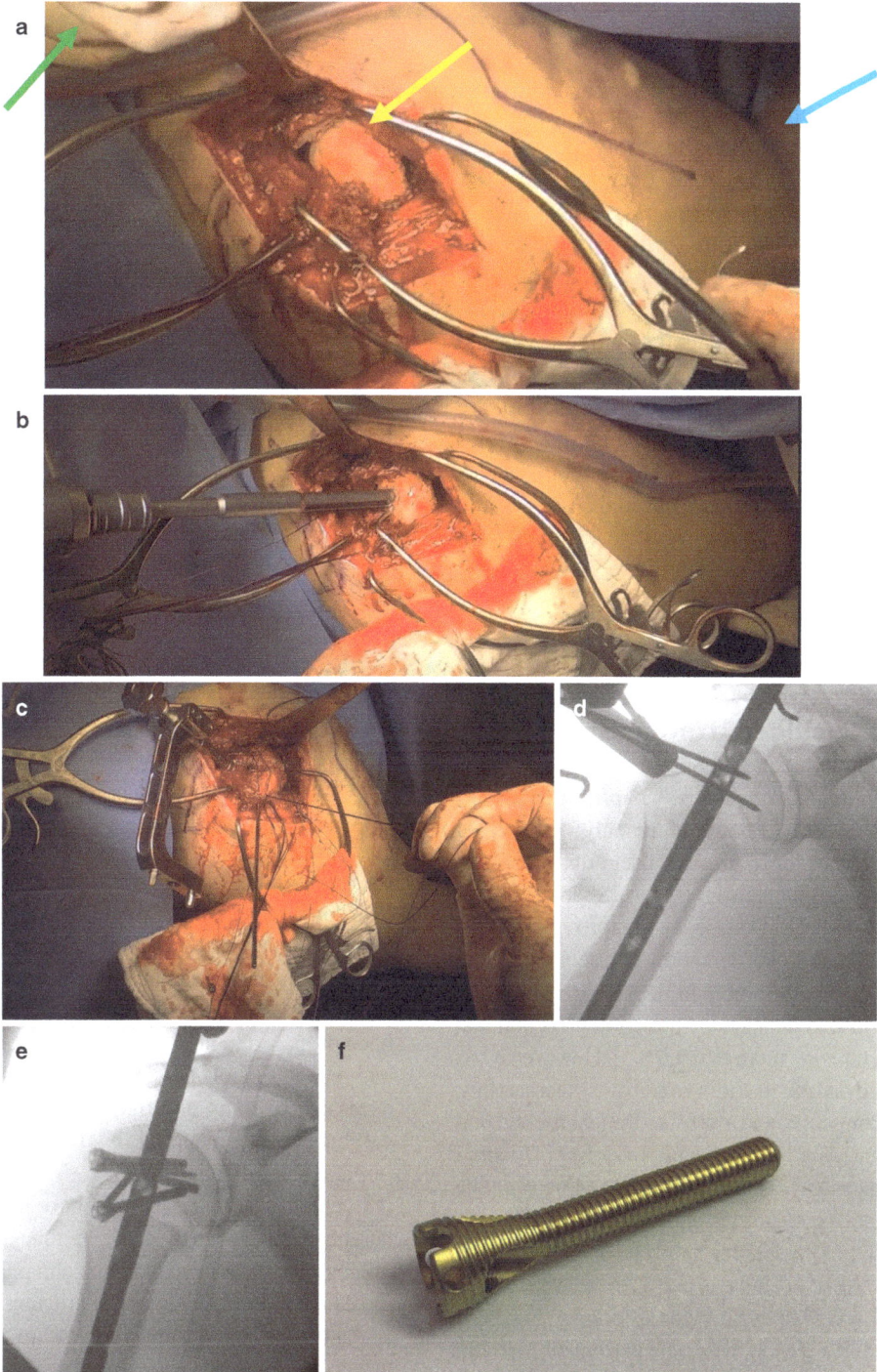

Fig. 4.17 (**a**) The humeral head is exposed by splitting the rotator interval along the biceps tendon. Yellow arrow: humeral head. Green arrow: Cephalic side. Blue arrow: Ipsilateral elbow. (**b**) Entry site preparation with cannulated reamer. (**c**) Humeral head and shaft relationship are restored and stabilized with nail insertion. Greater tuberosity and lesser tuberosity are tied to each other with strong non-absorbable sutures. (**d**) Head-shaft reduction is already achieved at this stage. (**e**) Intraoperative radiograph showing MultiLoc nail (Depuy Synthes) instrumentation. Proximal locking bolts with screw-in-screw options are inserted. (**f**) There are four suture holes per MultiLoc nail (Depuy Synthes) screw to allow rotator cuff attachment

4.9   Reverse Shoulder Arthroplasty

1. Patients with complex 3-part and 4-part fractures that cannot be stably fixed due to osteoporotic bone had been treated with hemiarthroplasty in the past. However, the results of hemiarthroplasty in these group of patients had been unreliable [40, 41]. Recently reverse shoulder arthroplasty had been introduced as an alternative treatment option. The main advantage of reverse shoulder arthroplasty is that the results are unaffected by tuberosity healing. Meta-analysis had shown improvements in forward flexion, clinical outcome scores, and risk of reoperation, with no difference in external rotation, tuberosity healing, and deep infection rate [42].

4.10   Controversies in Reverse Shoulder Arthroplasty

1. *Approach: Deltopectoral vs split deltoid*

    The two most commonly performed approaches for reverse shoulder arthroplasty are deltopectoral approach (Fig. 4.18) and split deltoid approach. Deltopectoral approach required either tendon peel, tenotomy or osteotomy of the subscapular insertion [43]. Also, visualization and instrumentation of posterior glenohumeral structures are more difficult [43]. However, it has the advantage that it is atraumatic, internervous, intermuscular, and extensile. Deltoid muscle bellies are not violated with less risk of deltoid dehiscence or weakening [43]. Moreover, the surgeon enjoyed an improved access and visualization of the inferior humeral osteophytes [43]. The risk of notching is less as there is better glenoid access to avoid high positioning or superiorly tilted glenoid baseplate placement [44, 45]. The split deltoid approach is limited distally due to the traversing axillary nerve with the advantage of better access to the greater tuberosity.

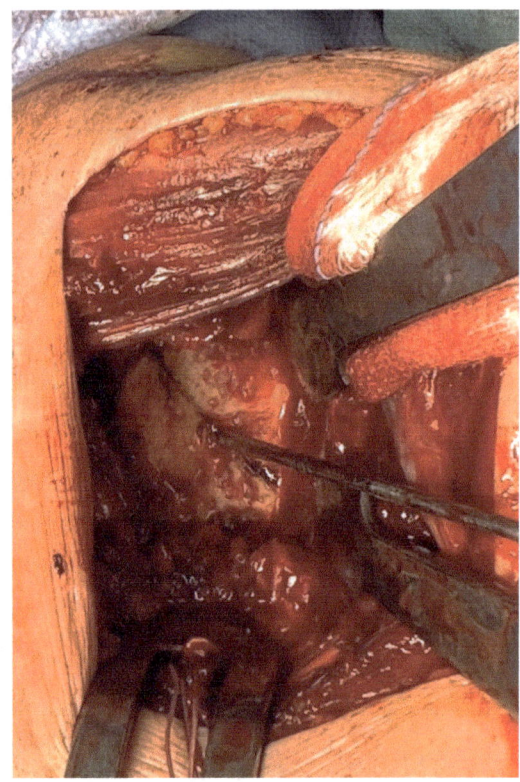

Fig. 4.18 Glenoid exposure obtained with deltopectoral approach

2. *Glenoid tilt*

    The benefits of inferior tilt remain controversial in the literature, and new evidence seems to suggest it may be worse than neutral tilt [46]. Inferior tilt of 10°–15° degrees has been proposed to improve the adduction range and reduce scapula notching [46] but requires excessive reaming and therefore its theoretical benefit is countered by bone loss and implant medialization.

    Previous researches [47–49] have found that baseplate location had an eight times greater influence on inferior scapular notching then tilt. Excessive reaming and neck shortening [50] to accommodate inferior tilt may lead to reduced head neck ratio, loss of strong subchondral bone stock and a higher likelihood of impingement with reduced range of motion on adduction and external rotation. In elderly patients with small

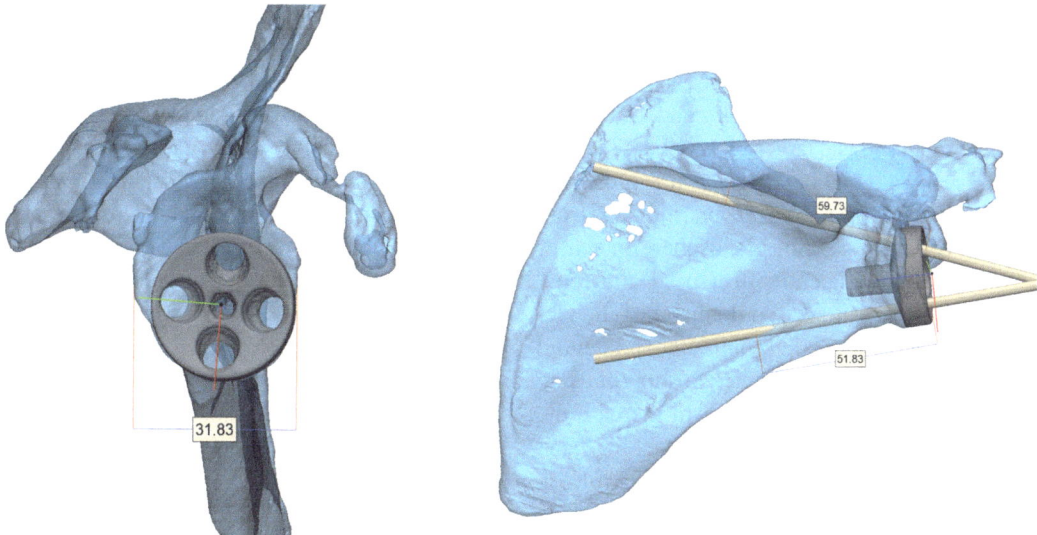

Fig. 4.19 Pre-operative planning. The baseplate is flush with the inferior margin of the glenoid and with neutral tilt to minimize the need for reaming (relative to native glenoid)

body build and small glenoid sizes routine inferior tilt is therefore not recommended (Fig. 4.19).

3. *Lateral offset*

Because of concerns about scapula notching, there was an increase in interest to increase the lateral offset [46]. Systematic review by Helmkamp et al. showed no clear difference in outcome scores between the lateralized and medialized centre of rotation groups. The lateralized centre of rotation group displayed increased postoperative ROM and lower reported incidence of scapular notching [51]. Increasing the lateral offset is commonly achieved by increasing the length of the scapular neck with bone graft (BIO-RSA) (Fig. 4.20) and is applicable to patients with glenoid bone loss with high rate of graft incorporation [52] but not applicable to those with acute humeral fracture and normal glenoid anatomy.

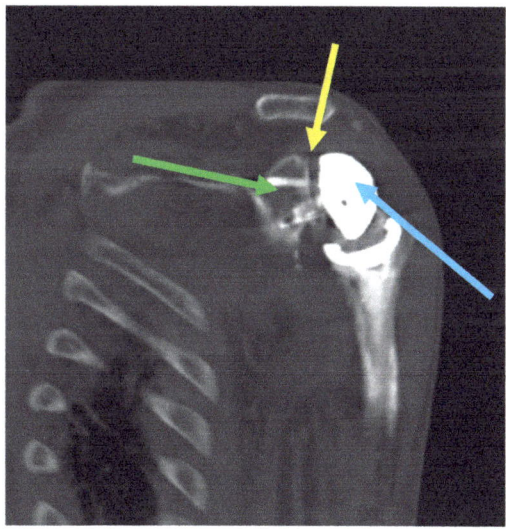

Fig. 4.20 Postoperative computed tomography after BIO-RSA surgery. Green arrow: scapula. Yellow: bone graft. Blue arrow: glenosphere

(a) Size of glenosphere: Data from cadaveric analysis showed improve impingement-free range of motion increases with larger glenosphere [53, 54], and computer model showed larger glenosphere reduced scapula notching because of prosthetic overhang [55]. However, moving from 36 mm to 42 mm glenosphere increases the global lateral offset by 1 mm only [56]. Also, increased diameter of the glenosphere increased joint load and deltoid force [57]. The evidence to support using a larger glenosphere size to increase the global lateral offset is lacking and required further research studies [46].

(b) Humeral lateralization: Lateralization of the humerus is largely achieved by stem design (straight vs. curved), whether humerus component is embedded in metaphysis (inlay) or sits above humeral cut (onlay) (Fig. 4.21), and the neck shaft angle [46]. While traditional Grammont design has a straight stem, some modern stems are curved stem with onlay system. The benefits of curved stem are multifold: to preserve the tuberosity and metaphyseal bone stock and decrease the risk of greater tuberosity fracture, to preserve the remaining rotator cuff insertion, to optimize the ease of insertion, and to allow the option of modularity between reverse shoulder arthroplasty and anatomic shoulder arthroplasty [58].

4. *Neck shaft angle*

Grammont's Delta III humeral stem has a neck-shaft angle of 155°, which compared with 135°–140° in normal shoulders [46].

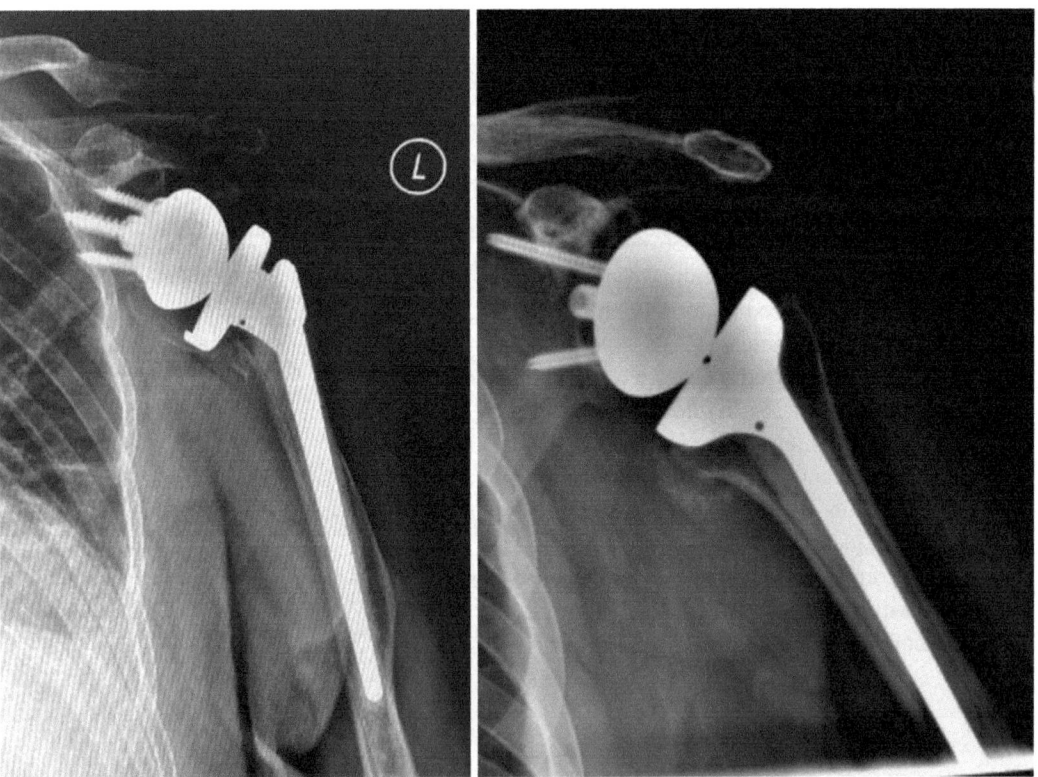

Fig. 4.21 X-ray of two different reverse shoulder arthroplasty systems. Right: onlay stem; Left: inlay stem

Erickson et al. [59] conducted a systematic review on the influence of humeral head inclincation in reverse shoulder arthroplasty. 2222 shoulders in 38 studies were included. 79.3% of used the 155° inclination prosthesis and 20.7% used the 135° prosthesis with a lateralized glenosphere. There are no difference in the dislocation rate but the rate of scapula notching was significantly higher with the 155° prosthesis.

5. *Humeral component version*

Kontaxis performed computer modelling on 30 shoulders and compared the effects of 40° retroversion to 40° anteversion [60]. Intra-articular and extra-articular impingement was calculated for 10 activities of daily living. Impingement free range of motion was also calculated across all motions. Although 40° retroversion produced the largest impingement-free range of motion, neutral version produced the least amount of impingement in activities of daily living. In Kontaxis' series, there was a large variability among subjects and 0° was not optimal for all 30 shoulders, which suggested that no single best optimal value exist for all individuals.

6. *Supraspinatus tenotomy*

Removal of the supraspinatus tendon can facilitate operative visualization of the superior glenoid and with no compromise in the outcomes as restoration of forward flexion and abduction independent of cuff status [61]. Bonnevialle et al. [61] in a retrospective multicenter study compared patients who underwent supraspinatus excision ($n = 117$) or supraspinatus preservation ($n = 33$). There was no difference in complication rate, mean constant score, simple shoulder value, active anterior elevation, internal rotation, and greater tuberosity healing rate. Active external rotation was better in those with suprasinatus excision. This was consistent with the results by Siebenburger et al. [62] ($n = 76$) who showed there was no significant differences between those with or without supraspinatus tenotomy regarding tuberosity integration, resorption or displacement. Supraspinatus tenotomy had a better constant score especially regarding mean active external rotation and active abduction.

7. *Subscapularis repair*

Repair of the subscapularis is recommended where there is insufficient stability and soft tissue tension after implant reduction. Lateralization of the humerus may render the tendon irreparable and on the other hand subscapularis repaired under excessive tension may limit the external rotation range. Meta-analysis by Matthewson et al. analysing 1306 patients from seven studies. Results demonstrated lower dislocation rate overall in the subscapularis repair group. For the subgroup of patients without subscapularis repair, lateralized centre of rotation resulted in lower dislocation rates then medialized centre of rotation [63].

4.11 Authors' Preferred Technique (Fig. 4.22a–o)

Fig. 4.22 (**a**) Patient is placed in a beach chair position under general anaesthesia. The arm is supported on a mayo tray independent of the operation table, which allowed shoulder hyper-extension to facilitate humeral preparation steps. The chief surgeon is positioned at the axilla position. The first assistant is opposite the chief surgeon and the second assistant is next to the chief surgeon. (**b**) Deltopectoral approach for reverse shoulder arthroplasty. The lateral Hohmann is placed between the deltoid muscle and greater tuberosity. The superior Hoffmann is placed over the coracoid process. Green arrow: Deltoid muscle. Yellow arrow: clavipectoral fascia. Blue arrow: pectoralis major muscle. (**c**) The long head of biceps tendon is unroofed from the intertubercle groove and elevated with an artery forceps. Tenodesis to pectoralis major is performed. The rotator interval is opened following the biceps tendon. The humeral head is removed. Tuberosities are tagged with strong non-absorbable sutures. Green arrow: Long head of biceps tendon. (**d**) The humeral head is removed. Tuberosities are tagged with strong non-absorbable sutures. Supraspinatus tenotomy is often performed if it is intact. Green arrow: sutures anchored to infraspinatus. Yellow arrow: cut long head of biceps tendon. Blue arrow: humeral head. (**e**) Circumferential labrectomy was performed. Subperiosteal elevation of tissue off the inferior glenoid neck to 0.5 cm from the inferior rim allow proper baseplate positioning. Green arrow: artery forceps holding excised labrum and remnant of long head of biceps tendon. Yellow arrow: Glenoid. (**f**) 3D printed patient specific instrumentation jig is used to position the glenoid baseplate guide. The jig positioned the baseplate to align with the inferior glenoid rim in neutral tilt. The glenoid is drilled and reamed to a flat surface. (**g**) Guide pin inserted at the centre of glenoid. Noted the glenoid retractor inferiorly allowed adequate exposure to position the baseplate to align with the inferior rim of glenoid. (**h, i**) The baseplate is impacted into the glenoid. 3D printed patient specific instrumentation jig guided locking screw trajectory for maximal bone purchase in small sized glenoids. Authors' case series showed 3D printed patient specific instrumentation jig facilitates long superior and inferior screw placement in the fixation of glenoid component. The mean screw lengths was 44.7 mm and 43 mm for superior and inferior screws, respectively [64]. (**j**) The shoulder is extended and "presented" to the wound. The humerus is prepared with serial canal reaming until cortical chatter is detected. A cemented humeral stem is typically chosen in a fracture setting. The stem version is set at 20° retroversion. (**k**) Humeral neck osteotomy is often not necessary with proximal humerus fracture. A trough is created in the metaphysis to accommodate the keel of the stem to increase the rotational stability of the stem. Green arrow: keel. Yellow arrow: bone trough. (**l**) Two 2.0 mm hole are created at direct lateral position of humerus metaphysis. (**m**) Fibretape suture out-in-out through the cuff tendon and bone. Green circle: greater tuberosity fragment. Blue circle: humerus. Purple line: fibre tape suture through infraspinatus tendon and bone. (**n**) The sutures are tied after shoulder joint reduction with shoulder in slight external rotation. Cement over the metaphysis is removed. Fibre tape sutures pass through the holes at the lateral fin of the implant and are tied to achieve a double row fixation. Bone graft are layed around the greater tuberosity to promote healing. Green arrow: cement in the metaphysis. Yellow arrow: lateral fin of the implant. (**o**) Patient is instructed to avoid active external rotation in the first 6 weeks to protect the infraspinatus repair. Strengthening is started at postop week 7. X-ray at 1 year showed reliable greater tuberosity healing

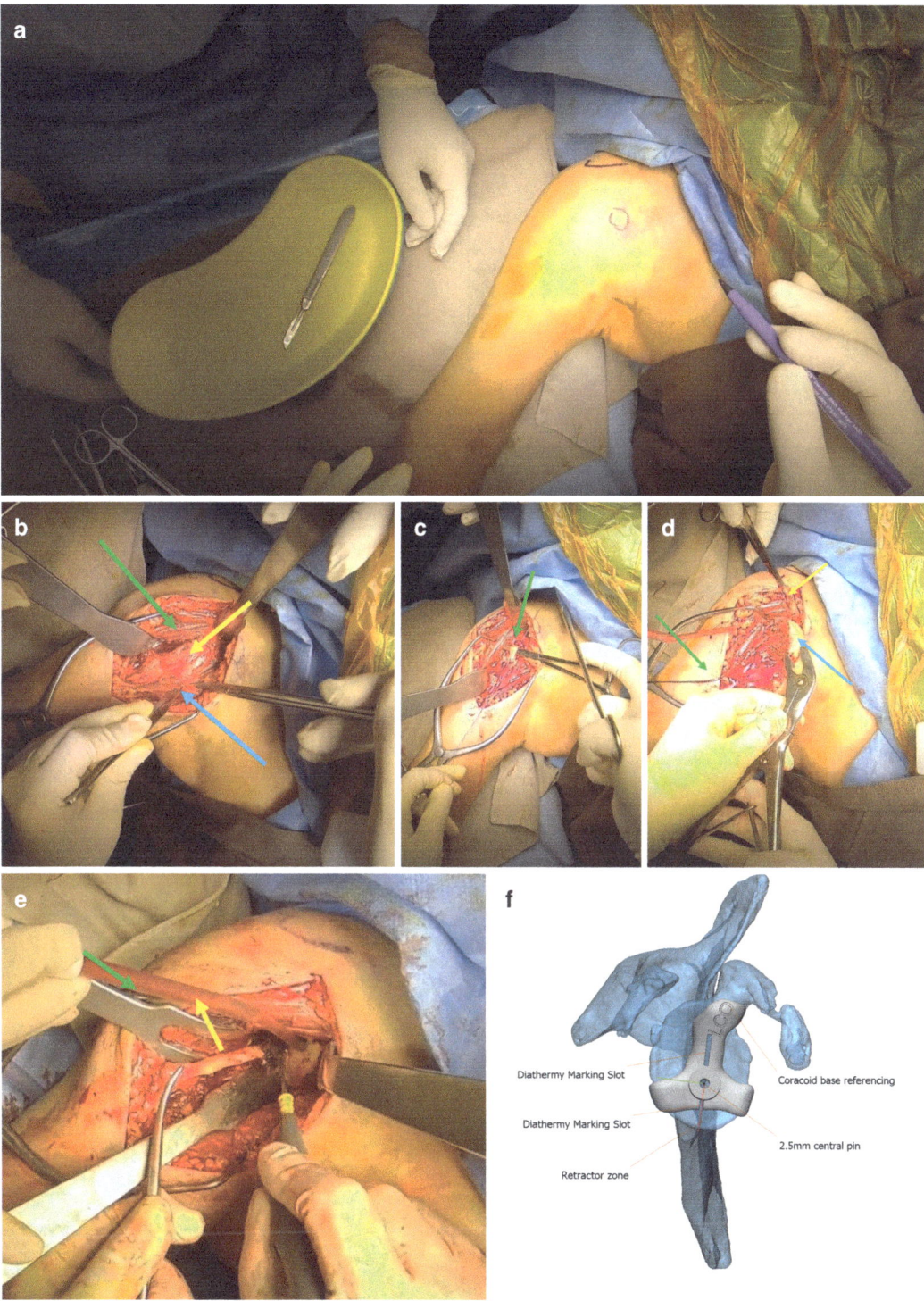

Diathermy Marking Slot

Diathermy Marking Slot

Retractor zone

Coracoid base referencing

2.5mm central pin

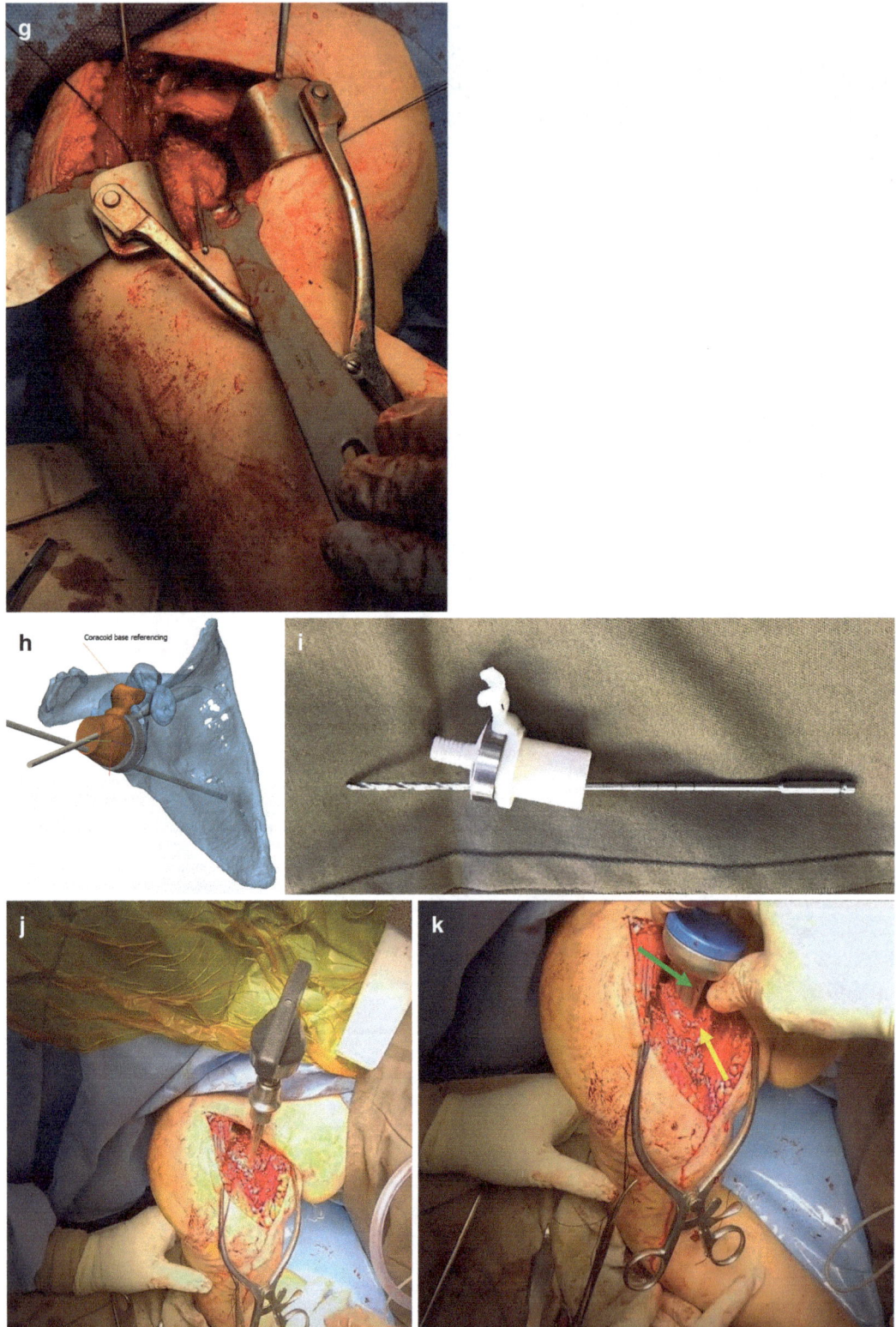

Fig. 4.22 (continued)

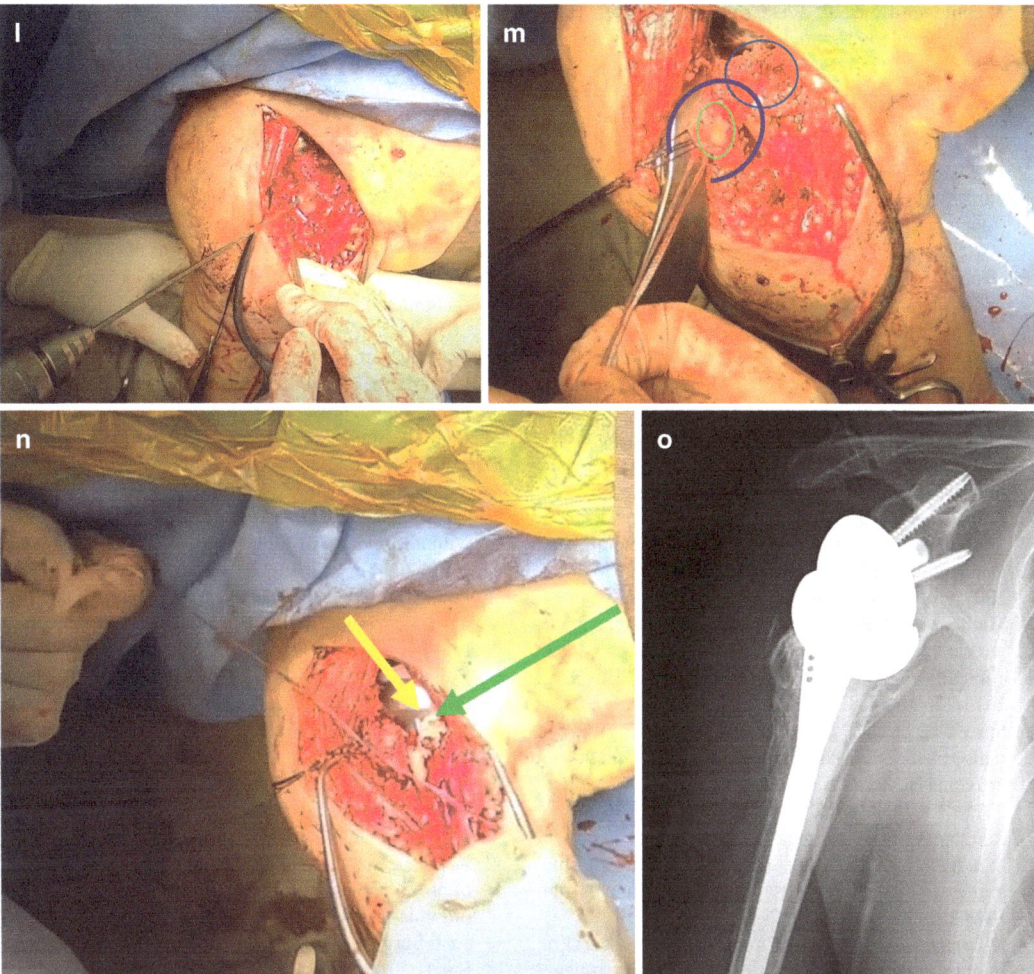

Fig. 4.22 (continued)

4.12 Conclusion and Summary

Plating or proximal humerus nails for proximal humerus fracture required specialized techniques. For irreparable proximal humerus fractures or failed fixation, reverse shoulder arthroplasty presented a good option for reliable functional restoration.

References

1. Court-Brown CM, Caesar B. Epidemiology of adult fractures: a review. Injury. 2006;37(8):691–7.

2. Calvo E, et al. Nondisplaced proximal humeral fractures: high incidence among outpatient-treated osteoporotic fractures and severe impact on upper extremity function and patient subjective health perception. J Shoulder Elb Surg. 2011;20(5):795–801.

3. Helmy N, Hintermann B. New trends in the treatment of proximal humerus fractures. Clin Orthop Relat Res. 2006;442:100–8.

4. Harrison JW, et al. Internal fixation of proximal humeral fractures. Acta Orthop Belg. 2007;73(1):1–11.

5. Brunner F, et al. Open reduction and internal fixation of proximal humerus fractures using a proximal humeral locked plate: a prospective multicenter analysis. J Orthop Trauma. 2009;23(3):163–72.

6. Hirschmann MT, et al. Clinical longer-term results after internal fixation of proximal humerus fractures with a locking compression plate (PHILOS). J Orthop Trauma. 2011;25(5):286–93.

7. Krappinger D, et al. Predicting failure after surgical fixation of proximal humerus fractures. Injury. 2011;42(11):1283–8.

8. Agudelo J, et al. Analysis of efficacy and failure in proximal humerus fractures treated with locking plates. J Orthop Trauma. 2007;21(10):676–81.

9. Barvencik F, et al. Age- and sex-related changes of humeral head microarchitecture: histomorphometric analysis of 60 human specimens. J Orthop Res. 2010;28(1):18–26.

10. Hepp P, et al. Where should implants be anchored in the humeral head? Clin Orthop Relat Res. 2003;415:139–47.

11. Saitoh S, et al. Distribution of bone mineral density and bone strength of the proximal humerus. J Shoulder Elb Surg. 1994;3(4):234–42.

12. Tingart MJ, et al. Three-dimensional distribution of bone density in the proximal humerus. Calcif Tissue Int. 2003;73(6):531–6.

13. Yamada M, et al. Age- and gender-related distribution of bone tissue of osteoporotic humeral head using computed tomography. J Shoulder Elb Surg. 2007;16(5):596–602.

14. Mather J, et al. Proximal humerus cortical bone thickness correlates with bone mineral density and can clinically rule out osteoporosis. J Shoulder Elb Surg. 2013;22(6):732–8.

15. Spross C, et al. Deltoid Tuberosity Index: a simple radiographic tool to assess local bone quality in proximal humerus fractures. Clin Orthop Relat Res. 2015;473(9):3038–45.

16. Rangan A, et al. Surgical vs nonsurgical treatment of adults with displaced fractures of the proximal humerus: the PROFHER randomized clinical trial. JAMA. 2015;313(10):1037–47.

17. O'Donnell JA, Gage MJ. Proximal humerus geriatric fracture care: fix, replace, or nonoperative treatment? J Orthop Trauma. 2021;35(Suppl 5):S6–S10.

18. Franz Kralinger MB. Proximal humerus. In: Michael Blauth SLK, Nicholas JA, editors. Osteoporotic fracture care. New York: Thieme; 2018.

19. Thanasas C, et al. Treatment of proximal humerus fractures with locking plates: a systematic review. J Shoulder Elb Surg. 2009;18(6):837–44.

20. Gerber C, Hersche O, Berberat C. The clinical relevance of posttraumatic avascular necrosis of the humeral head. J Shoulder Elb Surg. 1998;7(6):586–90.

21. Hettrich CM, et al. Quantitative assessment of the vascularity of the proximal part of the humerus. J Bone Joint Surg Am. 2010;92(4):943–8.

22. Hertel R, et al. Predictors of humeral head ischemia after intracapsular fracture of the proximal humerus. J Shoulder Elb Surg. 2004;13(4):427–33.

23. Strasser S, et al. Nail Versus Plate: a biomechanical comparison of a locking plate versus an intramedullary nail with an angular stable locking system in a shoulder simulator with active muscle forces using a two-part fracture model. J Orthop Trauma. 2021;35(3):e71–6.

24. Fuchtmeier B, et al. Proximal humerus fractures: a comparative biomechanical analysis of intra and extramedullary implants. Arch Orthop Trauma Surg. 2007;127(6):441–7.

25. Yoon RS, et al. A comprehensive update on current fixation options for two-part proximal humerus fractures: a biomechanical investigation. Injury. 2014;45(3):510–4.

26. Gracitelli ME, et al. Locking intramedullary nails compared with locking plates for two- and three-part proximal humeral surgical neck fractures: a randomized controlled trial. J Shoulder Elb Surg. 2016;25(5):695–703.

27. Plath JE, et al. Locking nail versus locking plate for proximal humeral fracture fixation in an elderly population: a prospective randomised controlled trial. BMC Musculoskelet Disord. 2019;20(1):20.

28. Zhu Y, et al. Locking intramedullary nails and locking plates in the treatment of two-part proximal humeral surgical neck fractures: a prospective randomized trial with a minimum of three years of follow-up. J Bone Joint Surg Am. 2011;93(2):159–68.

29. Laux CJ, et al. Current concepts in locking plate fixation of proximal humerus fractures. J Orthop Surg Res. 2017;12(1):137.

30. Boileau P, et al. Displaced humeral surgical neck fractures: classification and results of third-generation percutaneous intramedullary nailing. J Shoulder Elb Surg. 2019;28(2):276–87.

31. Lopiz Y, et al. Proximal humerus nailing: a randomized clinical trial between curvilinear and straight nails. J Shoulder Elb Surg. 2014;23(3):369–76.

32. Konrad G, et al. Open reduction and internal fixation of proximal humeral fractures with use of the locking proximal humerus plate. Surgical technique. J Bone Joint Surg Am. 2010;92(Suppl 1):85–95.

33. Bai L, et al. Effect of calcar screw use in surgical neck fractures of the proximal humerus with unstable medial support: a biomechanical study. J Orthop Trauma. 2014;28(8):452–7.

34. Zhang W, et al. The mechanical benefit of medial support screws in locking plating of proximal humerus fractures. PLoS One. 2014;9(8):e103297.

35. Hodgson S. Proximal humerus fracture rehabilitation. Clin Orthop Relat Res. 2006;442:131–8.

36. Platzer P, et al. Displaced fractures of the greater tuberosity: a comparison of operative and nonoperative treatment. J Trauma. 2008;65(4):843–8.

37. Sun Q, et al. Plate fixation versus arthroscopic-assisted plate fixation for isolated medium-sized fractures of the greater tuberosity: a retrospective study. Orthop Surg. 2020;12(5):1456–63.

38. Young AA, Hughes JS. Locked intramedullary nailing for treatment of displaced proximal humerus fractures. Orthop Clin North Am. 2008;39(4):417–28.

39. Rothstock S, et al. Biomechanical evaluation of two intramedullary nailing techniques with different locking options in a three-part fracture proximal humerus model. Clin Biomech. 2012;27(7):686–91.

40. Boileau P, et al. Tuberosity malposition and migration: reasons for poor outcomes after hemiarthroplasty for displaced fractures of the proximal humerus. J Shoulder Elb Surg. 2002;11(5):401–12.

41. Boileau P, et al. Can surgeons predict what makes a good hemiarthroplasty for fracture? J Shoulder Elb Surg. 2013;22(11):1495–506.

42. Austin DC, et al. Decreased reoperations and improved outcomes with reverse total shoulder arthroplasty in comparison to hemiarthroplasty for geriatric proximal humerus fractures: a systematic review and meta-analysis. J Orthop Trauma. 2019;33(1):49–57.

43. Gillespie RJ, et al. Surgical exposure for reverse total shoulder arthroplasty: differences in approaches and outcomes. Orthop Clin North Am. 2015;46(1):49–56.

44. Levigne C, et al. Scapular notching in reverse shoulder arthroplasty. J Shoulder Elb Surg. 2008;17(6):925–35.

45. Melis B, et al. An evaluation of the radiological changes around the Grammont reverse geometry shoulder arthroplasty after eight to 12 years. J Bone Joint Surg Br. 2011;93(9):1240–6.

46. Sabharwal S, Bale S. The biomechanics of reverse shoulder arthroplasty. J Arthrosc Joint Surg. 2021;8(1):7–12.

47. Simovitch RW, et al. Predictors of scapular notching in patients managed with the Delta III reverse total shoulder replacement. J Bone Joint Surg Am. 2007;89(3):588–600.

48. Kempton LB, et al. A radiographic analysis of the effects of glenosphere position on scapular notching following reverse total shoulder arthroplasty. J Shoulder Elb Surg. 2011;20(6):968–74.

49. Edwards TB, et al. Inferior tilt of the glenoid component does not decrease scapular notching in reverse shoulder arthroplasty: results of a prospective randomized study. J Shoulder Elb Surg. 2012;21(5):641–6.

50. Patel M, et al. Inferior tilt of the glenoid leads to medialization and increases impingement on the scapular neck in reverse shoulder arthroplasty. J Shoulder Elb Surg. 2021;30(6):1273–81.

51. Helmkamp JK, et al. The clinical and radiographic impact of center of rotation lateralization in reverse shoulder arthroplasty: a systematic review. J Shoulder Elb Surg. 2018;27(11):2099–107.

52. Boileau P, et al. Bony increased-offset reversed shoulder arthroplasty: minimizing scapular impingement while maximizing glenoid fixation. Clin Orthop Relat Res. 2011;469(9):2558–67.

53. Berhouet J, Garaud P, Favard L. Evaluation of the role of glenosphere design and humeral component retroversion in avoiding scapular notching during reverse shoulder arthroplasty. J Shoulder Elb Surg. 2014;23(2):151–8.

54. Berhouet J, Garaud P, Favard L. Influence of glenoid component design and humeral component retroversion on internal and external rotation in reverse shoulder arthroplasty: a cadaver study. Orthop Traumatol Surg Res. 2013;99(8):887–94.

55. de Wilde LF, et al. Prosthetic overhang is the most effective way to prevent scapular conflict in a reverse total shoulder prosthesis. Acta Orthop. 2010;81(6):719–26.

56. Werthel JD, et al. Lateralization in reverse shoulder arthroplasty: a descriptive analysis of different implants in current practice. Int Orthop. 2019;43(10):2349–60.

57. Langohr GD, et al. The effect of glenosphere diameter in reverse shoulder arthroplasty on muscle force, joint load, and range of motion. J Shoulder Elb Surg. 2015;24(6):972–9.

58. Lädermann A, et al. Effect of humeral stem design on humeral position and range of motion in reverse shoulder arthroplasty. Int Orthop. 2015;39(11):2205–13.

59. Erickson BJ, et al. The influence of humeral head inclination in reverse total shoulder arthroplasty: a systematic review. J Shoulder Elb Surg. 2015;24(6):988–93.

60. Kontaxis A, et al. Humeral version in reverse shoulder arthroplasty affects impingement in activities of daily living. J Shoulder Elb Surg. 2017;26(6):1073–82.

61. Bonnevialle N, et al. Should the supraspinatus tendon be excised in the case of reverse shoulder arthroplasty for fracture? Eur J Orthop Surg Traumatol. 2020;30(2):231–5.

62. Siebenbürger G, et al. Supraspinatus tenotomy in reverse shoulder arthroplasty for fractures: a comparative cohort study. Geriatr Orthopaed Surg Rehabil. 2021;12:21514593211019973.

63. Matthewson G, et al. The effect of subscapularis repair on dislocation rates in reverse shoulder arthroplasty: a meta-analysis and systematic review. J Shoulder Elb Surg. 2019;28(5):989–97.

64. Yat YCS, Lau CFF. Surgeon-designed patient-specific instrumentation improves glenoid component screw placement for reverse total shoulder arthroplasty in patients with small glenoid dimensions. Int Orthop. 2021;47(5):1267–75.

Geriatric Elbow Fractures and Dislocations

5

Christian Fang

5.1 Introduction

Fractures around the elbow are common in the elderly population with low energy injury mechanisms. The most common being isolated olecranon fractures and radial head fractures, followed by distal humerus supracondylar and intercondylar fractures. "Terrible Triad" proximal radioulnar fracture dislocations and Monteggia proximal ulna fracture dislocations are challenging injuries of the elbow region. Modern treatment of elbow fractures demand a thorough understanding of the anatomy and biomechanics of the elbow. Successful treatment strategies include non-operative treatment, plate internal fixation, ligamentous stabilization procedures, arthroplasty, and combination of these, or complementary procedures for complications. Importantly, all elbow fractures demand early rehabilitative training if favourable outcomes are to be expected. Partnership between the surgeon and the rehabilitation therapist should be encouraged with protocols and feedback mechanisms worked out.

5.2 Anatomy

The elbow joint is a hinged joint in the ulno-humeral articulation and a pivot joint at the proximal radioulna articulation. The ulno-humeral joint is stabilized by primary bony and ligaments constraints. The important bony constraints are the shape of the proximal ulna at the olecranon and the coronoid process. The hook shaped olecranon disallows for any anterior subluxation of the proximal ulna through all ranges. The medial sublime tubercle of the proximal ulna and the coronoid process resists both varus and posterior translocation during pronation and internal rotation. The articular surface of the radial head and the lateral half of coronoid resist valgus and posterior displacement of the elbow joint at supination and external rotation. The ligamentous stabilizers act together with the bony stabilizers throughout the elbow range of motion. These are the anterior and posterior medial ulna collateral ligaments which resists opening of the medial joint. The lateral ulna collateral ligament (LUCL) is an important and commonly injured structure which resists opening of the lateral joint and posterolateral displacement of the radial head. Finally, the annular ligament and the forearm interosseous membrane stabilizes the radioulnar relationship (Fig. 5.1).

Prolonged immobilization of the elbow joint beyond 4 weeks following injury or surgery invariably results in stiffness. This is considerably

C. Fang (✉)
Department of Orthopaedics and Traumatology,
Queen Mary Hospital, The University of Hong Kong,
Pokfulam, Hong Kong

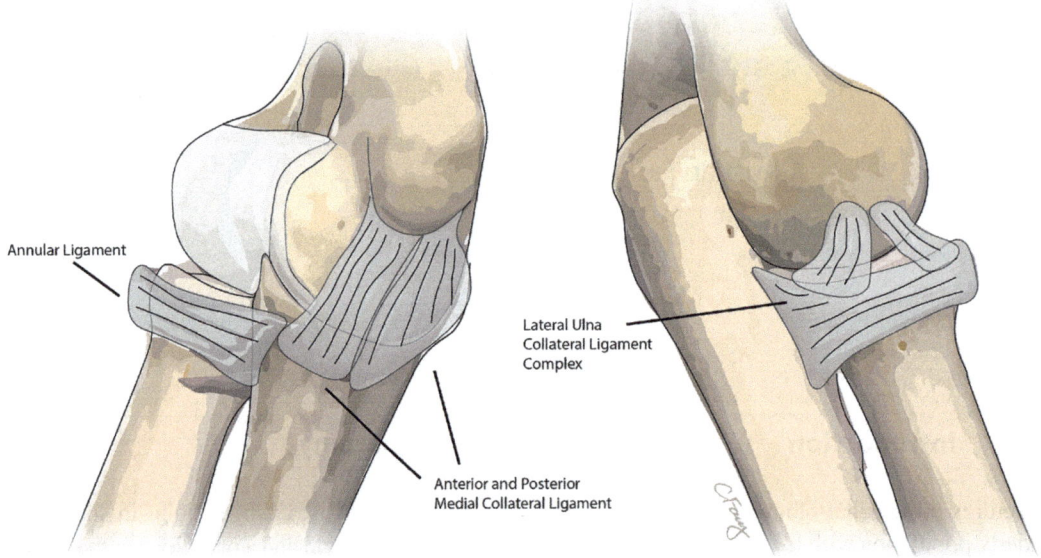

Annular Ligament

Lateral Ulna
Collateral Ligament
Complex

Anterior and Posterior
Medial Collateral Ligament

Fig. 5.1 Important ligamentous stabilizers structures on the medial aspect of the elbow joint is the anterior and the posterior medial collateral ligament (AMCL & PMCL) and on the lateral side is the lateral ulna collateral ligament (LUCL) which blends with the ulna origin of the annual ligament

debilitating to the elderly because an adequate elbow flexion-extension arc is physiologically important for critical self-care activities. Specifically, elbow flexion at 100–120° is required for feeding. Extension to 20–30° is necessary for perineal care. Hence, the objective of any treatment following elbow injuries is to restore this physiological arc of motion in a pain free and stable manner.

5.3 Surgical Approaches

The choice of surgical approach to the elbow joint is dependent on the type of injury. These approaches could be from lateral, medial, posterior or anterior. The principle is to allow adequate exposure while minimizing risk to neurovascular structures and preservation of biology via the use of natural internervous, fascial, and subcutaneous planes. Table 5.1 lists out the typical use of the above surgical approaches to access various regions of the elbow [1].

Table 5.1 List of common surgical approaches to the elbow useful in the elderly

Orientation	Name of approach	Plane between	Access to	Dangers and pitfalls
Lateral	Kocher	Anconeous and Extensor Carpi Ulnaris (ECU) internervous interval	Radial head fractures (posterior half), LUCL repair and reconstruction	Posterior interosseous nerve (PIN) (4–5 cm from radio-capitellar joint)
	Kaplan	Extensor Digitorum Communis EDC and Extensor Carpi Radialis Brevis (ECRB) internervous interval	Radial head fractures (anterior half)	PIN
	Lateral column procedure	Variation of above with detachment of ECRL and ECRB	Release of capsular contracture, lateral part of coronoid tip and proximal radial ulna joint, capitellum	PIN
Medial	Hotchkiss (over-the-top)	Flexor carpi radialis (FCR) and Palmaris Longus (PL)	Coronoid tip, anterior elbow capsule contractures	Medial antebrachial cutaneous nerve, median nerve
	Flexor Carpi Ulnaris (FCU) split	Along ulna nerve into the FCU muscle	Sublime tubercle of coronoid, medial collateral ligament	Ulna nerve, medial antebrachial cutaneous nerve
Anterior	Henry	Brachial artery—ulna artery—biceps tendon and median nerve—pronator teres	Anterior part of coronoid and trochlea	All neurovascular structures, scar contracture—need for a curvilinear incision
Posterior	Olecranon osteotomy/transolecranon approach	Olecranon chevron osteotomy or through fracture into elbow joint	Excellent for all distal humeri with olecranon and triceps reflected proximally. Transolecranon fracture approach to radial head and coronoid tip for Monteggia like injuries	Ulna nerve, posterior cutaneous nerve of forearm. Non-union of osteotomy
	Triceps reflecting variations	Triceps turndown, triceps splitting, triceps elevation	Distal humerus while avoiding osteotomy	Triceps weakness, poor view of anterior distal humerus, ulna nerve
	Para-triceps	Medial and lateral border of triceps	Distal humerus (extraarticular/supracondylar region)	Ulna nerve, posterior cutaneous nerve of forearm
	Boyd	Anconeus and ulna border	Lateral collateral ligament complex, posterior capitellum proximal ulna and radial head	PIN

5.4   Olecranon Fractures

Olecranon fractures are the most common elbow fractures, accounting for 10% of all upper extremity fractures [2]. They are commonly displaced and unstable due to the pull of the triceps. Surgical fixation and early mobilization have been the standard of care for young patients but the optimal treatment is more debated in the elderly. The complication rate of surgically treated olecranon fractures is high in the elderly, with a reoperation rate between 18 and 53% [2]. For those with low functional demand, non-operative treatment is reported to have low rate of functional weakness and high satisfaction despite an 80% radiological non-union rate [2].

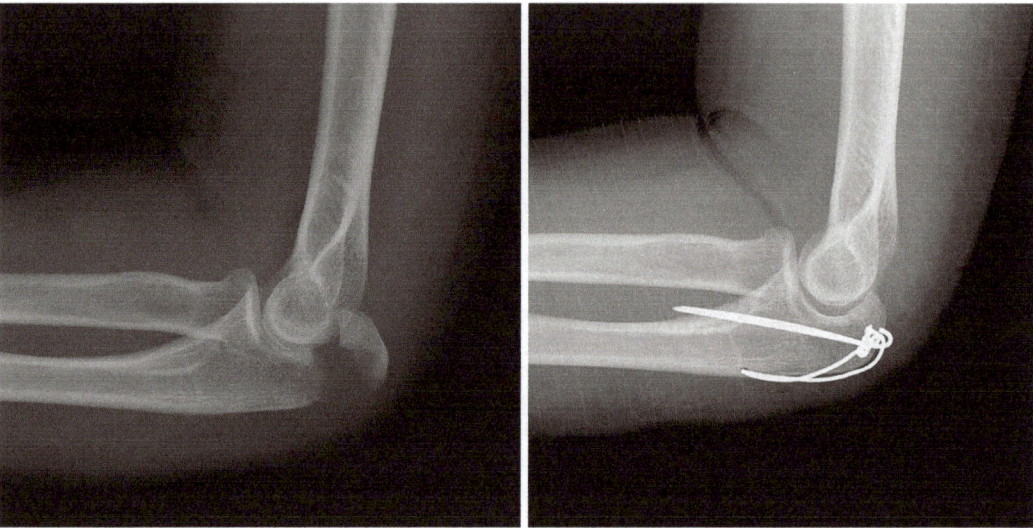

Fig. 5.2 Simple avulsion type fractures of the olecranon process is readily managed by tension band wiring and interfragmentary K-wires. The K-wires should engage the opposite cortex for sufficient stability

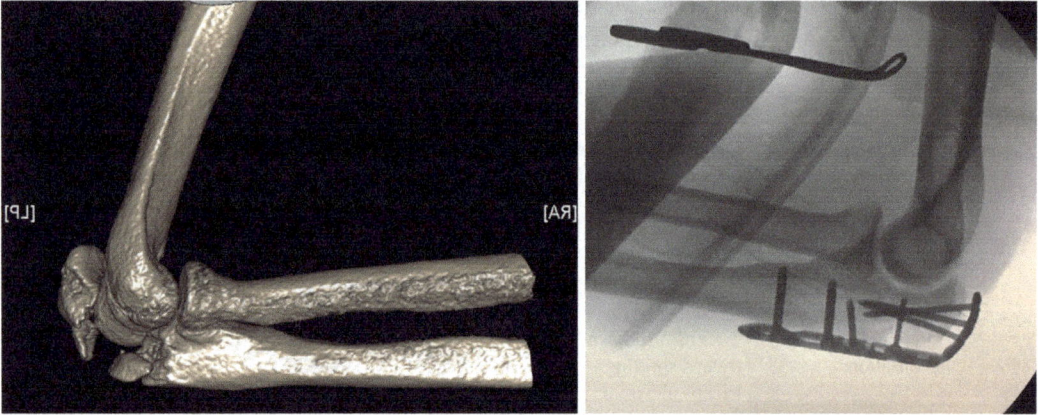

Fig. 5.3 Angular stable locking plate internal fixation with "home-run" screws is indicated for more comminuted olecranon fractures with articular comminution

When operative treatment is decided, the surgeon should differentiate between three types of olecranon fractures, each with increasing propensity for complications. The first type being simple displaced fractures without elbow subluxation. The second type is those with articular surface comminution and depression without joint subluxation and lastly, the transolecranon fracture subluxations. There is a strong indication for surgery when the elbow joint is subluxated.

The surgical principle is anatomical reduction and stable internal fixation. Simple fractures in patients with strong bone is to be managed by tension band fixation. The use of simple tension band in olecranon fracture requires the articular compression side to be non-comminuted and the fracture line should be transverse (Fig. 5.2). Comminuted olecranon articular fractures and fracture subluxations are best repaired with plate fixation and subarticular "home-run" screws (Fig. 5.3). Tricalcium phosphosphate granules can provide modest early and intraoperative mechanical support to comminuted articular fragments (Fig. 5.4). Plate fixation is more com-

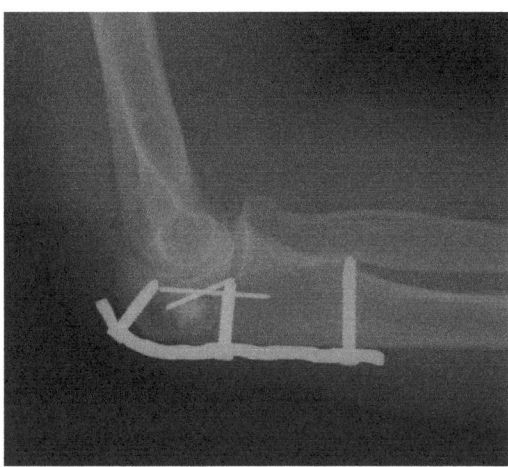

Fig. 5.4 In olecranon fracture with articular surface comminution and depression, the fixation can be enhanced by subarticular buried K-wires and tricalcium sulphate bone substitute along with a locking plate

monly associated with post-operative wound problems. Anatomically contoured plates may still cause triceps insertional irrigation and interference to the olecranon fossa resulting in limitation to elbow extension. Olecranon tip avulsion fractures following plate fixation at the proximal screw holes is occasionally encountered and maybe prevented by supplementing the plate fixation with a strong non-absorbable suture loop anchored to the triceps insertion.

5.5 Isolated Radial Neck and Head Fractures

Isolated radial neck and head fractures are caused by axial loading and valgus injury to the elbow. If the medial collateral ligament and the ulno-humeral articulation is intact, a dislocation would not occur. The most often used classification for radial head fractures is the Mason classification. Mason I fractures are undisplaced and best managed non-operatively with 2–3 weeks of immobilization. Mason II fractures are displaced more than 2 mm. They are often managed non-operatively in the elderly. A CT scan of Mason II fracture provides information on their location with relationship to the proximal radioulnar joint (PRUJ). Occasionally, the fracture may hinge on

the joint causing joint instability and rotation blockage when examined under anaesthesia. Large Mason II fractures that are unstable or interfering with PRUJ motion can benefit from open reduction and internal fixation by small 2.4 mm headless compression screws. For neck fracture with significant angulation >45°, the option is to perform closed reduction under fluoroscopy and local anaesthesia with intra-focal leverage by a larger diameter K-wire (Fig. 5.5). In this procedure, the surgeon should note the proximity of the posterior interosseous branch of the radial nerve which is anterior to radial head at the neck level and avoid iatrogenic damage.

Mason III fractures which are comminuted involving the neck can be managed by early or delayed resection on low demand patients. In patients with higher physical demand, prosthesis replacement may be required as it provides superior outcomes. This prevents proximal radial migration and late-onset distal radioulnar problems. The long-term results of patient receiving a radial head replacement is clinically satisfactory with low complication and revision rates [3]. Up to 40% of patients may show evidence of radiological loosening using both cement and cement-less designs after 2–3 years [4], yet, the presence of loosening may not directly negatively impact the clinical outcome of the patients and is therefore not an absolute indication for revision. "Loose-fit" radial head prosthesis has become an increasing popular alternative with satisfactory mid-term performance [5]. Modern locking plates anatomically contoured for the proximal radius are available for the treatment of radial head fracture but are technically challenging and fraught with high rates of non-union, stiffness, and avascular necrosis and are less suitable for use in osteoporotic patients. Management of Mason I to III fracture should accompany with the examination of mechanical pain and joint instability specifically for the medial collateral ligament. Resection of the radial head is a feasible option for the elderly patient lower functional demand with intact medical collateral ligament and a stable ulno-humeral articulation [6], unlike in younger patients who may sufferer from progressive proximal migration of the radius and late

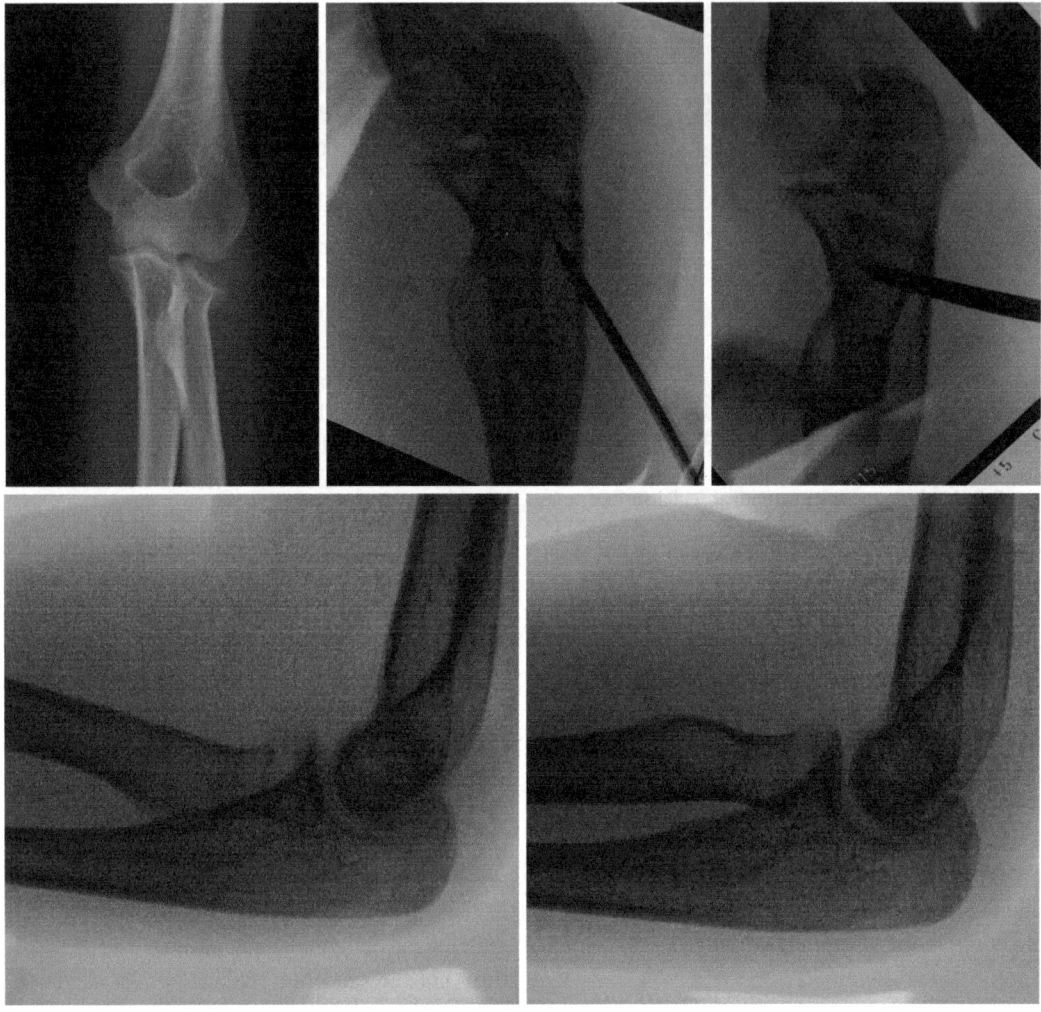

Fig. 5.5 Patient with a 45-degree angulated radial neck fracture. Closed reduction of the impacted radial head with two Intra-focal 2.0 mm K-wires under fluoroscopy at the plane of maximum deformity. Full supination and pronation screening after the procedure shows full correction of the deformity

distal radioulnar joint symptoms [7]. Mason IV fractures are accompanied by dislocation of the elbow joint and are associated with "terrible triad" injuries discussed below. Resection of the radial head is contraindicated in these injuries, and replacement is the treatment of choice.

5.6 Distal Humerus Fractures

Extraarticular and intraarticular distal humerus fractures are common injuries. In the elderly, healing is prolonged and immobilizing of the elbow joint is associated with stiffness. Serial displacement and malunions are common after conservative management of undisplaced or minimally displaced fractures [8]. Other complications include delayed union, non-union and joint stiffness after prolong immobilization. Bi-column fixation with angle stable locked implants arranged in either perpendicularly or parallel configurations, both provide good mechanical stability and should be the standard for most displaced osteoporotic distal humerus fractures. A stable fixation should be followed by early mobilization. The incidence of heterotopic ossification is around 9% using modern locking implants [9, 10].

The parartriceps approach is technically reliable and provides sufficient visibility for extraarticular fractures. The flexion angle of the distal humerus should be maintained. On the lateral radiograph, the anterior humeral cortical margin or the anterior humeral line should bisect the articular centre (Fig. 5.6). Fracture reduction is performed with the posterior fracture gap under direct vision and easily opposable. However, mal-reduction of the distal humerus in extension with opening of the anterior fracture line is possible. This leads to the loss of flexion range beyond 90° and hence impaired functional results.

Intercondylar fractures have varying degrees of articular extension and involvement. A CT scan is necessary in the initial evaluation. Multiplanar and joint subtraction 3D reconstruction are valuable modern assessment techniques to accurately define the fracture pattern. 3D printing is inexpensive and provides the surgeon a tactile and intuitive assessment for preoperative planning and patient explanation. T shaped fractures or comminuted AO/OTA type C3 fractures with good bone stock can be managed by open reduction and internal fixation using locking plate osteosynthesis. While various non-osteotomy approaches to the humeral articular surface have been proposed with success, the chevron olecranon osteotomy approach remains to be the standard and offers the best visualization for accurate restoration of articular surface congruity (Fig. 5.7). Repair of the osteotomy is reliably performed using tension band wire loop and subchondral K-wires, axial compression screws may have inadequate purchase in the porotic cancellus bone. In patients with severe osteoporosis, plate repair of olecranon osteotomy provides better stability at slightly increased risk of implant prominence and wound complications. Routine transposition of the ulna nerve is not recommended in distal humerus fractures as this is shown to increase the likelihood of ulna nerve neuropathy [11, 12]. The

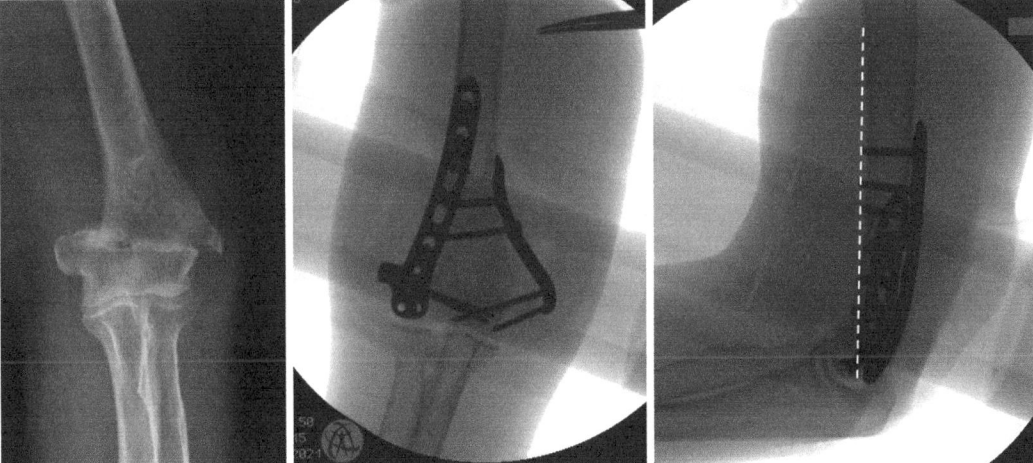

Fig. 5.6 Extraarticular supracondylar fracture with a small remaining distal fragment. Using the para-triceps approach, orthogonal fixation with bicondylar locking plates with distal clustered screws provides sufficient stability for immediate mobilization. The flexion angle of the distal humerus is restored as indicated by the anterior humeral line which bisects the distal condyles

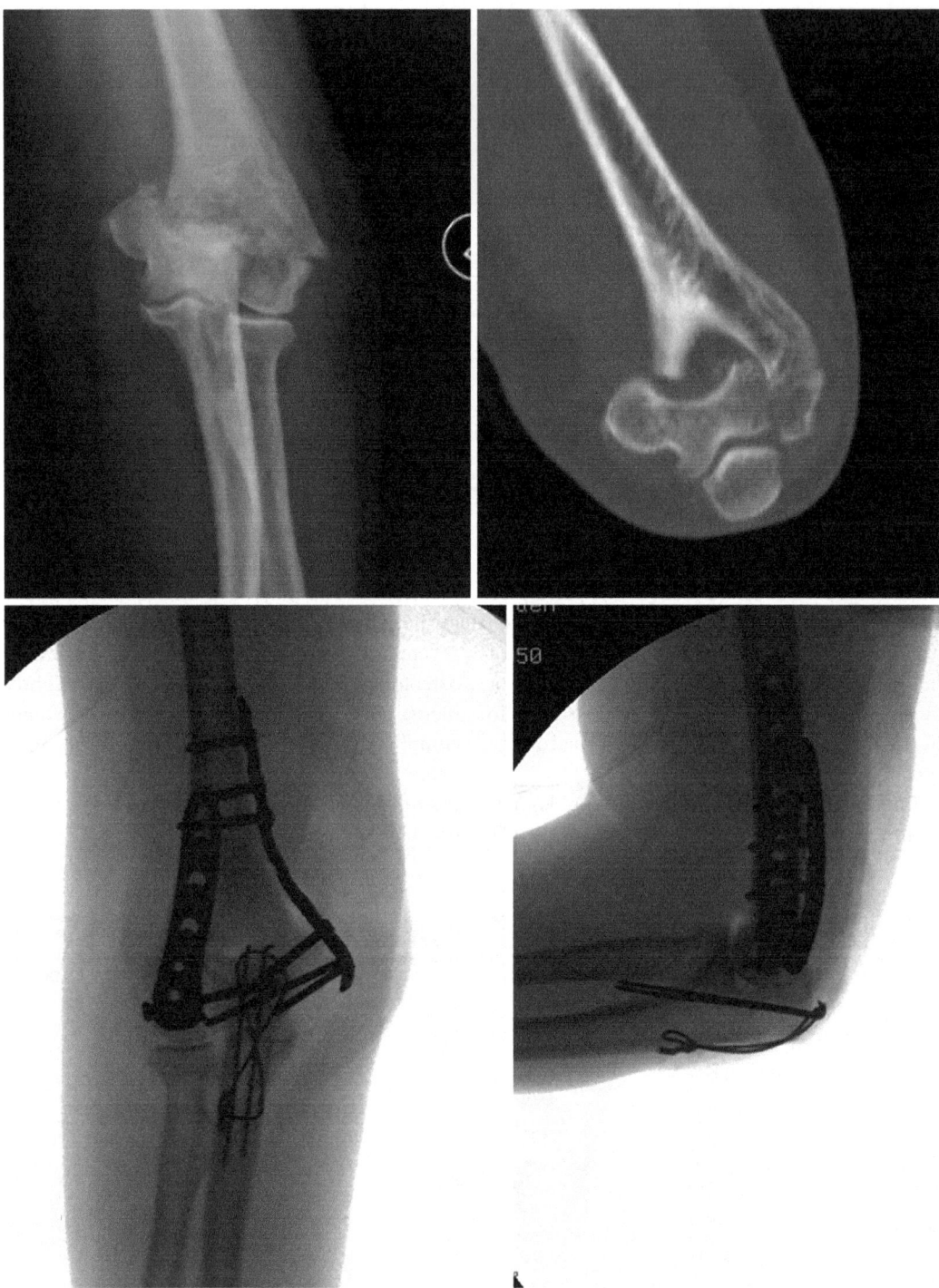

Fig. 5.7 Intraarticular distal humerus fracture with an intraarticular step. The olecranon osteotomy approach provides the best visualization and bicondylar fixation by locking plate is the most standard surgical treatment

cubital tunnel ligament overlying the ulna nerve is released so that the nerve is mobilized for fracture visualization and implant placement. Perineural tissue is repaired to its original location to prevent nerve subluxation with elbow flexion and extension.

Patients with highly comminuted distal humerus fractures with osteoporosis which are deemed unreliable for surgical repair are excellent candidates for primary total elbow replacement (TER). The Coonrad-Morry linked semi-constrained prosthesis offers excellent early recovery and mid to long-term results in elderlies suffering from complex elbow fractures [13].

5.7 Proximal Radioulnar Fracture Dislocations

The "Terrible Triad" consists of posterior elbow dislocation, proximal radius, and proximal ulna fracture [14]. These injuries once poorly understood are now better managed with the detailed understanding of elbow biomechanics on the collaborative stabilizing effects of bone and ligamentous structures. The more common posterolateral rotatory instability (PLRI) is caused by axial load, valgus, and external rotation forces at injury [15]. The radial head subluxates or dislocates posteriorly with supination and opening up of the lateral ulno-humeral joint space. The distal humerus impacts against the anterior half of the radial head and the coronoid, the LUCL and part of the common extensor is detached from the lateral condyle. This is the most common injury pattern. The hallmark injuries are fractures of the anterior half of the radial head, the coronoid process, complete rupture of the lateral ulna collateral ligament, and the anterior elbow capsule (Fig. 5.8). There can be varying degree of injury to the medial ulnar collateral ligaments and medial portions of the coronoid contributing to global and varus instability. For the rarer posteromedial rotatory instability (PMRI) pattern, the elbow dislocates with relative pronation, varus, and extension of the forearm. The hallmark injuries are fracture of the sublime

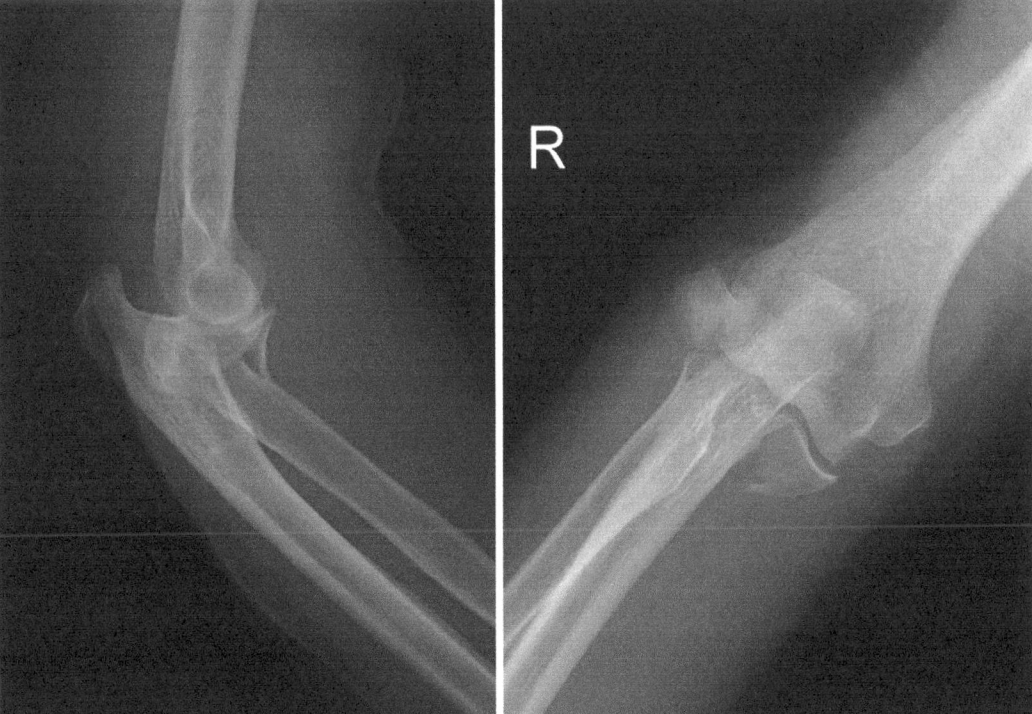

Fig. 5.8 "Terrible triad injury" with elbow dislocation, radial head fracture and large coronoid fracture. The elbow joint is unstable because of the loss of bony buttress and concomitant injury to the collateral ligaments

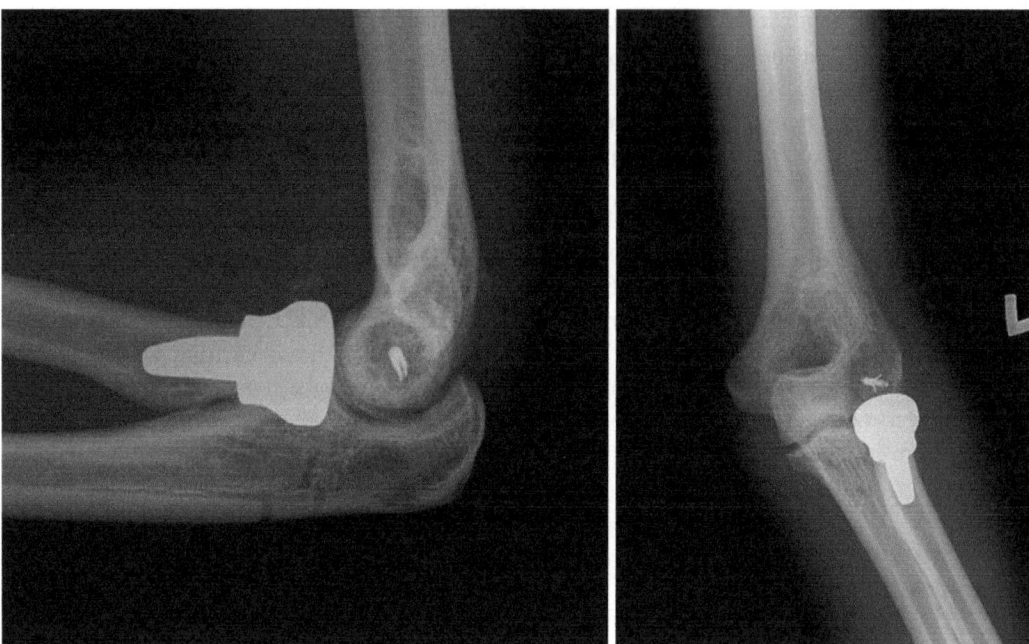

Fig. 5.9 Terrible triad injury stabilized by radial head replacement, and reattachment of anterior capsule by anterior to posterior pull through sutures in the ulna, and repair lateral ulna collateral ligament and common extensor origin complex using a suture anchor

tubercle of the anteromedial coronoid together with rupture of the posterior bundle of medial collateral ligaments (PMCL) [16]. There can be varying degree of injury to the radial head and involvement of the lateral ulna collateral ligament thus also contributing to global and valgus instability.

The objective of treatment is to restore concentric and joint stability throughout a functional arc of motion immediately following surgery. For PLRI, the radial head is commonly replaced. Suture or suture anchors are used for reattachments of anterior capsule and lateral ligamentous structures (Fig. 5.9). Due to osteoporosis and poorer soft tissue healing potential, small articular fragments are at time not amenable to surgical fixation. This applies to elderlies with PMRI, where sublime tubercle fixations and medial ligamentous repairs are sometimes attempted but found very difficult. Therefore, primary total elbow replacement should be reserved as one of the treatment options.

The usual post-operative protocol is to allow mobilization of the elbow joint at ranges of 60° to full flexion using a hinged elbow brace with avoidance of 'gravity varus' by shoulder abduction following stable restoration of the bony and ligament elbow stabilizers. However, the elbow joint may still be subjected to instability and subluxation when at extension beyond 45 degrees and the patient should be aware of the risks at this position.

5.8 "Monteggia Like" Fracture Dislocations

We group under this category of injuries a variety of patterns ranging from simple transolecranon fractures with mild joint subluxation to comminuted proximal ulna fractures with associated radial head fracture and ligamentous injuries. The hallmark features differs from terrible triad in that the radial head and the fractured proximal ulna is typically dislocated anteriorly. The injury is typically a low energy mechanism in the elderly caused by elbow hyperextension. These injuries are perceived to be of a major surgical challenge

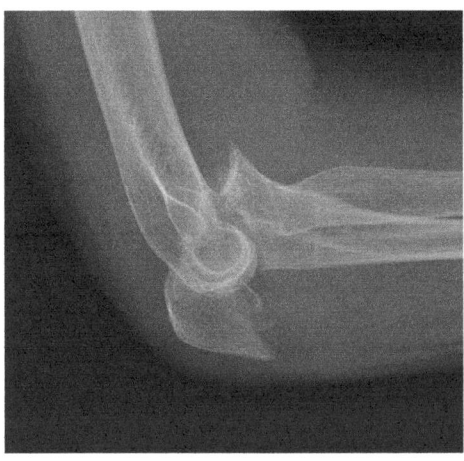 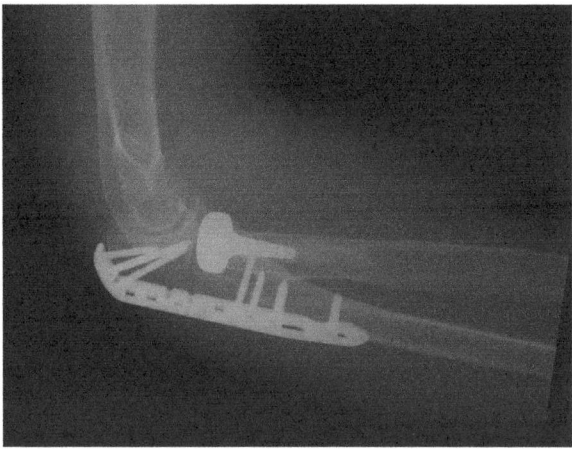

Fig. 5.10 A patient with simple transolecranon fracture dislocation and radial head comminuted fracture. Note anterior displacement of the forearm in relation to the humerus due to the direction of the muscle pull. Ligamentous attachment to the proximal pole of the olecranon remains intact. Stable fixation by anatomically contoured locking plate and radial head replacement provides stability for immediate mobilization

due to the lack of clinical studies with high level of evidence. As with other types of complex elbow injuries, CT scan and 3D imaging assessment is essential. The management of "Monteggia like" fracture dislocations depend on the status and size of the proximal ulna articular fragments, radial head, and ligamentous status. The ulnar fracture can be extraarticular or intraarticular, associated with varying degrees of comminution of the coronoid and olecranon. Those associated with comminution of the sublime coronoid tubercle and ulnohumerus subluxation is at higher risk of loss of fixation and poor outcomes.

Monteggia like proximal ulna fractures are best approached posteriorly using a single posterior "global" incision in the elderly. Presence of a comminuted coronoid articular fragment can be approach intraarticularly through the olecranon fracture (Fig. 5.12). Small coronoid fragments and the anterior elbow capsule is retrieved and stabilized by sutures. Associated radial head fractures is preferentially replaced when comminuted (Figs. 5.10, 5.11, and 5.12). Wedge fragments of the ulna metaphysis can be reduced and stabilized with suture cerclages placed from the posterior aspect back to the shaft (Fig. 5.13), this is especially beneficial when a large fragment is associated with the coronoid. A long anatomical locking plate can be used to bridge the proximal ulna and the olecranon (Figs. 5.11 and 5.12). Anterior metaphyseal fragments may be stabilized with posterior to anterior lag screws and additional cerclage loops (Fig. 5.11). The author finds reliable results using a single posterior approach with and minimal chance of nerve neurapraxia as opposed to using a separate anterior approach for the coronoid.

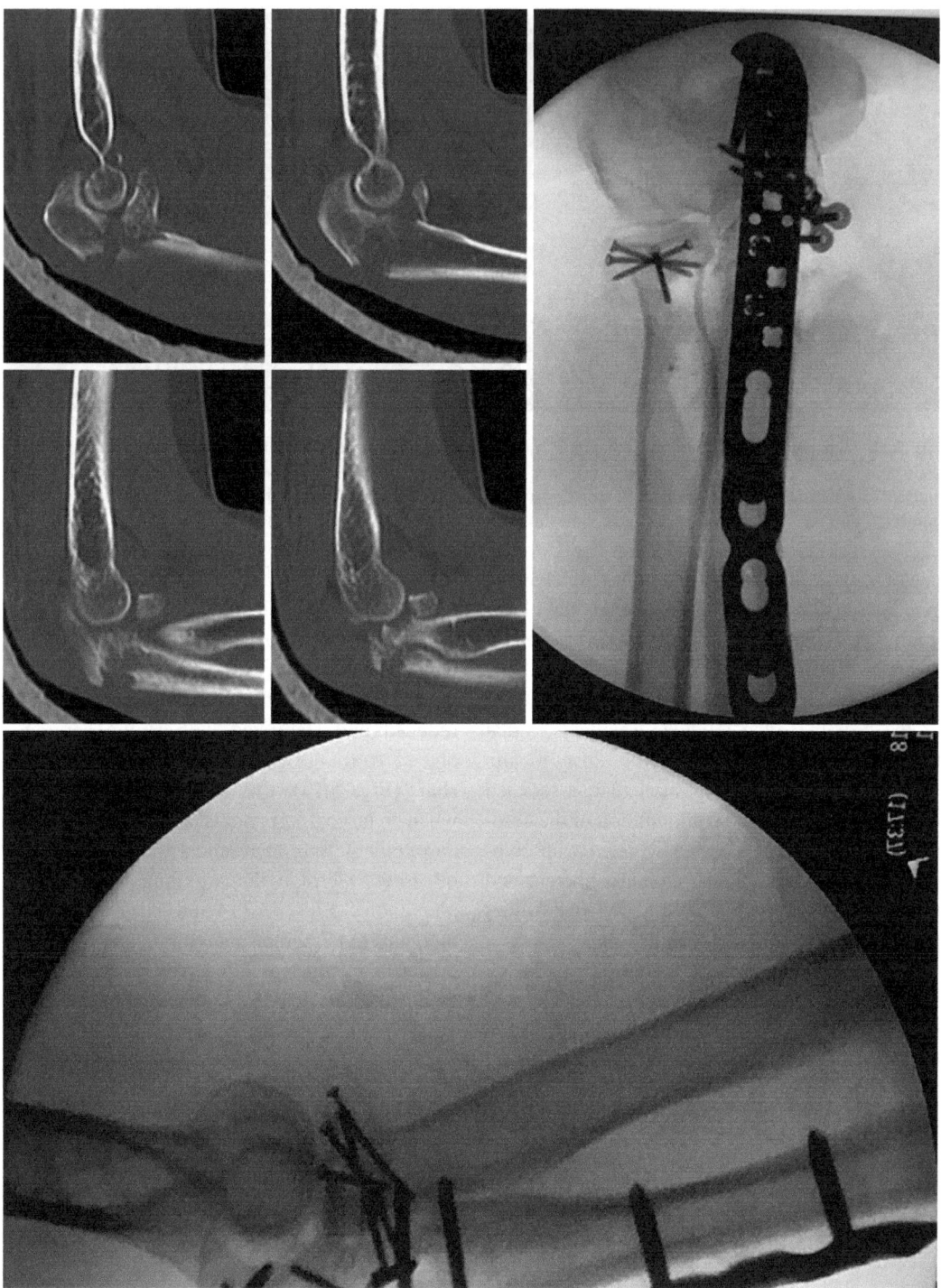

Fig. 5.11 62-year-old female with Monteggia variant transolecranon fracture dislocation. Management by plate internal fixation of the coronoid and the olecranon. The relatively large size of the radial head fragment is amenable to multiple screw fixation

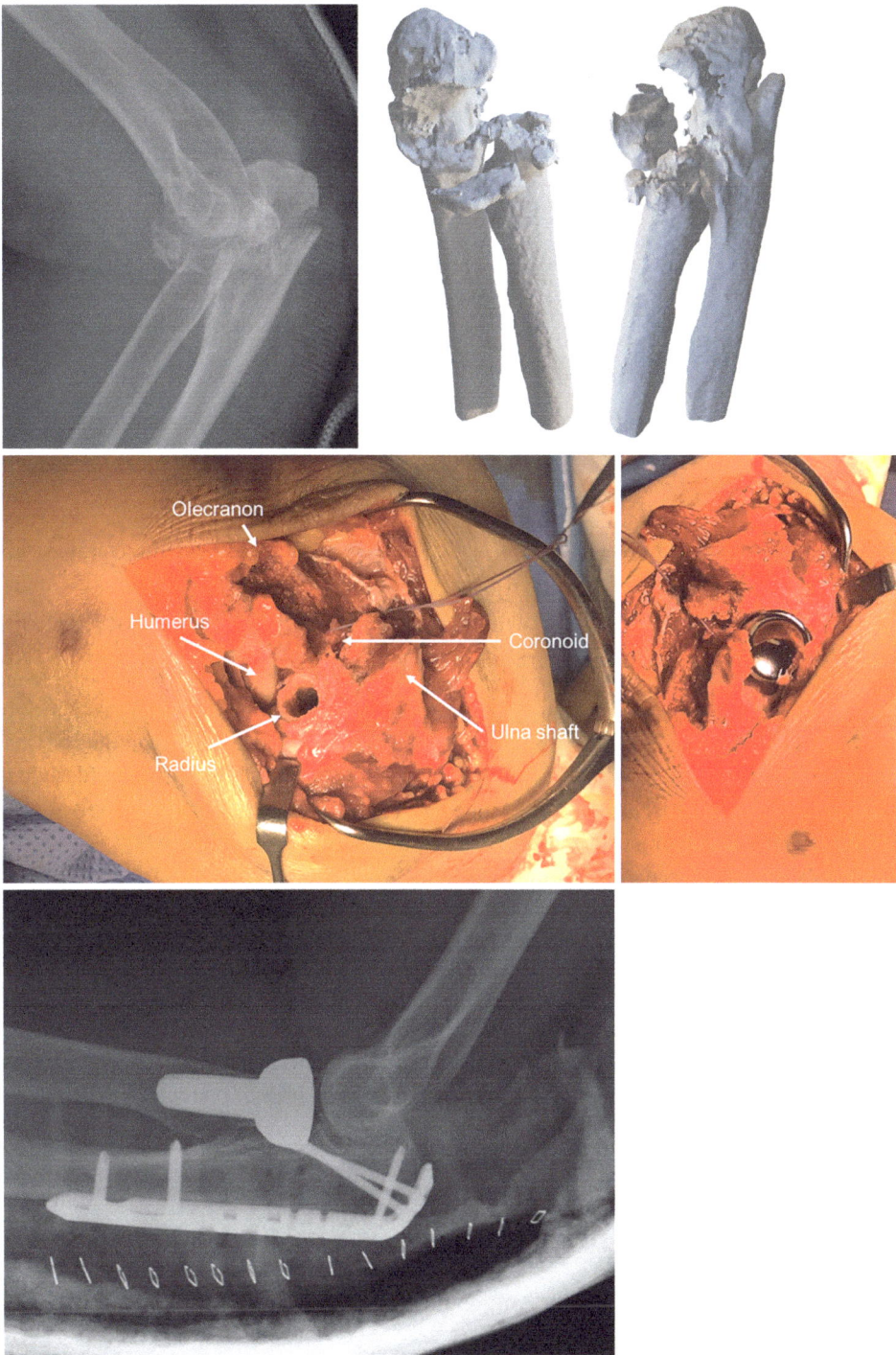

Fig. 5.12 83-year-old female with transolecranon fracture dislocation. A 3D reconstruction is shown. The coronoid and radial head are highly comminuted and not amenable to internal fixation. For the above situation, suture reattachment of coronoid fragments with the anterior capsule is performed via and radial head replacement is performed via the olecranon fracture window posteriorly. The patients regained good function and range of motion 3 months after surgery

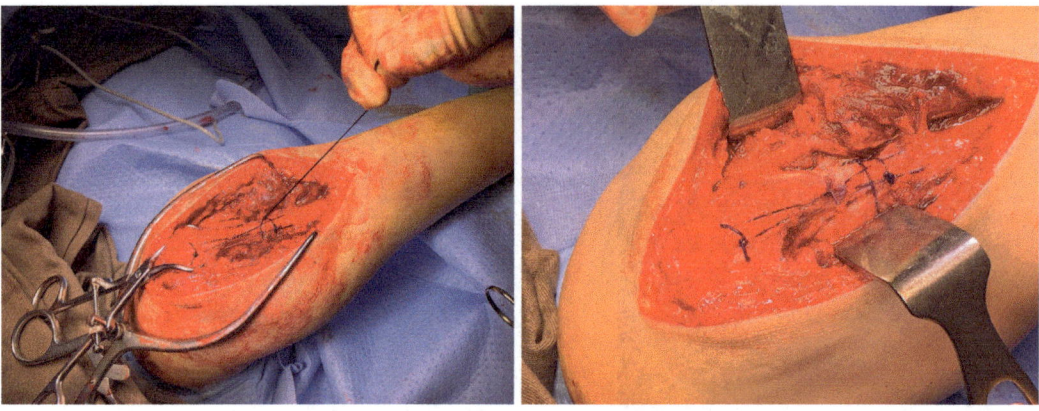

Fig. 5.13 Sutures can provide temporary reduction of proximal ulna comminuted fragments before plate fixation in osteoporotic bone, the technique is useful in Monteggia variants with metaphyseal wedges

5.9   Total Elbow Replacement

Primary total elbow replacement (TEA) should be considered in all types for fractures which are not amenable to reliable surgical repair in the elderly. Randomized study have demonstrated superior functional outcomes over ORIF from immediate post-operative to 2 years [17]. The surgical approach favoured by the author is the medial and lateral para-olecranon triceps sparring approach using a cemented Coonrad–Morrey semi-constrained prosthesis. This approach eliminates the need to protect the extensor mechanism repair and immediate full range of motion is encouraged. The approach is uniquely useful in fracture patients with non-arthritic elbow and minimal joint contractures. Furthermore, in distal humerus fractures, the fractured medial and lateral condyles can be removed entirely, this facilitates visualization and the insertion of the ulno-humeral connecting pins and eliminating the need for post-operative protection (Fig. 5.14). Removal of the condyles and common extensor and flexor origins is shown to not impact the hand and wrist flexor and extensor muscle function in elderly patients (Fig. 5.15). In young patients, condyle resection maybe associated with a higher risk of implant loosening and bushing wear [18]. Loosening of prosthesis leading to the need for revision is uncommonly encountered (<2%) in post-traumatic TER. Other reported common complications of TEA in the elderly are ulna nerve deficits, wound complications and stiffness related to heterotopic ossification, each occurring in up to 10% of patients [17, 19].

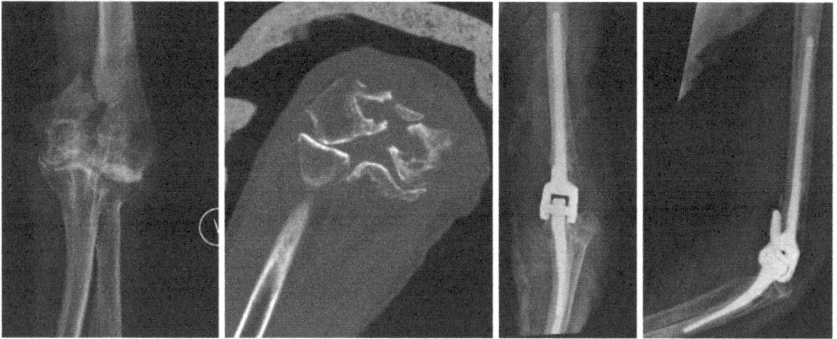

Fig. 5.14 90-year-old with prexisting elbow osteoarthritis and a comminuted distal humerus fracture with poor bone quality. Primary total elbow replacement with removal of the condyles allows for immediate mobilization

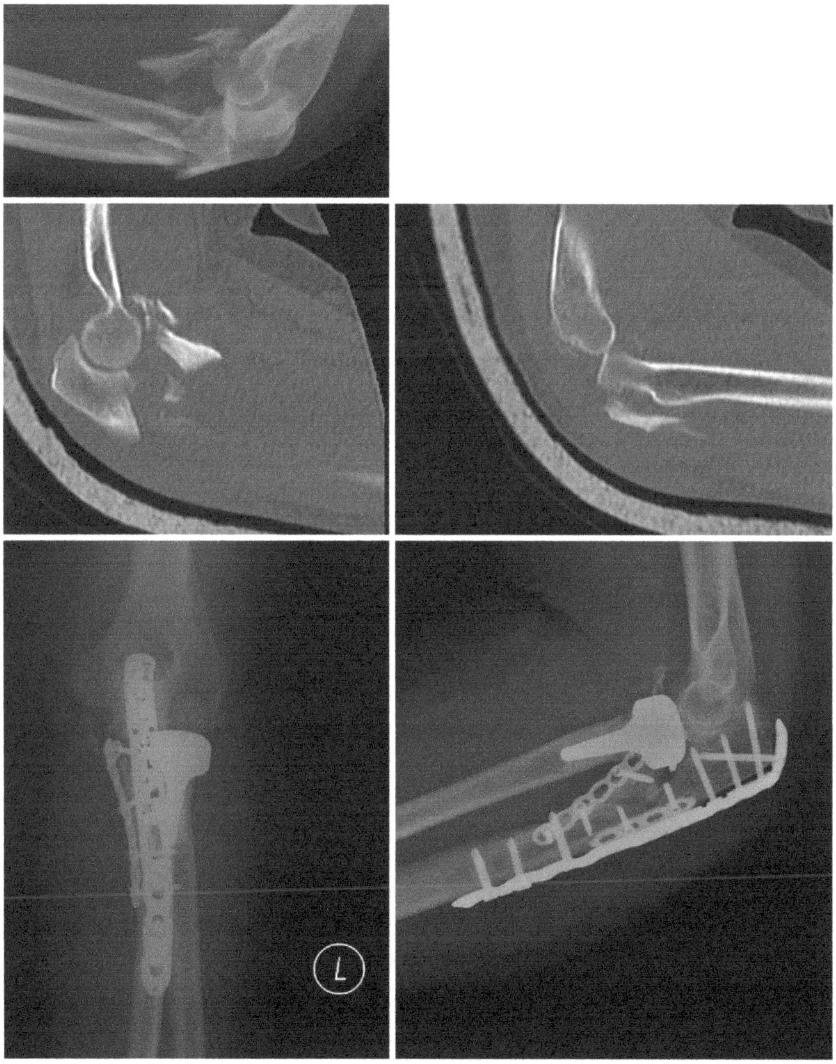

Fig. 5.15 71-year-old female with transolecranon injury. Attempted repair of the highly comminuted coronoid failed, resulting in stiffness and pain. Conversion to a semi-constrained Coonrad–Morry total elbow arthroplasty resulted in good range of motion and outcome despite noting a fracture of the medial epicondyle

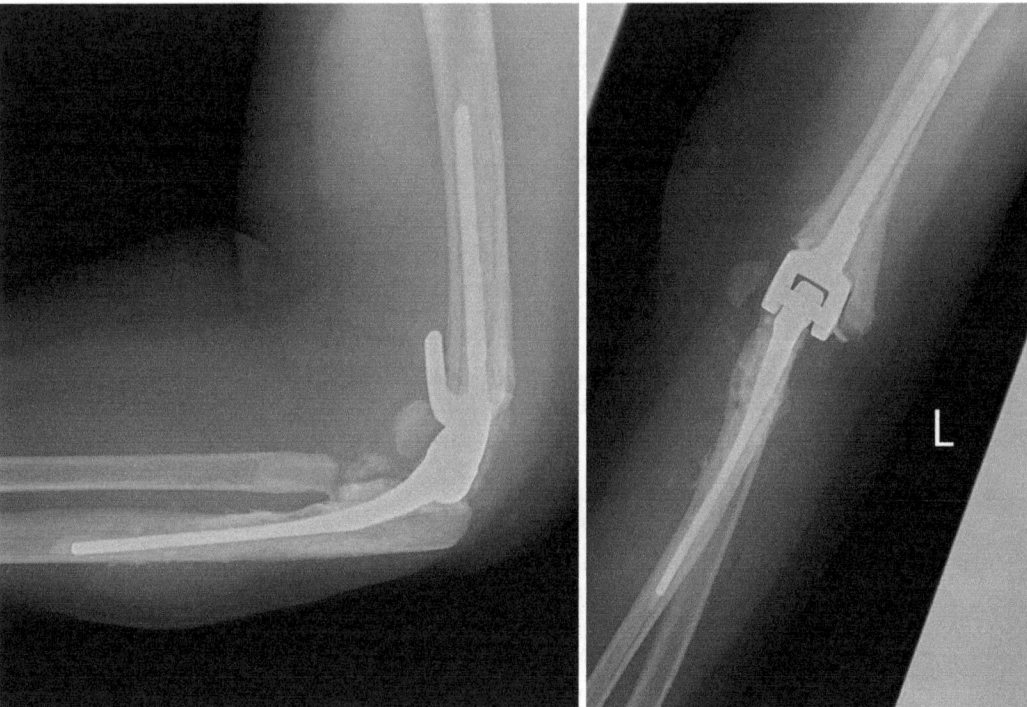

Fig. 5.15 (continued)

5.10 Post-traumatic Elbow Stiffness

Joint stiffness from soft tissue contracture and heterotopic ossifications are commonly encountered. For all types of elbow fractures in the elderly, early mobilization should be encouraged immediately following surgery when there is sufficient mechanical stability. The incidence of heterotopic ossifications occurring in elderly with lower energy and isolated elbow trauma managed with modern locked osteosynthesis is lower than young adults with high energy trauma [20]. Six weeks of non-steroidal anti-inflammatory drugs (NSAID) is shown to reduce the incidence of heterotopic ossifications [20] but long-term NSAID therapy in elderly is associated with significant morbidities such as peptic ulcers and kidney impairment.

The physiologic motion arc of the elbow is from 20 degrees of extension to 110 degrees of flexion. Surgical release of elbow stiffness is usually successful if proper preoperative workup and

consensus with the patient regarding rehabilitation and expectation is accomplished. The proper workup should include a CT scan to determine whether fracture healing is complete and to locate areas of osteophytes and heterotopic ossifications. Surgical timing is an important consideration especially in patients with heterotopic ossification. The optimal timing for surgery is 6 months following injury [21], during which all heterotopic ossification has matured and is no longer enlarging in serial radiographs. A 3D reconstruction of the CT images or 3D printing can help accurate evaluation of the regions of bony abutment (Fig. 5.16).

Elbow release can be performed open or arthroscopically, both with good outcomes [22]. The regions which improve elbow extension are excision of the anterior capsule and removal of para-olecranon osteophytes posteriorly. For improvement in flexion range, posterior joint capsule release, posterior medial collateral ligament release, removal of anterior osteophytes around the coronoid fossa, radial head fossa and

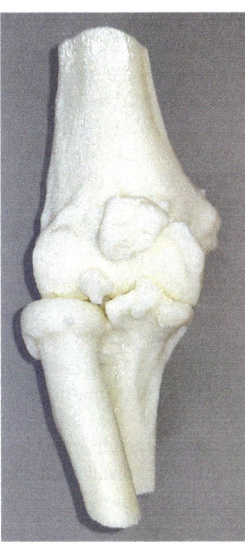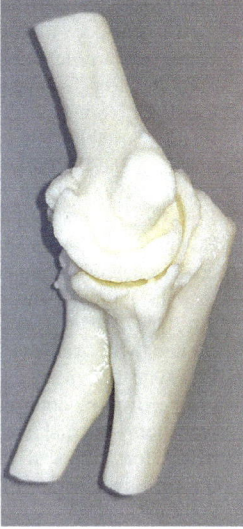

Fig. 5.16 3D Printed models are useful in assessing the location of interfering osteophytes in patients with elbow stiffness for preoperative planning of elbow release and osteophyte removal

capitellum, all help to various degrees. Fixation implants are best removed after conclusion of the elbow release as re-fractures may commonly occur during manual manipulation in osteoporotic bone.

5.11 Other Complications

Peripheral nerve injury occurring with elbow fractures and dislocation are most likely to be iatrogenic. Prevention is by good surgical panning and meticulous technique. Injuries from neuropraxia invariably recovers after a period of observations. A nerve conduction study performed early can provide useful information whether there is axonal regeneration or whether the nerve disruption is complete.

Malunions and non-unions maybe associated with high grade elbow injuries with failed internal fixation. Except in selected distal humerus malunions in active patients with well-preserved articular integrity, corrective osteotomies are generally not indicated in the elderly. Post-traumatic arthritis from malreduced or displaced distal humerus fracture, proximal radioulna frac-ture dislocations with elbow subluxation are best managed by elbow arthroplasty using a semi-constrained prosthesis with good clinical outcome [23] (Fig. 5.15).

Isolated ligamentous injuries are less common in the elderly as injuring forces are transmitted through osteoporotic bone. Elbow instability in the elderly is therefore a consequence of fracture dislocations or previously missed injuries. Isolated late instability due to deficient lateral ulna collateral ligament or medial ulna collateral ligament can occasionally present following PLRI injuries and elbow dislocations. Ligamentous reconstruction using the palmaris longus or split flexor carpi radialis graft supplemented by heavy suture internal bracing provides good outcomes in active patients [24, 25] but clinical reports are lacking in the elderly.

5.12 Conclusion

The elbow is commonly involved in fragility fractures. Listed above are various injuries with distinct pathoanatomy and treatment options. The objective for nearly all surgical treatments is to reconstruct a congruent joint which is mechanically stable to tolerate early motion. Joint subluxation resulting from failed bony and/or ligamentous integrity can lead to stiffness, pain, and long-term disability. The surgeon must be familiar with the various surgical approaches to the elbow joint and avoid iatrogenic neurological compromise. Late release of elbow stiffness is successful in selected patients. The final option of arthroplasty is a good salvage option for non-reconstructable and late injuries.

References

1. Aggarwal S, Paknikar K, Sinha J, Compson J, Reichert I. Comprehensive review of surgical approaches to the elbow. J Clin Orthop Trauma. 2021;20:101482.
2. Savvidou OD, Koutsouradis P, Kaspiris A, Naar L, Chloros GD, Papagelopoulos PJ. Displaced olecranon fractures in the elderly: outcomes after non-operative treatment - a narrative review. EFORT Open Rev. 2020;5(7):391–7.

3. Davey MS, Davey MG, Hurley ET, Galbraith JG, Molony D, Mullett H, et al. Long-term outcomes of radial head arthroplasty for radial head fractures—a systematic review at minimum 8-year follow-up. J Shoulder Elb Surg. 2021;30(10):2438–44.

4. Levy JC, Formaini NT, Kurowicki J. Outcomes and radiographic findings of anatomic press-fit radial head arthroplasty. J Shoulder Elb Surg. 2016;25(5):802–9.

5. Laumonerie P, Raad M, Tibbo ME, Kerezoudis P, Bonnevialle N, Mansat P. Midterm outcomes of 146 EVOLVE Proline modular radial head prostheses: a systematic review. Should Elb. 2021;13(2):205–12.

6. Solarino G, Vicenti G, Abate A, Carrozzo M, Picca G, Moretti B. Mason type II and III radial head fracture in patients older than 65: is there still a place for radial head resection? Aging Clin Exp Res. 2015;27(Suppl 1):S77–83.

7. Kiechle M, Thannheimer A, Hungerer S, Friederichs J, Bühren V, Von Rüden C. Long-term outcomes after primary radial head resection arthroplasty vs. acute radial head resection vs. secondary prosthetic removal in comminuted radial head fractures. Arch Bone Jt Surg. 2019;7(2):112–7.

8. Pidhorz L, Alligand-Perrin P, De Keating E, Fabre T, Mansat P. Distal humerus fracture in the elderly: does conservative treatment still have a role? Orthop Traumatol Surg Res. 2013;99(8):903–7.

9. Patel SS, Mir HR, Horowitz E, Smith C, Ahmed AS, Downes K, et al. ORIF of distal humerus fractures with modern pre-contoured implants is still associated with a high rate of complications. Indian J Orthop. 2020;54(5):570–9.

10. Shin SJ, Sohn HS, Do NH. A clinical comparison of two different double plating methods for intraarticular distal humerus fractures. J Shoulder Elb Surg. 2010;19(1):2–9.

11. Dehghan N, Nauth A, Hall J, Vicente M, McKee MD, Schemitsch EH. In situ placement versus anterior transposition of the ulnar nerve for distal humerus fractures treated with plate fixation: a multicenter randomized controlled trial. J Orthop Trauma. 2021;35(9):465–71.

12. Ahmed AF, Parambathkandi AM, Kong WJG, Salameh M, Mudawi A, Abousamhadaneh M, et al. The role of ulnar nerve subcutaneous anterior transposition during open reduction and internal fixation of distal humerus fractures: a retrospective cohort study. Int Orthop. 2020;44(12):2701–8.

13. Ali A, Shahane S, Stanley D. Total elbow arthroplasty for distal humeral fractures: Indications, surgical approach, technical tips, and outcome. J Shoulder Elb Surg. 2010;19(2):53–8.

14. Stambulic T, Desai V, Bicknell R, Daneshvar P. Terrible triad injuries are no longer terrible! Functional outcomes of terrible triad injuries: a scoping review. JSES Rev Rep Techniques. 2022;2(2):214–8.

15. Camp CL, Smith J, O'Driscoll SW. Posterolateral rotatory instability of the elbow: part I. Mechanism of injury and the posterolateral rotatory drawer test. Arthrosc Tech. 2017;6(2):e401–e5.

16. Bellato E, Kim Y, Fitzsimmons JS, Hooke AW, Berglund LJ, Bachman DR, et al. Role of the lateral collateral ligament in posteromedial rotatory instability of the elbow. J Shoulder Elb Surg. 2017;26(9):1636–43.

17. McKee MD, Veillette CJH, Hall JA, Schemitsch EH, Wild LM, McCormack R, et al. A multicenter, prospective, randomized, controlled trial of open reduction—internal fixation versus total elbow arthroplasty for displaced intra-articular distal humeral fractures in elderly patients. J Shoulder Elb Surg. 2009;18(1):3–12.

18. Celli A, Paroni C, Bonucci P, Celli L. Total elbow arthroplasty for acute distal humeral fractures with humeral condyle resection or retention: a long-term follow-up study. JSES Int. 2021;5(4):797–803.

19. Mansat P, Nouaille Degorce H, Bonnevialle N, Demezon H, Fabre T. Total elbow arthroplasty for acute distal humeral fractures in patients over 65 years old – results of a multicenter study in 87 patients. Orthop Traumatol Surg Res. 2013;99(7):779–84.

20. Agarwal S, Loder S, Levi B. Heterotopic ossification following upper extremity injury. Hand Clin. 2017;33(2):363–73.

21. Sun C, Zhou X, Yao C, Poonit K, Fan C, Yan H. The timing of open surgical release of post-traumatic elbow stiffness: a systematic review. Medicine. 2017;96(49):e9121.

22. Kodde IF, van Rijn J, van den Bekerom MP, Eygendaal D. Surgical treatment of post-traumatic elbow stiffness: a systematic review. J Shoulder Elb Surg. 2013;22(4):574–80.

23. Pogliacomi F, Aliani D, Cavaciocchi M, Corradi M, Ceccarelli F, Rotini R. Total elbow arthroplasty in distal humeral nonunion: clinical and radiographic evaluation after a minimum follow-up of three years. J Shoulder Elb Surg. 2015;24(12):1998–2007.

24. Finkbone PR, O'Driscoll SW. Box-loop ligament reconstruction of the elbow for medial and lateral instability. J Shoulder Elb Surg. 2015;24(4):647–54.

25. Ellwein A, Lill H, Smith T, DeyHazra R-O, Warnhoff M, Jensen G. Internal bracing in the treatment of elbow instabilities. Obere Extremität. 2021;16(3):192–7.

Management of Distal Radius Fractures in the Elderly Population

6

Terence Cheuk Ting Pun

6.1 Introduction

Distal radius fracture is the most common upper extremity fracture and second most common fracture in the elderly population [1]. There is a steady increase in incidence from age 45 to 60 years, followed by a plateau. Older patients tend to fall on their hips because they lose the ability to break a fall with outstretched hands [2]. Distal radius fracture tends to occur with relatively more active and healthy elderly individuals.

The number and life expectancy of elderly population are increasing in different parts of the world. With the improvement in medical treatment and health consciousness, many elderly and super-elderly (≥80 years old) persons remain active and demand high levels of wrist function for their vocational and avocational activities. On the other hand, many senior citizens are living alone or with their spouse marginally independently. They may easily lose their independence temporarily or permanently with any sudden drop in function after a distal radius fracture. Activities like preparing meals, performing housekeeping, climbing stairs, shopping and getting in and out of transportation all require a high

level of wrist function. There is both a greater number of distal radius fractures as well as an increased demand for surgical treatment that rapidly restores wrist function.

Among the different types of fragility fractures, the clinical and economic impact of hip and vertebral fractures have received most attention. While distal radius fractures are traditionally considered to be less significant than other osteoporotic fractures, with little functional decline and no effect on mortality, they are often associated with a poor outcome. There has been growing evidence to suggest the personal and public burden of distal radius fracture have been under-recognized. The occurrence of a distal radius fracture increases the odds of having a clinically important functional decline by 48% [3]. At 10 years follow-up, 15% of those surviving had an unsatisfactory outcome [4]. A particular complication is complex regional pain syndrome—a syndrome of pain, widespread tenderness, allodynia, vasomotor instability, diffuse swelling, and stiffness. Patients with complex regional pain syndrome often have poor results.

Distal radius fracture carries an increased risk of subsequent fractures and mortality. Data from osteoporosis epidemiology study suggests that all low-trauma fractures are associated with an increased mortality risk for 5 years [5]. Viewing elderly distal radius fracture as a sentinel event provides an opportunity for early diagnosis and intervention of underlying osteoporosis.

T. C. T. Pun (✉)
Department of Orthopaedics and Traumatology,
Queen Mary Hospital, The University of Hong Kong,
Pokfulam, Hong Kong

6.2   Classification

In the elderly population, the usual mechanism of injury is a low-energy level ground fall on an outstretched hand. The bending deforming force results in an extra-articular dorsally displaced metaphyseal fracture with tension failure of volar cortex, compression failure and comminution of the dorsal cortex (Fig. 6.1). With lower bone density and higher energy of trauma, the fracture pattern can be complex with various degrees of articular and metaphyseal comminution or depression. It is also common to have a concomitant distal ulna fracture, that may be an ulnar styloid or a metaphyseal fracture.

There are many classification systems for distal radius fracture. Gartland and Wesley incorporated three basic factors of fracture instability (metaphyseal comminution, intra-articular extension, and displacement of fragments) into their classification. Frykman's classification was based on the involvement of radiocarpal, distal radioulnar joints, and ulnar styloid [6]. Melone's four-part classification (radial shaft, radial styloid, dorsal medial, and volar medial fragment) emphasized on the involvement of the "die punch" intermediate column. Fernandez's classification was a mechanism-based system that addresses ligamentous injury, wrist fracture dislocation and gives insight to fracture reduction technique [7]. AO/OTA classification is currently the most used classification system, dividing fractures into extra-articular, partial articular, and complete articular fracture of increasing severity.

While these classification systems are comprehensive, they did not fully take some important factors in decision making (patient age, pre-injury functional level, magnitude of displacement, and bone quality) into account.

Rikli and Regazzoni introduced the three-column concept in 1996 [8]. It divides the distal radius and ulna into radial, intermediate, and ulna columns (Fig. 6.2). The radial column includes the radial styloid and scaphoid fossa. It supports the carpus and prevents radial translation of the carpus. It serves as an anchor for the radioscaphocapitate and long radiolunate ligament to prevent ulnar translation of the carpus. The length of the radial column is important as it holds the carpus out to length and allows more uniform distribution of load across the scaphoid and lunate fossa. The radial column is shortened under the pull of brachioradialis once fractured. The intermediate column encompasses the lunate fossa and sigmoid fossa. The volar lip of lunate facet

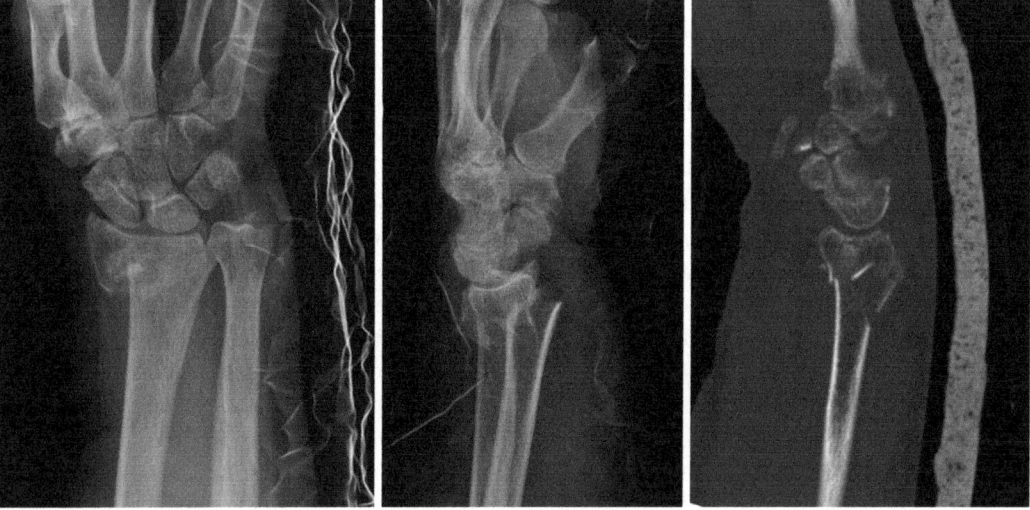

Fig. 6.1 This shows a typical deformity of a Colles' fracture. A large metaphyseal bone void is evident after closed reduction. This fracture tends to re-displace because of the metaphyseal comminution, old age, and osteoporosis

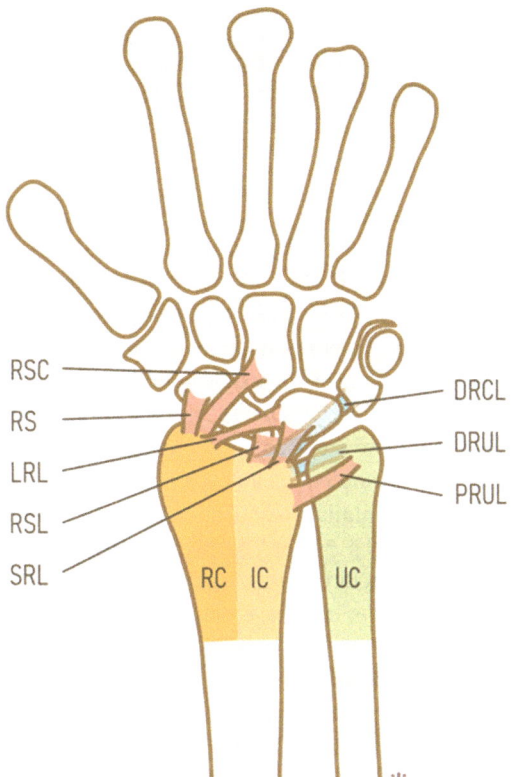

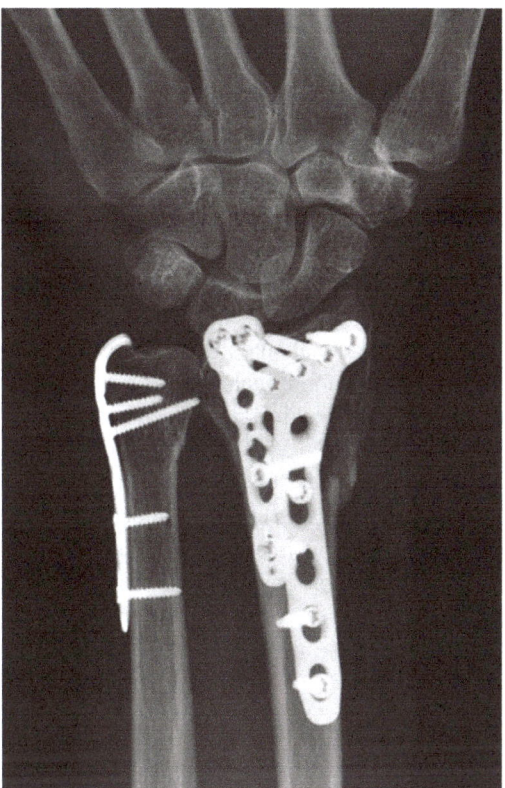

Fig. 6.2 Three-column theory of distal radius and ulna. The attachment of stabilizing radiocarpal and distal radioulnar ligaments in each column is shown

Fig. 6.3 When a volar locking plate does not provide the adequate dorsal side control by ligamentotaxis effect, additional surgical approach is needed for reduction, and fragment-specific plates are needed for fixation. All three-columns are addressed in this unstable distal radius and ulna fractures

gives origin to the short radiolunate ligament that prevents volar carpal subluxation. The intermediate column serves as an anchor for distal radioulnar and dorsal radiocarpal ligaments that prevent dorsal subluxation of carpus. Both radial and intermediate columns transmit load from the hand to forearm. The ulnar column includes the ulnar head and triangular fibrocartilage complex. It maintains the distal radioulnar joint stability and forearm rotation.

While most surgically treated distal radius fractures in the elderly can be managed with a single volar locking plate, understanding the three-column concept is useful for surgeons to identify the need for fragment-specific reduction and fixation in exceptional cases (Fig. 6.3).

6.3 Decision-Making on Surgical Management

Like other extremity fractures, the decision of treatment of distal radius fracture with surgery is based on patient age, physical activity level, comorbidities, functional demand, fracture pattern, and soft tissue condition.

In young adults, restoration of normal morphological parameters is an important factor in predicting good functional outcomes. The parameters are derived from clinical studies of young adults and biomechanical studies with cadaver models.

Acceptable radiographic parameters for distal radius fracture in active young patients		
	Normal	Acceptable
Radial height/ulnar variance	13 mm	<5 mm shortening
Palmar tilt	11°	<5° loss
Radial inclination	23 °	Neutral, 0°
Intra-articular step-off	Congruous	<2 mm step-off

After closed reduction of distal radius fracture, if the alignment falls out of this acceptable range, the fracture will heal with malunion and risks poor functional outcome. Even if the alignment is restored to normal, there is a risk of secondary displacement in a cast. Fracture instability is defined as a failure to hold the reduced position within the forearm cast with a loss of reduction at 1–2 weeks. Lafontaine et al. developed criteria to predict distal radius fracture instability [9]. Malaligned or unstable distal radius fracture is an indication for open reduction and internal fixation in adults.

Lafontaine criteria: ≥3 criteria are predictive of fracture instability and need for surgical fixation
Substantial initial deformity—Dorsal angulation >20° or >5 mm radial shortening
Dorsal metaphyseal comminution
Intra-articular involvement
Concomitant distal ulna fracture
Age > 60

6.4 Special Considerations in the Elderly Patients

There has been a lot of success with volar locked plating in geriatric distal radius fracture fixation. Many case series have documented excellent results of internal fixation with very low complication rates [10].

It is important to recognize that defining indication of surgery by morphological deviation is based on studies that included young, healthy patients whose bone characteristics and physical performance do not resemble an elderly and osteoporotic population. In the elderly patients, fracture reduction and anatomical alignment do not correlate with functional outcomes.

Despite the potential for cosmetic deformity, and an initial decline in independence, older patients are able to adapt and regain much of their functionality. DASH score, VAS function, strength, wrist motion at 1 year are not inferior in patients with fractures treated non-surgically.

In a systematic review of unstable distal radius fractures in elderly patients, worse radiographic outcomes were reported in patients with fractures treated non-surgically; however, functional outcomes were similar to patients who were treated surgically [11]. Major complication rates were higher for fractures treated surgically. Surgically treated patients may have hardware based problems warrant secondary operations and implant removal. Conservatively treated patients may have symptomatic malunion and neurological deficits such as carpal tunnel syndrome and complex regional pain syndrome. As a result, some researchers suggest that unstable distal radius fracture in geriatric population should be treated conservatively.

In a randomized control trial in 2011 compared volar locking plate with cast treatment in patients older than 65 years old. The surgical group showed better wrist function in the early post-operative period, at 6 and 12 weeks. However, at 6 and 12 months, there was no significant difference in wrist function or pain between groups. At all timepoints, grip strength was considerably better in the surgical group [12]. This study highlights the benefit and limitation of surgical treatment.

Many geriatric patients are living alone or living with their spouse who also has marginal physical reserve. They have a high demand on being able to perform and retain independence. If they are to suffer from a distal radius fracture, they will benefit from a quicker and more predictable clinical course following surgical treatment. The rate of recovery of performance of activity of daily living may be more important than the final functional outcome in this group of patients.

Overall, the indications of surgery in elderly are more controversial. Aside from radiographic parameters of displacement and angulation, the decision to operate depends on the patients' functional activity level and their need for rapid return of wrist function. The approach to management is patient- and fracture-specific and one should remain focused on the primary goal of restoring a functional hand and forearm.

6.5 Indication of Surgery in Geriatric Distal Radius Fracture

In my institution, the common indications of surgery in distal radius fracture in elderly populations are:

Open distal radius fracture
Radiocarpal fracture dislocation including displaced Barton fractures
Bilateral distal radius fractures
Concomitant fracture in the upper and lower limb (e.g., hip and distal radius)
Distal radius and distal ulna comminuted metaphyseal fracture (3 columns)
Patient who demands early return of function
Patient who refuses conservative treatment

6.6 Conservative Treatment

Most distal radius fracture can be treated conservatively in the elderly population. Closed reduction is performed under hematoma block with local anesthetic agent, followed by maintenance of reduction in a short arm cast or slab with "three-points molding." The wrist is kept in slight palmar flexion and ulnar deviation. The cast is kept for 4 weeks. In the elderly population, particular attention should be paid to skin quality as skin tears are possible when performing close reduction.

The patient is reviewed in 2 weeks with a repeated radiography. The fracture is considered stable when fracture alignment can be maintained with minor displacement in 1–2 weeks. Secondary fracture displacement is common in elderly patients and is reportedly as high as 89% [13]. Repeated closed reduction and casting are unlikely to be successful. Most patients and surgeons will choose to continue with conservative treatment by accepting the malunion, understanding that most elderly patients tolerate wrist deformity well and that radiological outcome does not correlate with functional outcome in this elderly population. A small number of conservatively treated patients may choose to receive surgical fixation after discussion. Surgery at this 2–3-week time point is still relatively straightforward. Few conservatively treated patients (about 1%) may eventually require salvage procedure for symptomatic malunion [14].

Other than secondary displacement of fracture, complication of casting includes muscle atrophy and stiffness. They can be avoided by early mobilization of the thumb and fingers. This should be emphasized in every patient visit. Active and active-assisted motion of the wrist and grip strengthening can be safely started at weeks after cast removal. Poorly applied short arm cast may cause soft tissue complications such as skin necrosis and carpal tunnel syndrome.

6.7 Surgical Treatment

Surgical options include volar locking plate, fragment-specific plate, combined internal and external fixation or dorsal bridge plating. Traditional methods of closed reduction and percutaneous pinning or external fixation alone do not lead to satisfactory outcomes in the literature.

Among the surgical options, volar locking plating has become popular with excellent results in elderly patients. It has shown superior recovery rates and minor complication rates compared with other surgical methods [15]. While both dorsal and volar locking plate may achieve adequate reduction and comparable functional outcome, studies suggest that patients with volar locking plate have better grip strength, less pain, and less complication.

Most geriatric distal radius fractures can be fixed with volar locking plate alone. However, certain fracture patterns are more appropriately addressed with alternate approach and fixation. Displaced dorsal fragments with an intact or non-displaced volar fracture is a strong indication for dorsal approach. A volar medial fracture of the intermediate column is addressed more strategically with a volar approach and fragment-specific plate. Fragment-specific fixation demonstrates greater stiffness than volar locking plate in maintaining the volar medial fragment, especially in the presence of osteoporotic bone [16].

6.7.1 Surgical Approach

The modified Henry's approach is a versatile approach to address both intra-articular, extra-articular, dorsally- or palmarly displaced fracture (Fig. 6.4). After mobilizing flexor pollicis longus ulnarly, the pronator quadratus is elevated from its radial border in one piece to protect the flexor pollicis longus and median nerve. Although it is not repaired routinely at the end of the procedure, it serves as a cushion between implant and flexor tendons.

6.7.2 Reduction

Open reduction is achieved by clearing hematoma and periosteum from the fracture site, exaggeration of dorsiflexion deformity, longitudinal traction, followed by palmar translation, flexion, and pronation of the distal fragment (Fig. 6.5). Radial translation and loss of radial inclination is corrected by a radially directed vector from a Hohmann retractor on the medial border of the proximal shaft fragment. This radial translation of the shaft fragment is important not only for reduction of the volar cortex, but also to restore tension to the distal oblique bundle of the interosseous membrane. This is important for distal radioulnar joint stability and forearm rotation range of motion.

Sometimes, the volar cortex of the distal fragment remains dorsal to that of the proximal fragment. An intra-focal K-wire can be used to lever the volar cortex out so that it is flushed or slightly over-reduced to the proximal fragment. The maneuver must be gentle or an iatrogenic fracture of the volar cortex may result.

The reduction is maintained by a pad at the hand dorsum to keep the wrist flexed for the dorsally angulated fracture. An extra-focal K-wire is

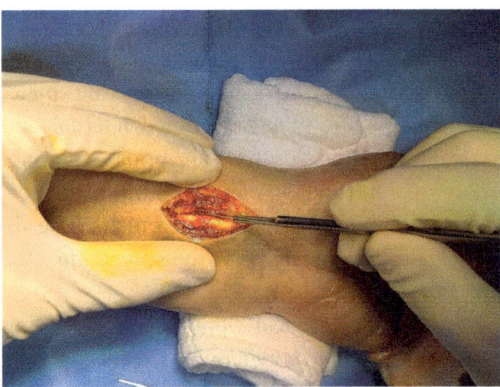

Fig. 6.4 It is our practice to divide the FCR tendon sheath radial to the tendon, rather than denuding the FCR tendon front and back, in the hope of lessening post-operative pain

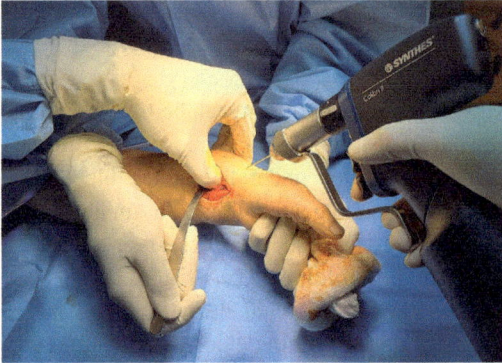

Fig. 6.5 With a Hohmann retractor on the ulnar border of the radial shaft, the assistant delivers a radially directed force to reduce translation. The assistant provides palmar flexion, ulnar deviation and usually pronation with the other hand. The surgeon can fine-tune the reduction with his thumb on the fracture site. The surgeon feels the volar and dorsal cortices so that a K-wire can be introduced accurately from the radial styloid to the ulnar border of the radial shaft

inserted obliquely from the radial styloid. Reduction is checked under fluoroscopy. In lateral alignment, elevating the wrist by 20° toward the beam of the fluoroscopy unit removes the radial inclination and gives a straight down view of the radiocarpal joint.

In the presence of dorsal comminution, volar tilting of the distal fragment may be difficult to be maintained with a single K-wire. One intrafocal or extra-focal K-wires can be inserted dorsally from the distal fragment to the volar cortex. External pressure on the K-wire also helps to maintain the volar tilt (Fig. 6.6). In the presence of radial comminution, loss of radial inclination, or ulnar translation of shaft fragment, an intrafocal K-wire is inserted through the radial side of fracture site and levers the distal fragment to a proper location. By the end, with a well-reduced volar cortex, one can proceed to plate fixation or further reduction of sagittal mal-reduction with plate reduction technique.

Reduction by plate is a powerful and indirect technique to correct dorsal tilting of distal fragments (Fig. 6.7). Yet, it is more predictable to have the fracture reduced to near neutral tilt before application of such technique. It can be achieved by lifting the proximal end of plate off the shaft at a certain angle, inserting fixed-angle distal locking screws, followed by reduction of the plate to the shaft with a cortical screw in the oblong hole. To gain length, the plate can be advanced distally before insertion of a second locking screw at the shaft.

In cases of very distal fractures with a short distal fragment, the previously mentioned method does not work well because the screws will not be placed close enough in the subchondral bone. As an alternative, reduction is done by first insertion of a distal row of variable angle locking screws. They are not inserted fully and are left unlocked. Subsequently the proximal end of the plate is lifted off the shaft at a certain angle. Final reduction is achieved by locking the variable angle screws, followed by reduction of the proximal plate to the shaft with a cortical screw.

When reducing palmarly displaced partial articular fractures, the direction of reduction is primarily wrist hyper-extension. The metaphyseal spikes are tentatively stabilized by K-wires in a volar-to-dorsal direction. K-wires can penetrate and be withdrawn from the dorsal wrist. K-wires should be carefully placed in a site that do not interfere with the subsequent volar plate implantation.

6.7.3   Fixation

There are a number of commercially available locking plates specifically designed for fixation of distal radius fracture. Surgeons have to choose a locking plate with the correct design, size, and length. It has to be placed in a precise location to fit for a fracture pattern and patient's wrist anatomy. The number, length and location of locking screws also warrant special attention during surgery. Angular stable screws and locking plates have become standard implants for osteoporotic distal radius fracture fixation. Most modern volar locking plates go with 2.4 mm to 2.8 mm locking screws. They can be used for all types of distal radius fractures. For the older generation of 3.5 mm locking plate, they are used only in extra-articular fractures but not intra-articular fractures or fractures with small distal fragments.

6.7.3.1 Rim Plate Vs. Extra-Articular Plate

The most appropriate plate should be selected according to the fracture pattern. There is no single plate that is universally successful without complications. Extra-articular plates are placed in the pronator quadratus fossa, proximal to the pronator quadratus line and watershed line. Screws are inserted at an angle to support the distal fragment. Proper placement of extra-articular plates avoids flexor tendon irritation and the need of implant removal.

Rim plate or juxta-articular plates are placed beyond the pronator quadratus line or watershed line as it is pre-contoured to fit the volar rim of distal radius. Their distal row of screws, angled proximal to the articular surface, allow purchase of far distal intra-articular fracture fragments and provide subchondral support of the articular surface. They are particularly useful for C3 comminuted intra-articular fracture and B3 volar lip

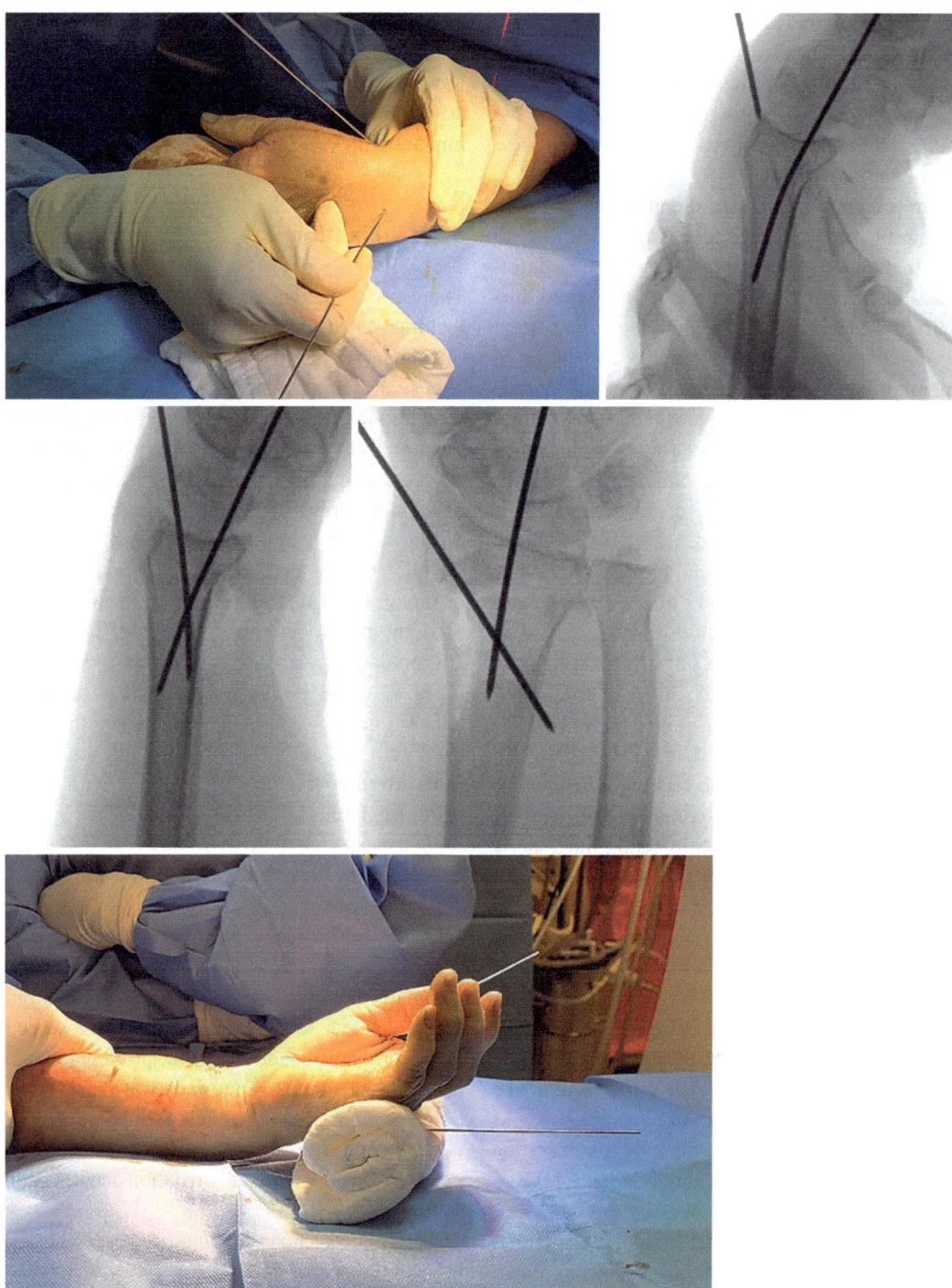

Fig. 6.6 In fractures that are inherently unstable, with residual dorsal angulation, with a sagittal split, a K-wire is inserted intra-focally or extra-focally through the dorsal cortex, to obtain and maintain the reduction before plate application. The K-wire can be first inserted by hand through the dorsal cortex, followed by driving through the volar cortex with an air-drive. A soft pad underneath the hand and dorsal K-wire help to maintain the volar tilt

Fig. 6.7 Reduction by plate is achieved by lifting the proximal end of plate off the volar cortex while inserting the distal row of locking head screws. One way of elevation is by inserting a locking head screw into the plate hole without prior drilling of bone. The magnitude of elevation is adjusted by the length of the screw. This way of reduction by plate does not work well in fractures with small distal fragments because the screws cannot engage the subchondral bone

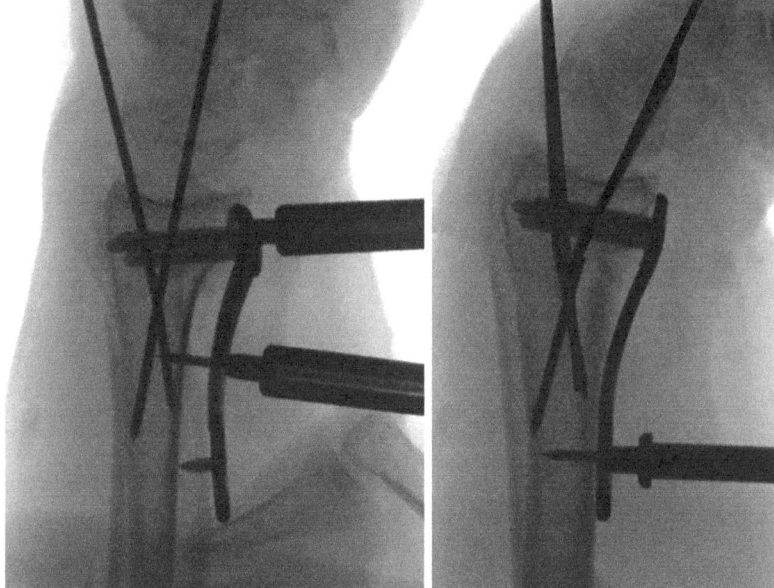

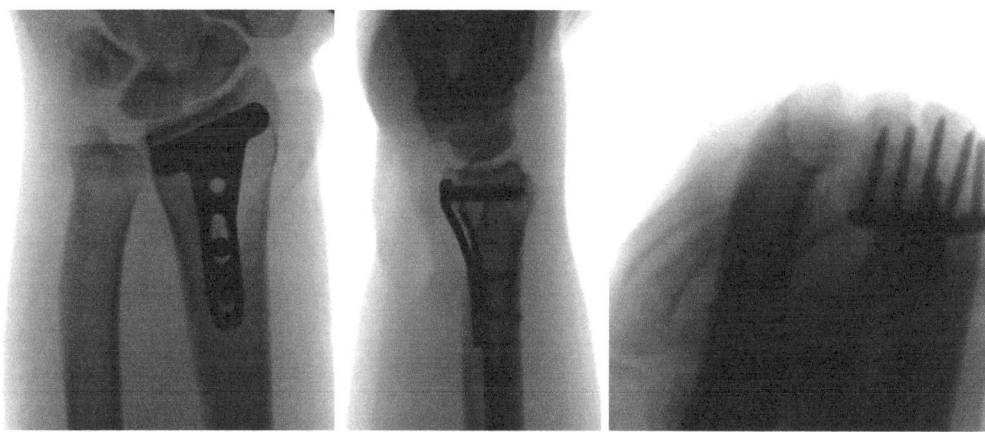

Fig. 6.8 Optimal plate positioning allows locking screws to engage subchondral bones along the sigmoid notch

fractures. Although rim plate has a contoured surface and low profile design, flexor tendon irritation may occur in the course of recovery. Plate removal may be necessary in future.

6.7.3.2 Location of Locking Plate

In osteoporotic distal radius, the strongest bone for fixation is at the subchondral bone [17]. The locking plate must be precisely placed in a location where fixed-angle distal locking screws are immediately beneath the subchondral bone (Fig. 6.8). Inappropriate proximal placement leads to the loss of reduction in the early post-

operative period, resulting in deformity, malunion, and flexor tendon irritation. Inappropriate distal placement, distal to the watershed line, risks radiocarpal joint screw penetration, and flexor tendon irritation.

It is common to place the plate too radially because of the surgical approach (Fig. 6.9). If the locking plate is placed too radially, the screw fails to capture the subchondral bone of the intermediate column. The plate also fails to capture volar medial corner fracture that is vital for palmar and axial stability. Radially placed plate creates abnormal contact between the plate and flexor pollicis longus,

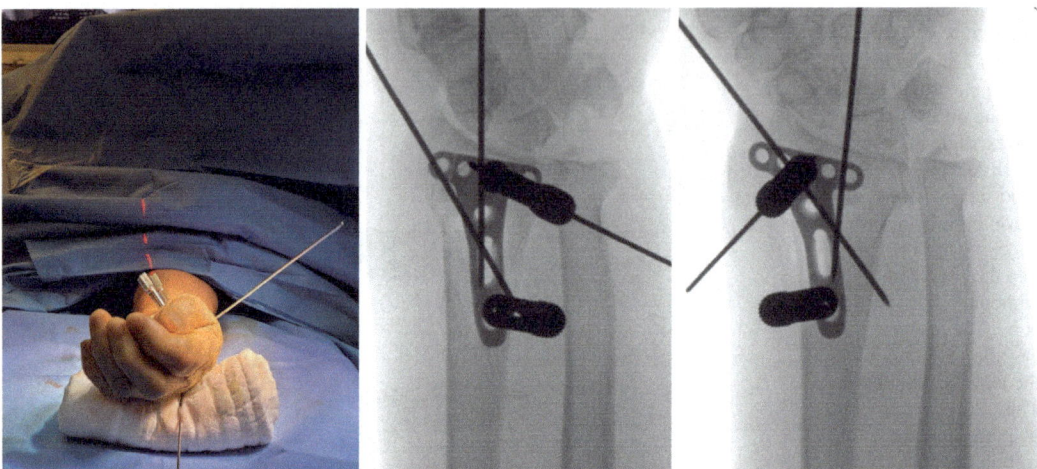

Fig. 6.9 Without external force, the forearm rests in slight pronation. If the volar plate position is adjusted under fluoroscopy in this forearm position, the plate ends up too radially placed, causing plate impingement radi- ally, flexor tendon irritation, and screws missing the strong subchondral bone in the intermediate column. With the forearm in full supination, the true sigmoid notch view of distal radius reveals the wrong plate position

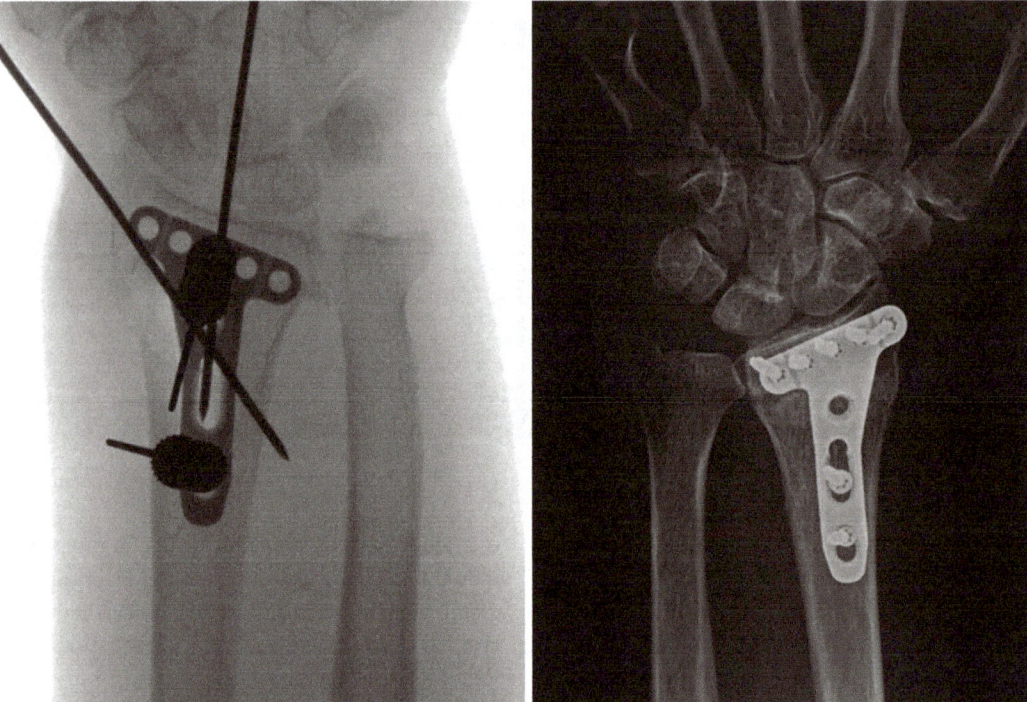

Fig. 6.10 The position of the locking plate should be guided by the sigmoid notch view. The most medial screw catches the strong subchondral bone of the volar medial corner and sigmoid notch, without violating the distal radioulnar joint

increasing the chance of flexor tendon rupture. The plate is felt to be prominent on the radial side by the patient. Erroneous placement may occur if the plate position is not fine-tuned under the fluoro- scopic sigmoid notch view (Fig. 6.10). The sig- moid notch view is obtained when there is cortical

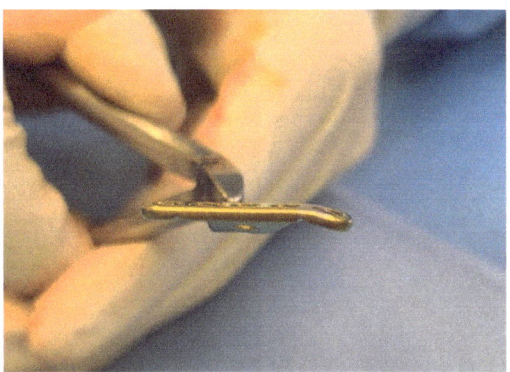

Fig. 6.11 The radii of curvature on the radial and ulnar volar radius are not the same. The ulnar volar radius projects more anteriorly. Contouring of the volar locking plate helps to prevent malrotation of distal fragment and implant impingement. Newer generation plates have built-in features respecting the difference in the two curvatures

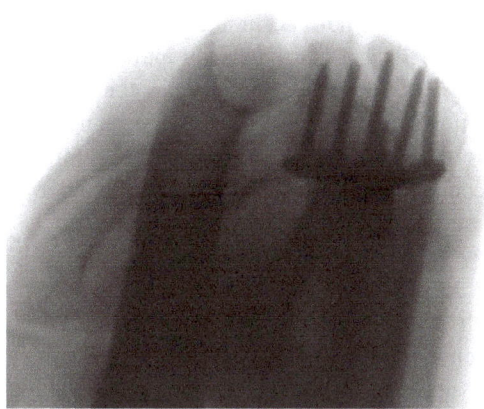

Fig. 6.12 Example of an intraoperative skyline view to detect screw penetration through the dorsal cortex

overlap of the sigmoid notch surfaces of the volar and dorsal lunate facet. It is the anteroposterior view of the distal radioulnar joint. The plate should be placed as ulnar as possible without screw violation of distal radioulnar joint (Fig. 6.11).

6.7.3.3 Length of Screw

A long screw that penetrates the dorsal cortex leads to extensor tendon rupture. It is recommended that surgeons should drill to but not through the dorsal cortex. The author's exception is on coronal plane fracture fixation. The dorsal cortex is penetrated by a drill bit but a shorter screw is inserted. The penetration is to prevent dorsal displacement of the dorsal fragment when a screw is inserted. Once the drill bit passes through the volar cortex, it should be advanced carefully with the "woodpecker" drilling technique. Reversing the direction of the drill bit enhances the tactile feedback of reaching the dorsal cortex. Surgeons can feel the impending cortical penetration with the finger on the wrist dorsum. Biomechanical study showed that a unicortical screw that traverses 75% length to the dorsal cortex has similar stiffness to a bi-cortical screw [18]. Length of screw higher than 20 mm warrants a check with depth gauge. An intraoperative dorsal horizon or skyline view helps to detect dorsal cortex penetration (Fig. 6.12).

6.7.3.4 Number of Screws

Theoretically as the number of locking screws used increases, more bone fragments are fixed and overall fixation stiffness increases. However, too many screws increases the operation cost and increases the risk of screw-related complications. Biomechanical study showed that four screws in the distal row and two screws in the shaft can provide sufficient stability for post-operative rehabilitation in dorsally comminuted, extra-articular non-osteoporotic distal radius fracture fixation [19]. In our practice, with a proper reduction of volar cortex, four locking screws in the distal row in the subchondral bone, two screws (one locking and one cortical, or two locking screws) in the shaft will provide sufficient stability for osteoporotic distal radius fracture fixation. The two shaft screws are adequately spaced out, with a one screw close to the fracture site and one screw at the end of the plate.

6.7.3.5 Avoiding Complications

Complications associated with surgery can negate any gains made by the improved alignment. Proper decision-making and execution in surgical approaches, reduction technique, plate and screw implantation are important to avoid complications. Injuries to medial nerve and its palmar cutaneous branch, radial sensory nerve, dorsal ulnar cutaneous branch of ulnar nerve can lead to painful neuromas and precipitate complex regional pain syndrome. Implants cannot securely maintain reduction, irritate and rupture tendons if not properly inserted. Surgery can contribute to additional trauma, swelling, scarring, and stiffness to the hand, wrist, and forearm. Nonunion is uncommon but sometimes occur with fixation in a distracted position.

6.7.3.6 Adjuncts to Volar Plate Fixation

With proper placement of locking plate and subchondral locking screws, volar locking plate can support comminuted fracture and metaphyseal bone loss. Additional bone augmentation by bone graft or bone substitute is usually not necessary. In selected cases, tricalcium phosphate granules help to provide structural support after elevation of depressed articular fragments. It is often required in old neglected malunion or nonunion cases. It is easy to use, relatively cheap, and carries no donor site morbidity. Minor degree fracture collapse may still occur, but it is usually well tolerated by elderly patients [20].

Dorsal wrist spanning plates are internal distraction plates that use ligamentotaxis to obtain reduction. It is particularly beneficial in patients with fractures extending into the radial diaphysis, in comminuted osteoporotic distal radius fracture, and in polytrauma patients who may require load bearing through the wrist for mobilization. The plate is removed after 12 weeks with good functional outcome [21].

External fixation and pin fixation cannot adequately maintain reduction in unstable distal radius fracture and has been shown to result in poor function. They are reserved for cases with soft tissue compromise. They are used as an intraoperative reduction tool and post-operative supplement to internal fixation (Fig. 6.13). Intraoperatively, external fixation can help to provide distraction force necessary to gain radial length. Traction alone may exaggerate the dorsal tilt of distal fragments because the stout volar radiocarpal ligaments are shorter. They pull out to

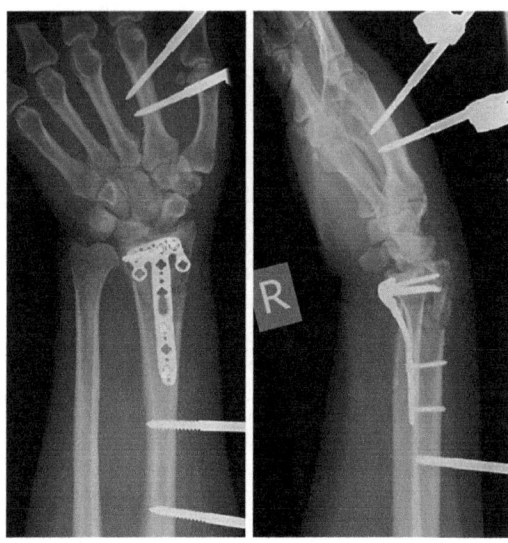

Fig. 6.13 An example of combined internal and external fixation

length before the dorsal ligaments. In distal radius fracture with very small, comminuted, osteoporotic distal fragments, leaving a cross-wrist external fixation after reduction and internal fixation helps to prevent early fracture displacement. It can be removed at 4 weeks. It is important not to maintain excessive distraction force, evident by distracted mid-carpal or radiocarpal joint, as it may cause complex regional pain syndrome.

6.8   Rehabilitation

Most elderly patients with distal radius fracture fixed with volar locking plate are allowed to mobilize their hand and wrist immediately. Active thumb, fingers, and wrist range of motion exercise is started immediately. The same applies to patients with concomitant ulnar styloid fracture. In patients with distal ulnar metaphyseal fracture, severe osteoporosis, distal radioulnar joint laxity, a static wrist splint can be applied for 2–4 weeks. Even in these cases, thumb and fingers mobilization should not be delayed. The hand is incorporated into all light daily activities. Whenever possible, forearm rotation is encouraged as supination and pronation are important in many daily functions in older patients.

6.9   Management of Concomitant Distal Ulnar Fracture

Distal ulna, the ulnar column in the three-column theory, is a key structure for load transfer across the wrist, attachment of stabilizing ligament of the wrist, and articulation with the sigmoid notch of radius for forearm rotation.

Distal ulnar fracture is present in 50—70% of distal radius fracture cases. It is most commonly an ulnar styloid fracture, less commonly a metaphyseal fracture or rarely a head intra-articular fracture. Accompanying distal ulnar fracture may affect the outcomes of distal radius fracture by disturbing the congruity and stability of the distal radioulnar joint. Inappropriately managed distal ulnar fracture leads to restriction of forearm motion, ulnar sided wrist pain and distal radioulnar joint instability.

Optimal management of distal ulnar fracture is as controversial as its distal radius counterpart. Some surgeons routinely treat it non-operatively after fixation of distal radius. Some surgeons treat it selectively by internal fixation if the distal ulnar fracture remains mal-aligned or unstable after fixation of distal radius. When facing a combined distal radius and distal ulna fracture, the distal radius fracture should be addressed first and then decisions are made regarding the treatment of distal ulna fracture.

6.10   Types of Distal Ulnar Fracture

Distal ulna fractures are classified according to location and pattern. According to the AO/OTA Classification, distal ulnar fractures associated with distal radius fractures are classified using the Q modifier, as follows: Q1, ulnar styloid base fracture; Q2, simple ulnar neck fracture; Q3, comminuted ulnar neck fracture; Q4, ulnar head fracture; and Q5, combined ulnar neck and head fracture. Ulnar styloid fracture an also be classified according to the Biyani classification [22].

6.10.1 Ulnar Styloid Fracture

More than half 50–70% of the distal radius fractures are combined with an ulnar styloid fracture. Considerable cases of ulnar styloid fractures result in nonunion. However, ulnar styloid nonunion usually does not cause any objective or subjective clinical problem to the wrist, especially when the distal radius, including the sigmoid notch, is anatomically restored and rigidly fixed with a locking plate. Rarely, symptomatic nonunion may give rise to pain at the nonunion site, ulnocarpal impaction, extensor carpi ulnaris tendinitis, or distal radioulnar joint instability.

After fixation of distal radius fracture, the distal radioulnar joint stability is tested by dorso-palmar ballottement with the forearm in neutral rotation, supination, and pronation. The laxity is compared with the contralateral wrist. Another way of testing is by compression of the ulna against the radius and passively rotating the forearm between full supination and full pronation to assess for "clunk" or instability. In the majority of cases with concomitant ulnar styloid fracture, the distal radioulnar joint is stable after reduction and fixation of radius. Fixation of ulnar styloid fracture, regardless of its size and displacement, does not provide a better outcome. Free mobilization of the wrist is allowed. Splintage is mainly for comfort [23].

When the distal radioulnar joint is unstable in one forearm position, the wrist can be immobilized in a stable position for 4 weeks. However, if the distal radioulnar joint is unstable in all positions, open reduction and internal fixation of ulnar styloid fracture with a tension band wiring construct are performed. On the other hand, the presence of an ulnar styloid fracture does not prevent a concomitant injury to the triangular fibrocartilage complex. If there is no ulnar styloid fracture, presence of a small styloid tip fracture or persistence of instability after styloid fixation, arthroscopic or open repair of triangular fibrocartilage complex could be performed.

6.10.2 Ulnar Head Fracture

Ulnar head fracture is rare. If the fracture is displaced, reduction and fixation with headless compression screws are indicated.

6.10.3 Ulnar Metaphyseal Fracture

Fractures from the ulnar neck to 5 cm proximal to the ulnar head are distal ulnar metaphyseal fractures. It is reported in 5–6% of distal radius fracture. Such a combination occurs more commonly in the older population.

Distal ulna fracture is more stable with there is anatomical restoration of distal radius anatomy. Ligamentotaxis effect of the triangular fibrocartilage complex and interosseous membrane will help to realign and stabilize the distal ulna fracture. Decision on surgical fixation distal ulnar metaphyseal fracture should be addressed after fixating the distal radius fracture [24]. If the distal ulna fracture is realigned and stable, short-term immobilization with a short arm slab for 3–4 weeks allows for bony union and avoids stiffness.

If the distal ulna fracture is mal-aligned, defined as >10° angulation, >3 mm ulnar variance change, or >1/3 translation of fracture surface, reduction, and fixation can be performed to restore the ulnar column of the wrist. Such degree of mal-alignment implies a disruption of interosseous membrane and confers longitudinal instability.

Fixation of distal ulna fracture is challenging because the fracture fragment is small, mostly covered by cartilage, comminuted, and osteoporotic. The surgery is usually performed with the elbow flexed at 90°. Care must be taken to avoid injury to the dorsal sensory branch of the ulnar nerve. The soft tissue envelope over the distal ulna is thin and placement of implant is poorly tolerated in this region.

Various methods of distal ulnar fracture fixation have been described. The 2.0 mm locking plate is our internal fixator of choice. For more proximal Q2 and Q3 fractures, locking plates can be inserted on the volar surface with distal locking screws engaging the distal fragments at an angle. On the volar surface, there is a flatter bone surface and thicker soft tissue envelope. For more distal Q2,Q3, and Q5 fractures, a locking plate can be inserted on the subcutaneous border with a hook on the ulnar styloid to enhance distal fixation (Fig. 6.14).

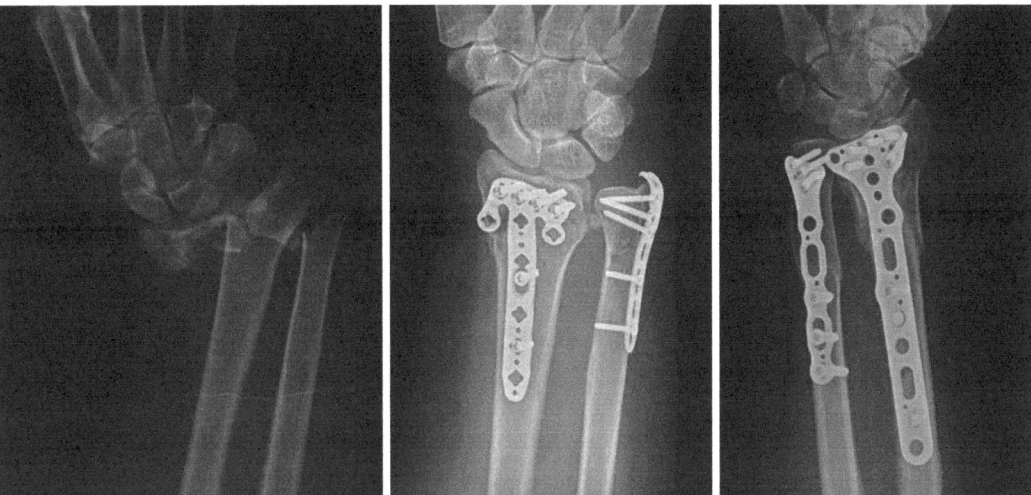

Fig. 6.14 Examples of concomitant distal ulna fracture fixed with a distal ulna locked hook plate and a volar precontoured plate

6.11 Salvage Options in Geriatric Distal Radius Malunion

Although it has been stated that elderly patients tolerate deformity well and functional outcomes do not correlate with radiographic outcome, there is a small subset of elderly patients who are suffering from symptomatic distal radius malunion. Treatment should be directed at symptoms rather than radiographs. Around 1% of conservatively treated patients have subsequent wrist surgery. Timing of intervention is controversial. Once a decision is determined to intervene in a malunion, surgery should generally be performed as soon as possible. Correction is easier to achieve when there is less soft tissue contracture. Structural bone graft may be spared. Most patients have surgery within the first year.

Wrist surgeries include joint-preserving and joint-sacrificing surgeries depending on the underlying pathoanatomy. Joint-preserving surgery includes early conversion to open reduction and internal fixation, opening and closing wedge radial osteotomy, ulnar shortening osteotomy, and distal radioulnar joint reconstruction. Joint-

sacrificing procedure includes limited radiocarpal arthrodesis, total wrist arthrodesis, distal radioulnar joint fusion, and distal ulna resection. In the adult population, the choice of procedure depends on the magnitude of radial deformity (shortening, volar and dorsal tilt, loss of inclination), the amount of positive ulnar variance, the presence of radiocarpal and distal radioulnar joint arthrosis incongruity and arthrosis.

Malunion of distal radius fracture often results in radial shortening as the main deformity. The positive ulnar variance lead to limited range of wrist and forearm range of motion, overloading of ulnocarpal compartment, ulnocarpal impaction with lesions of triangular fibrocartilage complex and ulnar carpal bones, and instability of distal radioulnar joint. Patient presents with ulnar sided wrist pain, limited ulnar deviation and forearm rotation, and decrease grip strength.

Radial or ulnar osteotomy can relieve symptoms by re-establishing a neutral radioulnar variance. Closing and opening wedge osteotomy of distal radius is a challenging surgery because of the difficulty in addressing both length and angular deformity at the same time, more extensive surgical dissection, longer operative time, and need of bone grafting. Not infrequently, there is incomplete correction of positive ulnar variance, leading to suboptimal results or need for additional ulnar shortening osteotomy (Fig. 6.15). Complications of radial osteotomy include delayed union, nonunion, infection, hardware failure, median nerve neuritis, superficial radial nerve neuritis, complex regional pain syndrome, bone graft donor site morbidity, and residual ulnar wrist pain from under-correction. It is undesirable in the elderly population.

Ulnar shortening osteotomy restores neutral ulnar variance reliably with comparable functional outcomes. It is a technically simpler surgery that involves a uniplanar correction, less surgical dissection, shorter operative time, fewer complications, fewer secondary surgeries, and shorter rehabilitation. With the development of an osteotomy guide with a cutting jig, 2.4 or 2.7 mm locking plate, volar plate placement with

better soft tissue coverage, complications of osteotomy nonunion and hardwire irritation are minimized.

Methods of ulnar shortening can be divided into intra-articular and extra-articular, subcapital and diaphyseal osteotomy. Our preference is to perform extra-articular diaphyseal oblique osteotomy, aiming at achieving 2 mm negative ulnar variance or within 2 mm of the contralateral wrist (Fig. 6.16). Fixation in this part of the bone is more secure. Healing of an oblique osteotomy in the diaphysis is possibly faster. Wrist arthroscopy can be done to tackle intra-articular pain generators such as triangular fibrocartilage complex tears.

Ulnar shortening osteotomy produces excellent outcomes in the short and medium term. That is particularly important in the elderly population. Leaving the loss of palmar tilt and radial inclination unchanged may result in radiocarpal degenerative arthritis in the long term, but it is less of a concern.

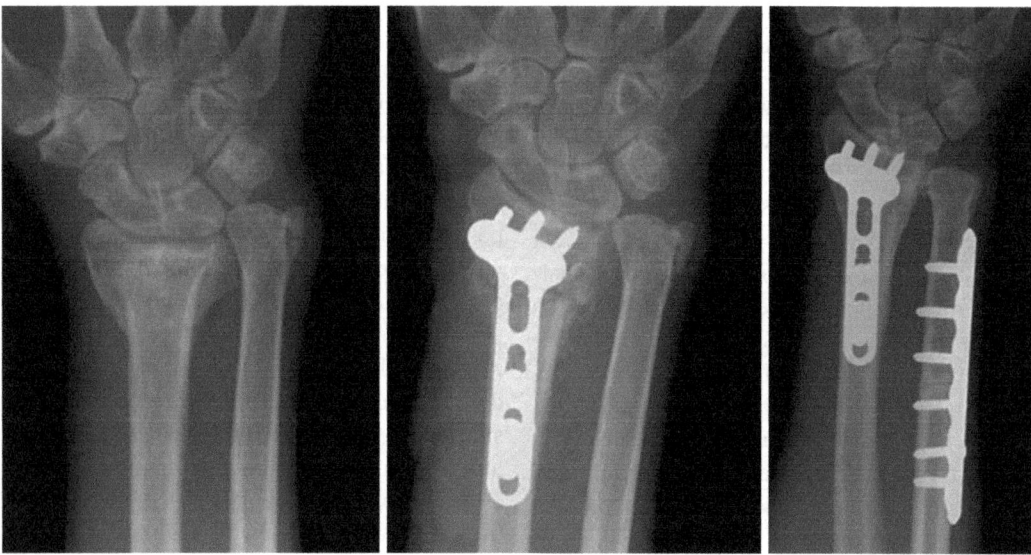

Fig. 6.15 Incomplete correction of positive ulnar variance after opening wedge radial osteotomy. A second surgery to shorten the ulna is required

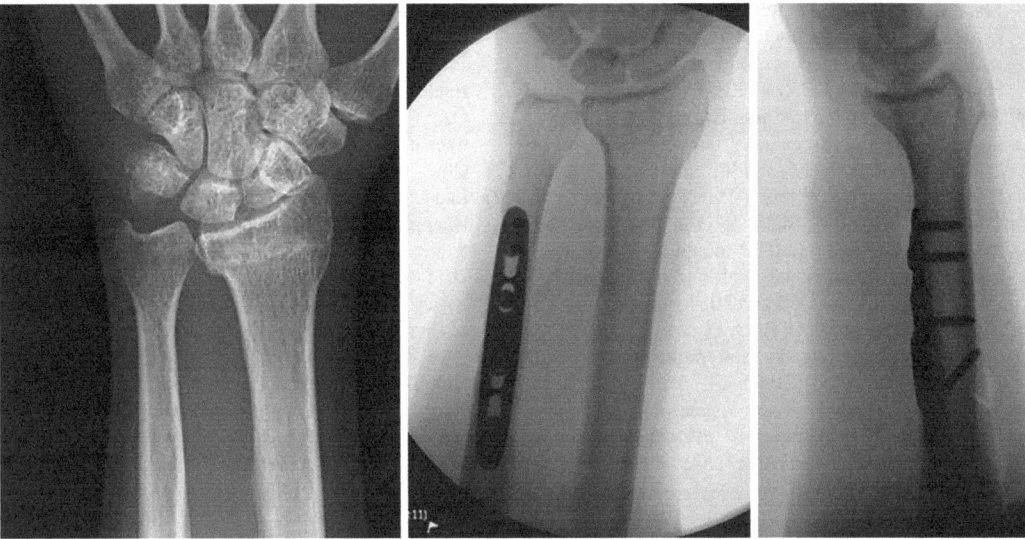

Fig. 6.16 An extra-articular diaphyseal oblique shortening osteotomy, fixed with a 2.7 mm locking plate on the volar surface, resulting in 2 mm negative ulnar variance

6.12   Conclusion

Distal radius fractures are common in the elderly population. The goal of treatment is restoration of wrist function to allow for rapid return of function. In surgical decision-making, special attention should be given to a patient's functional activity level. While most distal radius fractures can be treated non-operatively, fractures treated surgically have improved alignment, quicker recovery and better grip strength.

References

1. Nellans KW, Kowalski E, Chung KC. The epidemiology of distal radius fractures. Hand Clin. 2012;28(2):113–25.
2. DeGoede KM, Ashton-Miller JA, Schultz AB. Fall-related upper body injuries in the older adult: a review of the biomechanical issues. J Biomech. 2003;36(7):1043–53.
3. Edwards BJ, Song J, Dunlop DD, Fink HA, Cauley JA. Functional decline after incident wrist fractures—Study of Osteoporotic Fractures: prospective cohort study. BMJ. 2010;341:c3324.
4. Stern PJ, Derr RG. Non-osseous complications following distal radius fractures. Iowa Orthop J. 1993;13:63–9.
5. Bliuc D, Nguyen ND, Milch VE, Nguyen TV, Eisman JA, et al. Mortality risk associated with low-trauma osteoporotic fracture and subsequent fracture in men and women. JAMA. 2009;301:513–21.
6. Frykman G. Fracture of the distal radius including sequelae—shoulder-hand-finger syndrome, disturbance in the distal radio-ulnar joint and impairment of nerve function: a clinical and experimental study. Acta Orthop Scand. 1967;Suppl 108:3.
7. Fernández dl. Fractures of the distal radius: operative treatment. Instr Course Lect. 1993;42:73–88.
8. Rikli DA, Regazzoni P. Fractures of the distal end of the radius treated by internal fixation and early function. A preliminary report of 20 cases. J Bone Joint Surg Br. 1996;78:588–92.
9. Lafontaine M, Hardy D, Delince P. Stability assessment of distal radius fractures. Injury. 1989;20(4):208–10.
10. Jakubietz RG, Gruenert JG, Kloss DF, Schindele S, Jakubietz MG. A randomised clinical study comparing palmar and dorsal fixed-angle plates for the internal fixation of AO C-type fractures of the distal radius in the elderly. J Hand Surg Eur. 2008;33(5):600–4.
11. Diaz-Garcia RJ, Oda T, Shauver MJ, Chung KC. A systematic review of outcomes and complications of treating unstable distal radius fractures in the elderly. J Hand Surg Am. 2011;36(5):824–835.e2.
12. Arora R, Lutz M, Deml C, Krappinger D, Haug L, Gabl M. A prospective randomized trial comparing nonoperative treatment with volar locking plate fixation for displaced and unstable distal radial fractures in patients sixty-five years of age and older. J Bone Joint Surg Am. 2011;93(23):2146–53.

13. Makhni EC, Ewald TJ, Kelly S, Day CS. Effect of patient age on the radiographic outcomes of distal radius fractures subject to nonoperative treatment. J Hand Surg Am. 2008;33(8):1301–8.

14. Nicholas PS, Gopal RL, Sarah EM, Igor I. Incidence of corrective procedures after nonoperatively managed distal radius fractures in the elderly. J Am Acad Orthop Surg Glob Res Rev. 2019;3(11):e10.5435.

15. Chung KC, Kim HM, Malay S, et al. The wrist and radius injury surgical trial: 12-month outcomes from a multicenter international randomized clinical trial. Plast Reconstr Surg. 2020;145:1054e–66e.

16. Brogan DM, Richard MJ, Ruch D, et al. Management of severely comminuted distal radius fractures. J Hand Surg Am. 2015;40:1905–14.

17. Miyamura S, Oka K, Lans J. Cartilage and subchondral bone distributions of the distal radius: a 3-dimensional analysis using cadavers. Osteoarthr Cartil. 2020;28:1572–80.

18. Liu X, Wu W-d, Fang Y-f, Zhang M-c, Huang W-h. Biomechanical comparison of osteoporotic distal radius fractures fixed by distal locking screws with different length. PLoS One. 2014;9(7):e103371.

19. Jung HS, et al. Volar locking plating for distal radius fractures. Clin Orthop Surg. 2020;12(1):22.

20. Ozer K, Chung KC. The use of bone grafts and substitutes in the treatment of distal radius fractures. Hand Clin. 2012;28(2):217–23.

21. Lauder A, Agnew S, Bakri K, Allan CH, Hanel DP, Huang JI. Functional outcomes following bridge plate fixation for distal radius fractures. J Hand Surg Am. 2015;40(8):1554–62.

22. Biyani A, Simison AJ, Klenerman L. Fractures of the distal radius and ulna. J Hand Surg Br. 1995;20(3):357–64.

23. Kim JK, Kim JO, Koh YD. Management of distal ulnar fracture combined with distal radius fracture. J Hand Surg Asian Pac. 2016;21(2):155–60.

24. Logan AJ, Lindau TR. The management of distal ulnar fractures in adults: a review of the literature and recommendations for treatment. Strategies Trauma Limb Reconstr. 2008;3(2):49–56.

Fragility Fractures of Pelvis

7

Christian Fang and Frankie Leung

7.1 Introduction

Osteoporotic pelvic fractures or fragility fractures of pelvis (FFP) are the third most common fragility fractures after hip and distal radius fractures and the incidence is increasing [1]. As there is increasing awareness of this entity, the definition, diagnosis, classification, and the overall management need to be revisited. The definition of FFP is pelvic fracture occurring in patients over 60 years old after minimal trauma or loads experienced during daily living. The diagnosis of FFP can be difficult and the optimal treatment remains debated. Like other fragility fractures, the mechanism is typically a low energy fall. The management of FFP must take the consideration of the patient as a whole and considerably differs from high energy pelvic ring injuries. FFPs are associated with other fragility fractures such as hip fractures, upper limb fractures, and vertebral collapse fractures. Together these injuries contribute significantly to pain, short-term morbidity and difficulty in nursing. Patients are often in their 80s or 90s, with female predominance. Patients have multiple co-morbidities are at risk of developing complications and deterioration in mobility [2]. The treatment goals are prompt and adequate pain relief, early mobilisation, and eventual fracture union.

7.2 Diagnosis

The main presenting symptoms of FFP are pain in the back, hip, groin, or perineum on either side of the symphysis pubis. Most patients need to rest on bed or wheelchair and cannot stand or walk. The pain typically intensifies on change of body postures. The patients should be carefully examined and checked for tenderness located at the perineum and sacroiliac regions since posterior element fractures are not easily detected on radiographs [3].

Pelvis radiograph is the commonest method in detecting fractures. With the standard three views (anteroposterior, inlet and outlet) it is possible to detect displaced pubic rami fractures and posterior ring injuries. However, the severe bone loss at the sacral alae and bowel gas shadows add to the difficulty in detecting posterior injuries. The incidence of an additional posterior pelvic ring fractures in patients diagnosed with pubic rami fractures is 59–97% [3–5]. Routine advanced imaging such as CT scan, MRI, and bone scintigraphy is helpful when there is clinical suspicion [6]. Missed fractures may lead to inadequate treatment, fracture displacement, and subsequent prolonged pain and disability. We recommended a careful examination of the patients' back and

C. Fang · F. Leung (✉)
Department of Orthopaedics and Traumatology,
Queen Mary Hospital, The University of Hong Kong,
Pokfulam, Hong Kong
e-mail: klleunga@hku.hk

© The Author(s), under exclusive license to Springer Nature Singapore Pte Ltd. 2024
F. Leung, T. W. Lau (eds.), *Surgery for Osteoporotic Fractures*,
https://doi.org/10.1007/978-981-99-9696-4_7

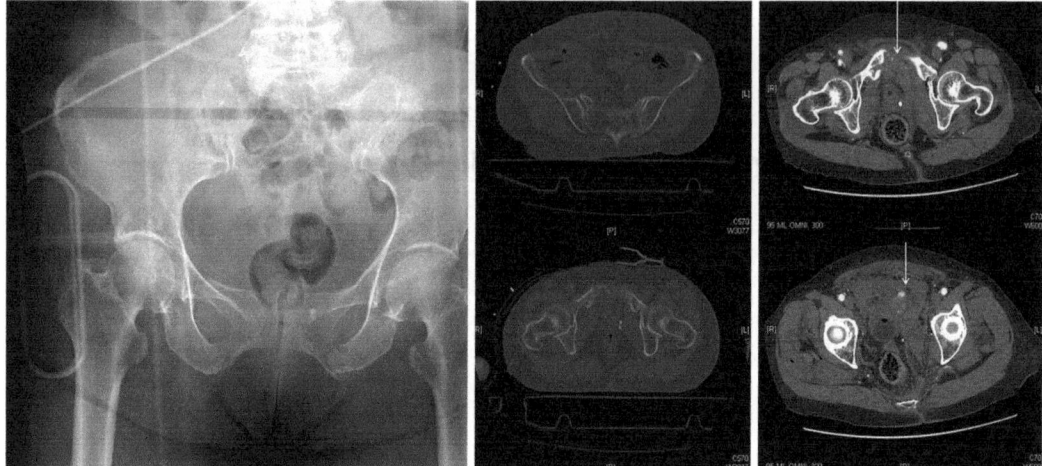

Fig. 7.1 An 87-year-old female pedestrian was injured by a low-speed vehicle. She was on anti-platelet therapy and beta-blockers for ischaemic heart disease. The initial radiograph and plain CT scan (FFP 1) showed an undisplaced pubic ramus fracture and no observable hematoma. She developed progressive hypotension but without tachycardia after admission. An immediate follow-up contrast CT scan demonstrated active contrast extravasation (arrow) from the corona mortis vessel. She was resuscitated and stabilized after an urgent arterial embolization

routine CT scan for all patients with X-ray showing a pubic rami fracture.

Pelvic insufficiency fractures are FFPs occurring with no history of prior trauma [7]. They occur thorough weak parts of the pelvic ring typically at the sacral alar in patients with severe osteoporosis. The diagnosis can be confused with lumbar spine pathologies. The fracture is painful but undisplaced and plain X ray examination is frequently negative. Compared to CT scan, which is more widely available, MRI has nearly 100% sensitivity by localization of high intensity T2 signals from bone oedema adjacent to the fracture. Additionally, MRI exam is invaluable in excluding pathological conditions such as infection and neoplasms. FFP patients almost invariably present with low energy trauma and haemodynamic compromise is rare. Yet, in the unlikely event that a patient presents with a higher energy of injury such as a motor vehicle accident, the clinician must stay vigilant that FFP

patients with benign looking radiographs may deteriorate rapidly from active exsanguination (Fig. 7.1).

7.3 Pathoanatomy and Classifications

The pelvic bone consists of anterior and posterior elements. Assessing FFP by its pathoanatomy according to the location of fracture is useful in evaluating the biomechanics and guiding further treatment. Anterior element fractures occur at the superior and inferior pubic rami and almost always occur in combination. Such fractures may occur in isolation or more commonly in combination with posterior element fractures. Low superior pubic rami fractures occur near the symphysis and high superior rami fractures occur near the anterior acetabulum margin. High rami fractures are shown to have poorer short-term outcomes possibly due to higher degree of pain and instability [8]. Inferior rami fracture is almost always associated with superior rami fractures. There is no reliable surgical fixation method for inferior rami fractures. Fortunately, the disability resulting from such injuries is usually minimal and recovery is often spontaneous. Non-operative management is generally recommended for patients with isolated anterior element fractures. The location of the posterior element injury varies, at the ilium body (crescent fractures), sacroiliac joint, and the sacrum alar or body. FFPs are almost universally low energy lateral compression (LC) injuries classifiable under the Young–Burgess Classification with LC-I and LC-II variants being most common. The presence of posterior element fractures means that the pelvic ring is rotationally or partially unstable. Uncommonly, patients with axial injuries may have isolated sacrum fractures presenting with U shaped or H shaped "jumper's fracture pattern" without anterior column involvement. These are unstable spinopelvic dissociation injuries associated with neurological compromise and are exquisitely painful.

The conventional Young and Burgess as well as Tile classifications are developed to address pelvic ring injuries in the younger adults. The Young–Burgess system [9] classifies pelvic fractures according to the predominant force vector and the Tile system [10] according to the degree of instability. Under these two systems, nearly all FFPs are lateral compression (LC) injuries and are partially/rotationally unstable resulting from low energy injuries. Anterior posterior compression (APC) or vertical shear patterns (VS) with gross instability are uncommon. With the unique clinical features of FFP, there is a need for another more specific classification. Based on analysis of radiographs and CT scans of 245 patients, Rommens and Hofmann [4] proposed a classification to guide the management of FFPs. The main differentiation among the fracture types is the degree of instability. Fracture displacement is the most important sign of fracture instability. Type I fractures are stable fractures involving anterior pelvic ring only. Types II to IV fractures involve posterior ring. Non-displaced posterior ring fractures are type II. Although there is no fracture displacement, some type II fractures can lead to prolonged disabling pain and slow rehabilitation. On the other hand, displaced posterior fractures are regarded as unstable. Unilateral displaced posterior fractures are type III and bilateral displaced fractures are type IV (Figs. 7.2 and 7.3).

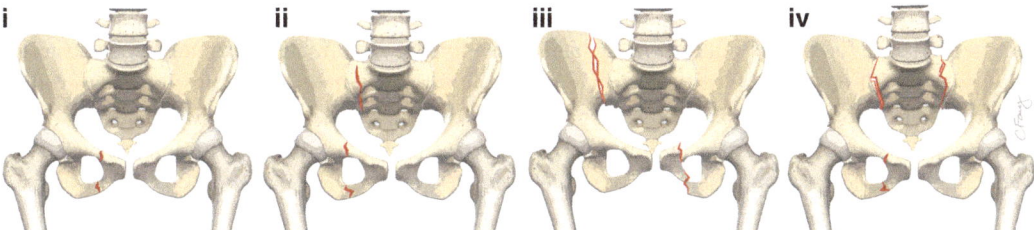

Fig. 7.2 The Rommens and Hoffmann classification of FFP. Type I—Involving only the anterior ring. Type II—Undisplaced/Impacted posterior ring involvement. Type III—Unilateral involvement of posterior ring with displacement. Type IV—Bilateral posterior ring involvement with displacement

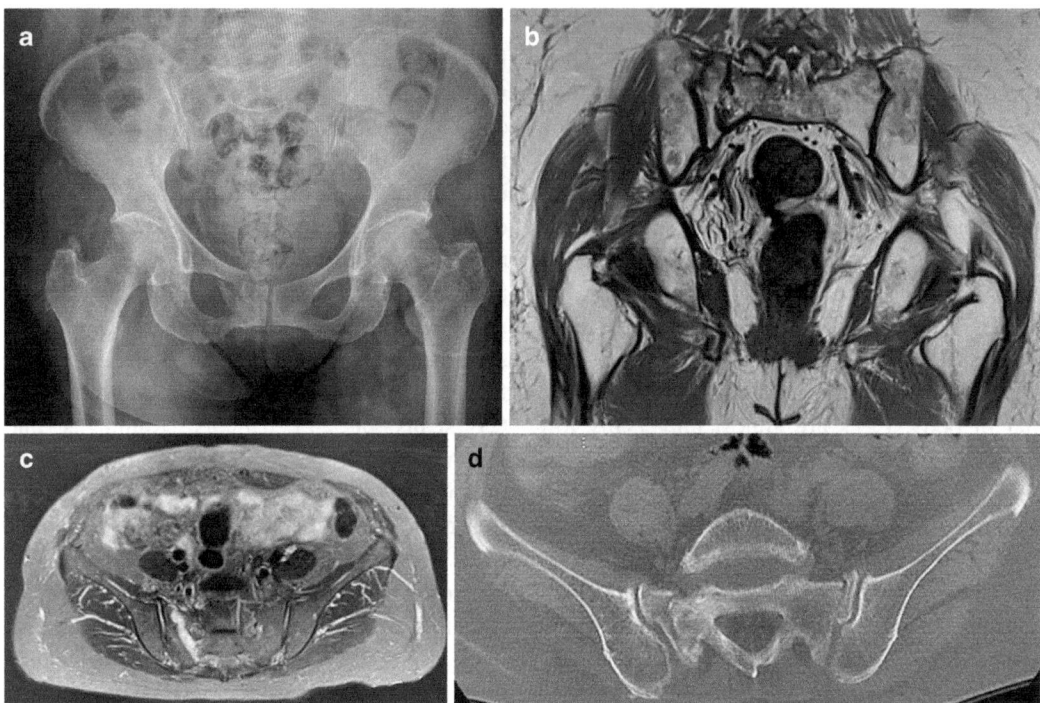

Fig. 7.3 An 82-year-old lady presented with groin and back pain after a trivial fall. (**a**) The initial radiograph just showed the displaced right pubic rami fractures. (**b**, **c**) An MRI scan was also performed which showed an undisplaced right sacral ala fracture. The fracture was classified as FFP type IIc. After an initial improvement with non-operative treatment, she experienced severe back pain, and a CT scan showed a new fracture of the left sacral ala (**d**). The fracture was re-classified as type IV

7.4   Management

The management strategy of FFP depends on the stability of the fracture. There are no universally accepted criteria for the definition of mechanically unstable FFPs. Type I fractures have no occult posterior injuries on CT scans. Type II fractures have some degree of instability associated with a posterior element fracture. Type IIa is an isolated non-displaced sacral fracture without anterior injury. In the presence of anterior injury, there is more instability. The sacral fracture pattern can vary from a sacral crush injury situated ventrally (FFP Type IIb) to a disruption of both ventral and dorsal cortices of sacral ala (FFP type IIc). The progression from a type with lower instability to a type with higher instability is possible if the fracture further propagates, or if there is inadequate treatment in cases of missed diagnosis.

Type III fractures have more significant instability as there is fracture displacement or gap formation between fracture fragments. The posterior injury can occur at the ilium (IIIa), sacroiliac joint (IIIb), or sacrum (IIIc). Patients with type III fractures typically have prolonged pain even at 4–6 weeks. Type IV fractures is the most unstable FFP type. The posterior injury can occur at the ilium (IVa), sacral ala (IVb), or fracture of the upper sacrum similar to a jumper's fracture. As complete dorsal disruptions occur bilaterally, there is in effect complete spinopelvic dissociation. As a result, the fixation method chosen needs to reconnect the lumbosacral spine with the pelvic ring. These injuries typically present with prolonged pain and difficult rehabilitation.

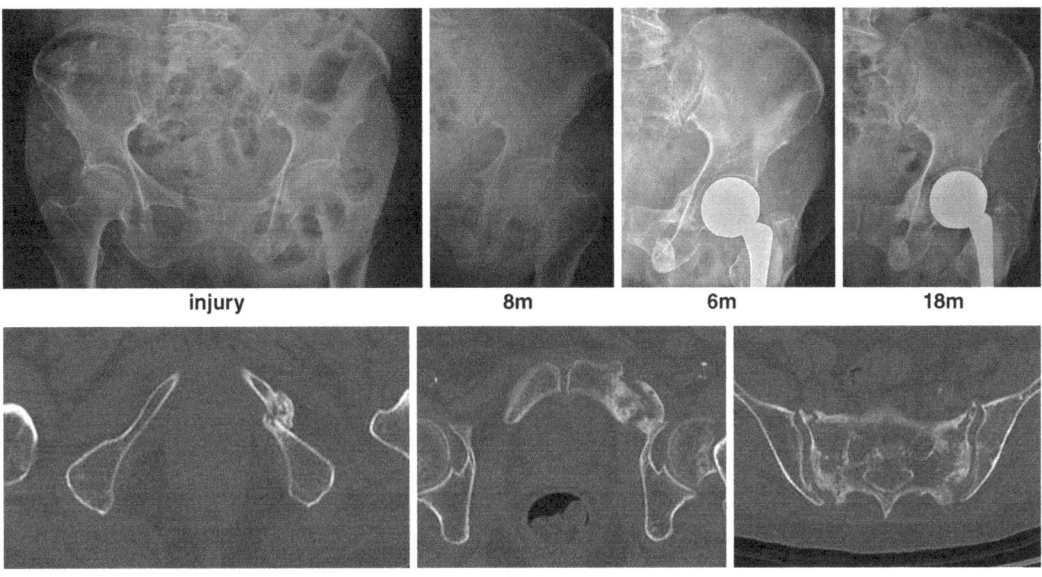

Fig. 7.4 Natural history of a patient with displaced FFP type III managed conservatively, demonstrating the natural history of prolonged healing by callus formation. The patient was able to tolerate the mild degree of pain and remained ambulatory outdoors. Note that the patient suffered a femoral neck fracture and received a hemiarthroplasty during recovery. A CT scan at 12 months demonstrates lack of union at the superior ramus and the contralateral sacral alar. Note the severe osteopenia and the lack of cancellous trabeculation

7.5 Non-Operative Treatment

There are no absolute contraindications to non-operative treatment. In most cases of FFP, conservative management is highly successful and therefore should be the primary method of treatment. All type I and most type II fractures and selected patients with FFP III and IV without significant mechanical pain can be successful managed non-operatively. Strong ligamentous connections contribute to the intrinsic stability. The pelvis is also rich in blood supply so fracture union can be obtained. In type I and II fractures, healing by robust callus formation is usually evident by 2 months and any associated mechanical pain is considerably reduced. Complete union of the fracture with callus formation is usually expected within 3 months.

An initial period of analgesics should relieve the symptoms. Bed rest should not be more than a few days. Patients undergoing non-operative treatment are safe to mobilise with weight bearing as tolerated even on the injured side. Early prescription of standing and walking exercises do not affect fracture healing. If the mechanical pain persists and remains intractable for more than 1–2 weeks, or if there is increasing pain during rehabilitation, the patient should be re-evaluated for fracture displacement or other missed injuries. Those with persistent mechanical pain hindering mobilization out of bed beyond 1–2 weeks can be considered for surgical stabilization.

Patients suffering from FFP are at high risk of developing a secondary fracture. Pharmacological and non-pharmacological management of osteoporosis must accompany the treatment of FFPs prevent future fractures (Fig. 7.4).

7.6 Surgical Treatment

Specific unstable FFPs are indicated for operative treatment including type II fractures failing non-operative treatment, as well as type III and IV fractures. Fixation should preferably be done via minimal invasive approaches. The benefits are better pain control and ambulation [11]. Due to a lack of high level of clinical evidence, the

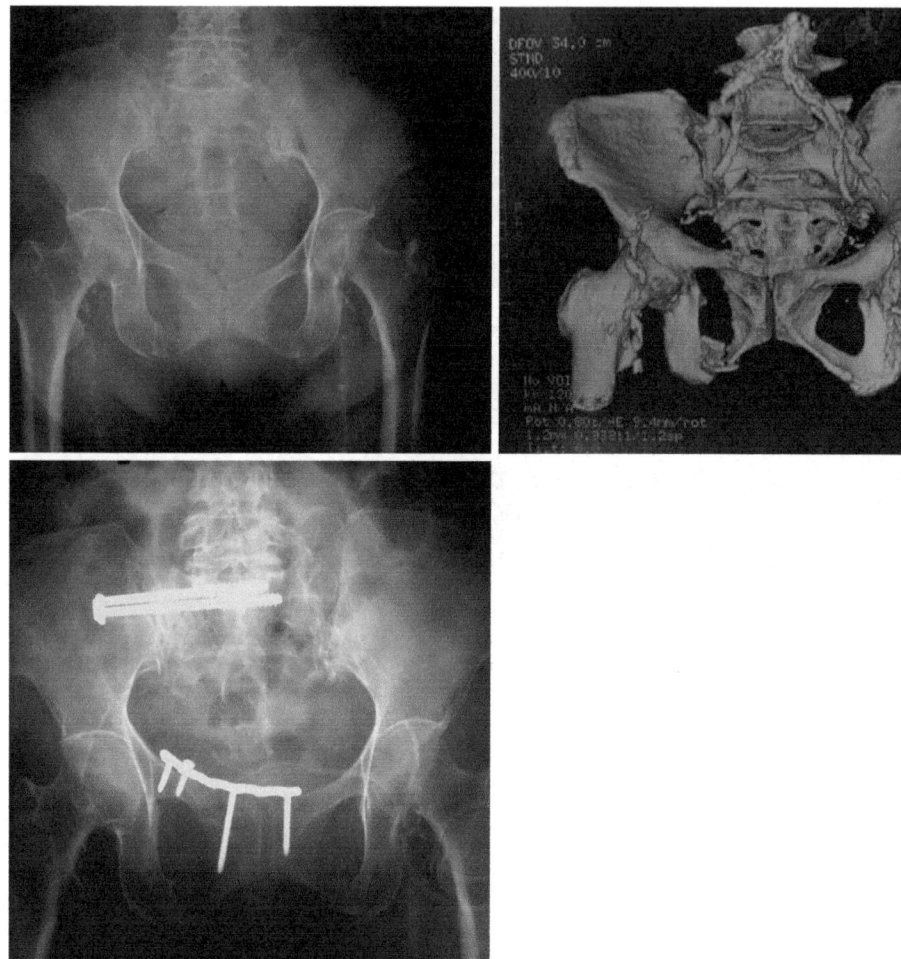

Fig. 7.5 An 85-year-old patient with 3 weeks history of groin pain and inability to mobilise. CT showed minimally displaced sacral alar fracture with right sided rami fractures. The fracture was classified as type IIc. Plating of pubic rami and iliosacral screw fixation were performed

optimal selection criteria remain a topic for debate.

The prime surgical indication is persistent and intractable pain resulting from mechanical instability. The main surgical goal is to alleviate pain by restoration of stability, thereby facilitating rehabilitation. Restoration of perfect anatomy is of lower priority. Prolonged bed rest related complications and deconditioning must be avoided following surgery. According to the severity and the fracture pattern, minimally invasive or minimal open fixation methods addressing the ante-

rior and posterior element can be chosen. Examination under anaesthesia is useful in determining the degree of anterior instability in LC injuries and guiding the extent of surgery needed [12] (Fig. 7.5).

7.6.1 Minimally Invasive Pelvic Fixation

Elderly patients often have significant comorbidities and poor cardiopulmonary reserves.

They cannot tolerate excessive blood loss associated with invasive open approaches to the pelvic ring. Proper preoperative planning is necessary regarding the 3-dimentional morphology of the pelvis and the fracture. There are various well described trajectories for screw osteosynthesis within the pelvic ring. These trajectories are straight cylindrical paths which offer medullary fixations within the pelvis. Multiplanar CT reformatting, 3D imaging, surgical navigation, and liberal use of fluoroscopy or intraoperative CT are invaluable in facilitating accurate intrapelvic screw placement. Minimal invasive stabilisation of the pelvic ring can be achieved with minimal blood loss and surgical morbidity. Early operative intervention by minimal invasive internal fixation has been shown to reduce pain and enhance patient recovery (Figs. 7.6, 7.7, 7.8 and 7.9).

7.6.2 Anterior Fixation

Fixation of anterior injury can be achieved with plate fixation or intramedullary screw fixation. High superior pubic rami fractures are reliably stabilized with screws. Non-cannulated 4.5 mm screws or preferably larger, cannulated 6.5 mm screws of 90–120 mm long can be placed antergrade or retrograde. The retrograde technique in supine position is preferred. Using a small incision over the parasymphiseal region, a drill bit or guide pin for cannulated screw is placed at the entry point over the pubic tubercle. A small incision may be necessary for minimal invasive reduction of an internally displaced pubic fragment using a pair of curved artery forceps. Passage of the guide pin can then be possible in the pubic canal. Insertion by gentle hammer strikes or manual wiggling provides tactile feedback during advancement compared to using powered instruments. There is less chance of creation of an unintended, extraosseous and potentially dangerous trajectories. Liberal use of fluoroscopy is usually necessary. The Pfannenstiel incision and Stoppa approach is useful for plate fixation of lower superior rami fractures and segmental fractures (Fig. 7.10).

7.6.3 Ilium Fractures

Ilium body fractures are typically displaced and are a common component in FFP III and IV injuries. Open reduction and internal fixation by plating is associated with significant bleeding and surgical morbidity. These fractures may not need anatomical reduction and healing by callus formation is usually rapid. Patients indicated for surgery due to pain and persistent instability are best stabilized by iliac screws inside the iliac crest and the supraacetabular cancellous corridors (Fig. 7.11).

7.6.4 Sacroiliac Joint and Sacral Injuries

S1 and S2 Sacroiliac screws provide stable fixation of the sacroiliac joint and lateral Denis zone 1 (alar) and 2 (transforaminal) fractures. However, partially threaded screw purchase maybe insufficient in the sacral vertebral body. Trans-sacroiliac bar fixation is promoted by Rommens but requires special instrumentation not widely available. Posterior ilium bridge plating requires more extensive dissection and is associated with long-term implant prominence and is indicated in the elderly with highly unstable posterior ring injuries. Minimally invasive iliac screw and rod systems placed to the ilium or using sacral-alar-iliac route are recently favoured less invasive method which have less implant prominences. There is also a developed technique of placing the posterior plate via a minimally invasive approach [13] (Fig. 7.12).

Percutaneous Screw Options for the Pelvis and special views

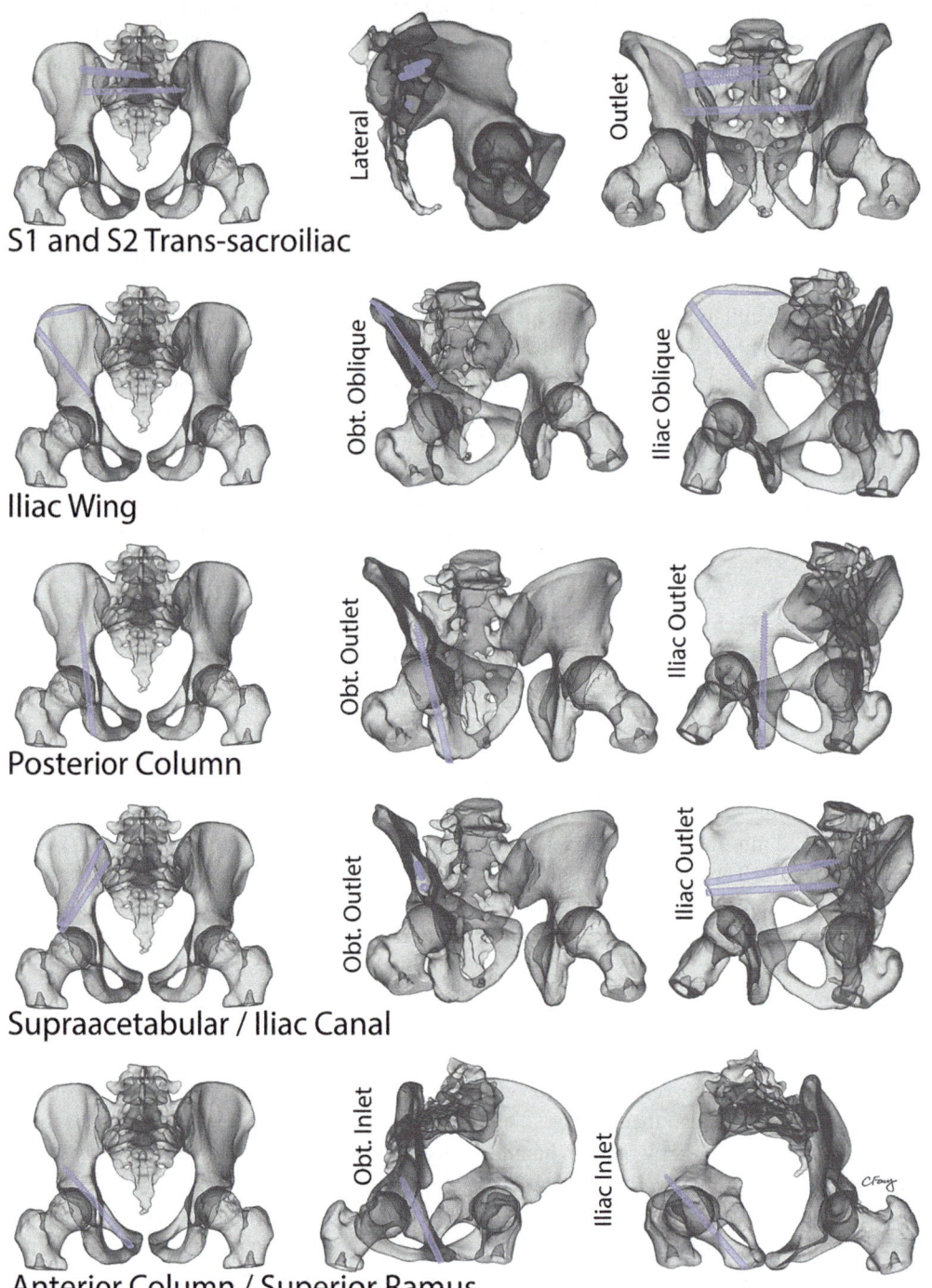

Fig. 7.6 Various paths for percutaneous screws in the pelvis and associated special fluoroscopic views. The prerequisite for choosing minimally invasive fixation is a properly reduced fracture. The name of the screw trajectory is on the left most column. Two supplementary orthogonal fluoroscopic view for the 3D pelvis to best assess the screw trajectory is provided in the two following columns. The prerequisites for a successful minimal invasive screw fixation are minimal displacement of the fractures or successful reduction by closed methods

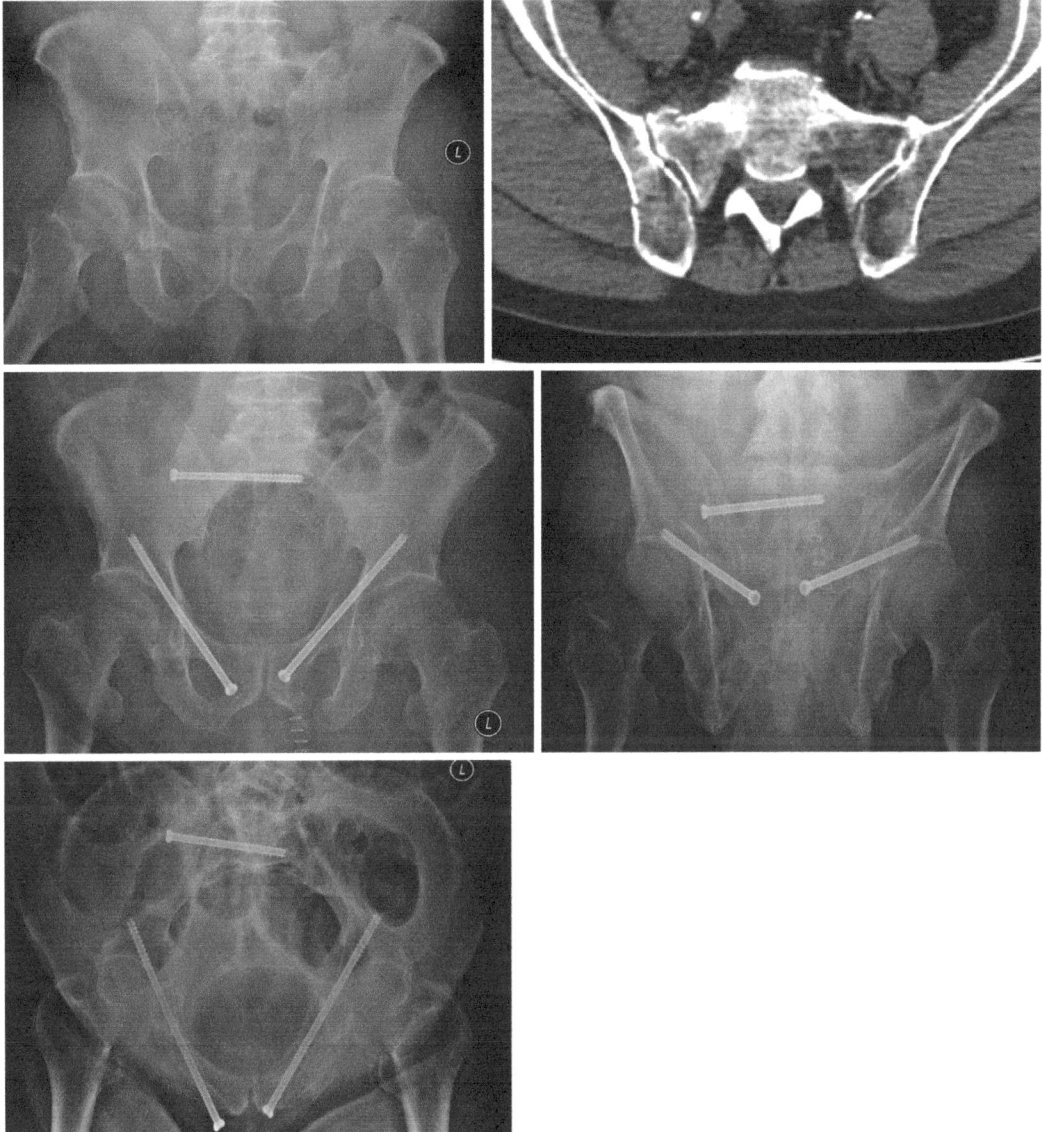

Fig. 7.7 79-year-old male pedestrian involved in a low-speed vehicle crash. The injury is a FFP III pattern. Percutaneous screw internal fixation to both superior rami and right sacroiliac joint was performed to facilitate early mobilization

7.6.5   Internal Fixator (INFIX)

An alternative method of minimal invasive stabilization for the anterior pelvic ring is the INFIX [14]. This involves off labelled use of a spinal pedicle screw and rod system. Long (>60 mm) monoaxial or polyaxial pedicle screws of 5–7 mm dimeters screws are inserted into the supraacetabular corridors at both anterior interior iliac spine.

They are then interconnected with a subcutaneous spinal instrumentation rod to maintain reduction of the anterior pelvic ring. The indication for INFIX is anterior pelvic ring instability in partial and completely unstable patterns (AO/Tiles B/C types). In the elderly, patients with intractable pain hindering mobilization may benefit from this minimal invasive treatment while avoiding formal open reduction and internal fixation or

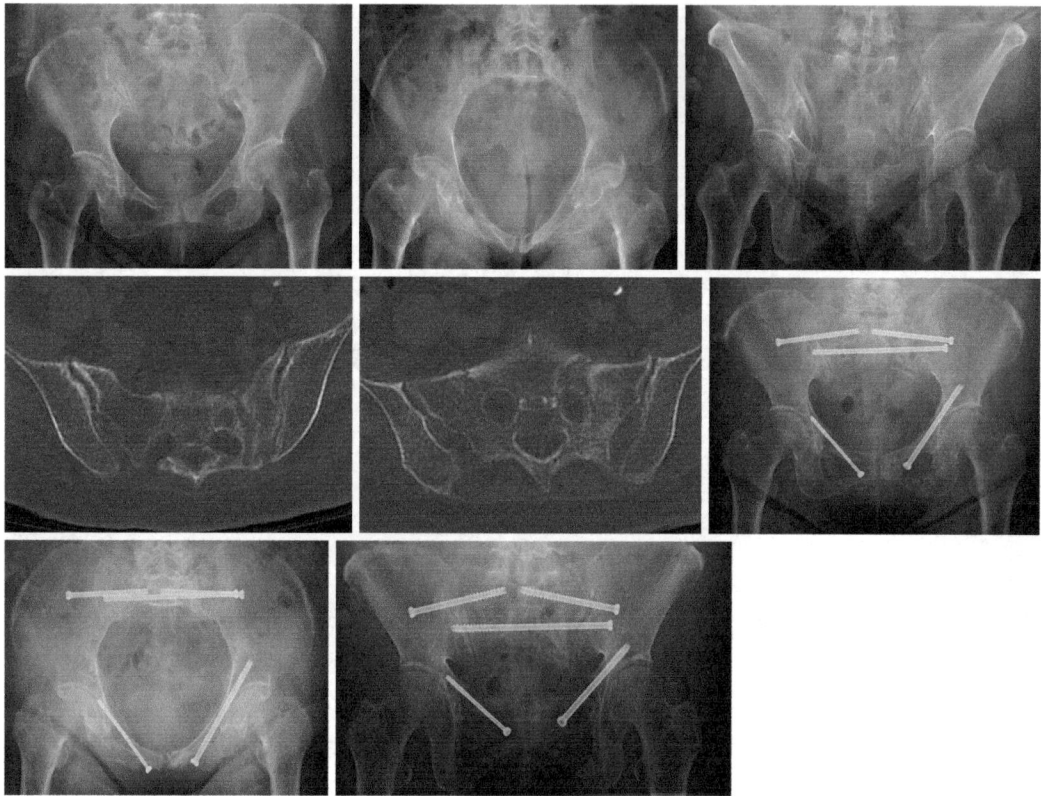

Fig. 7.8 74-year-old female with FFP IV (Bilateral posterior ring sacral alar fractures) and bilateral rami fractures shown in comprehensive preoperative AP, inlet and outlet views. She was treated with retrograde percutaneous screws to both superior rami, and bilateral S1 and S2 sacroiliac screws

external fixation. The proposed benefits are minimal invasiveness, reduced risk of pin tract infections and compatibility with patient mobilization, providing mechanical strength comparable to a two-rod anterior external fixator construct. The patient can be turned prone for other essential surgical procedures with the INFIX.

The most common adverse effects include lateral femoral cutaneous nerve injuries (up to 47%) [15]. Open identification of the nerve is recommended to prevent such injuries. To avoid compression to the femoral neurovascular structures under the interconnecting rod, the supraacetabular screws must stay 2 cm proud at the insertion site. The rod is contoured to overly in the inguinal sub-

cutaneous tissue, superficial to the deep fascia and cranial to the distal rectus abdominis muscle insertion. Some studies also recommend a routine postoperatively duplex ultrasound scan to ensure patency of the femoral vessels during hip flexion. In patients with posterior pelvic ring instability, addition posterior ring fixation is necessary as the INFIX cannot provide sufficient mechanical strength and partial implant loosening is common. In most patients, the INFIX will require implant removal due to hardware impingement and this can be performed 3 months after the initial injury. When considering the use of the INFIX, its benefits should be weighed against potential risks (Fig. 7.13).

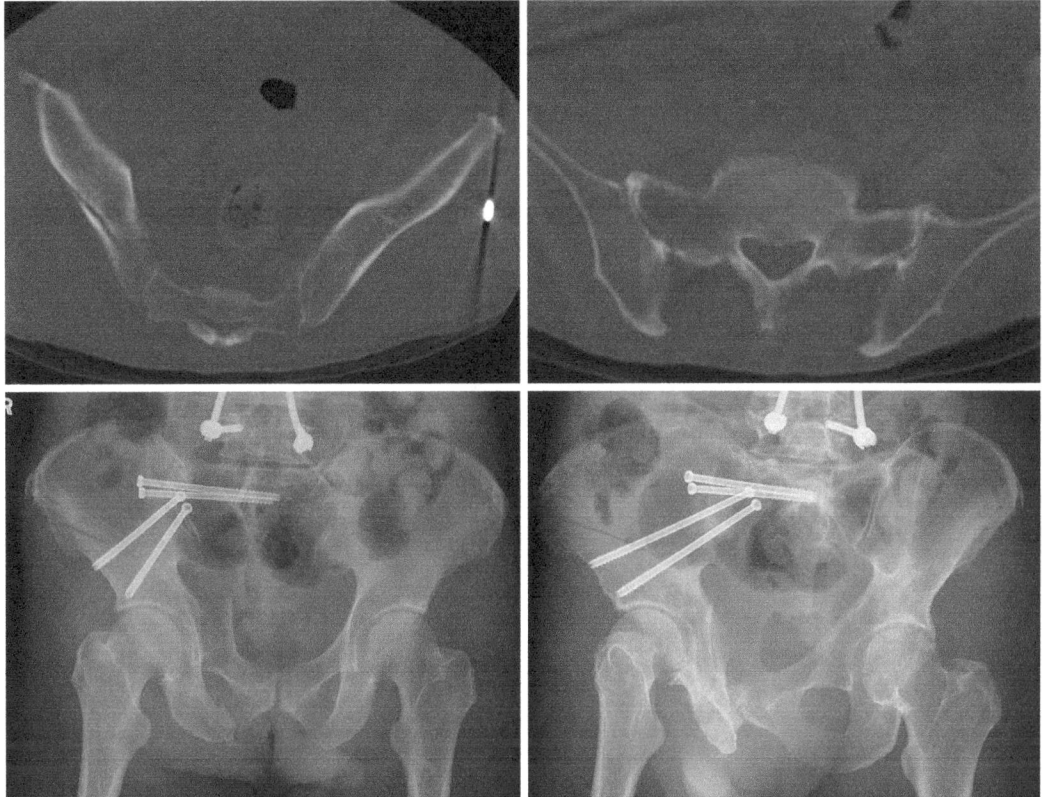

Fig. 7.9 Patient with FFP III pattern. The right iliac wing and sacral alar fractures are minimally displaced and readily stabilized by supraacetabular column and sacroiliac screws. The screws are inserted antegrade percutaneously in prone position as the patient also had a concomitant spinal burst fracture requiring instrumentation

7.6.6 Cement Sacroplasty

Poly Methyl Methacrylate (PMMA) cement sacroplasty is an emerging minimal invasive treatment for patients with unstable sacral alar/sacral insufficiency fractures with mechanical instability and pain persisting beyond 3 weeks after injury. Typically, up to 6 ml of high viscosity cement is injected under CT guidance carefully avoiding nearby nerve root irritation.

With cement interlocking the fracture zone, micromotion and mechanical pain can be significantly reduced. Studies have reported satisfactory pain control with low rate of complications [16]. Similarly, cement augmentation of sacroiliac screw can significantly increase mechanical strength in patients with severe osteopenia [17]. Sacroplasty may be useful in patients with highly unstable spinopelvic dissociations.

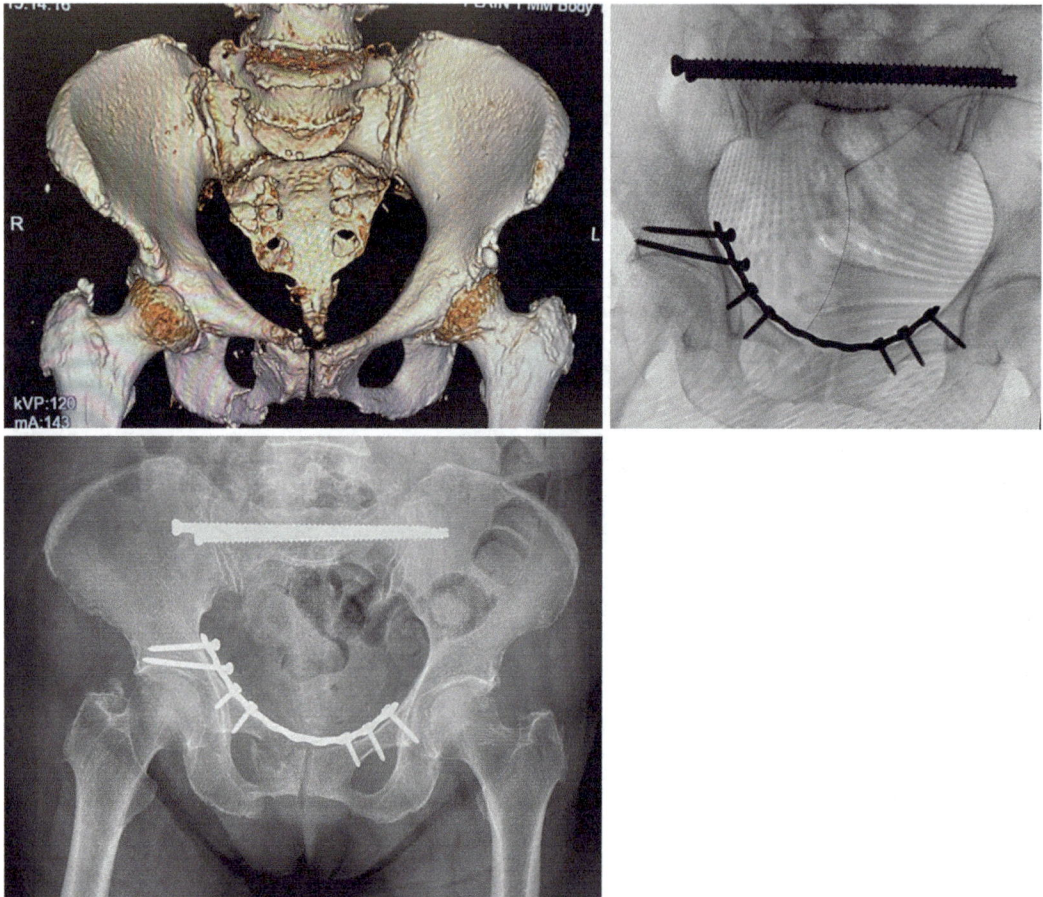

Fig. 7.10 An FFP type IV fracture was highly unstable. The anterior injury was fixed with a contoured pelvic plate through a modified Stoppa approach. The posterior injury was then fixed with two large percutaneously inserted trans-sacroiliac cannulated screws

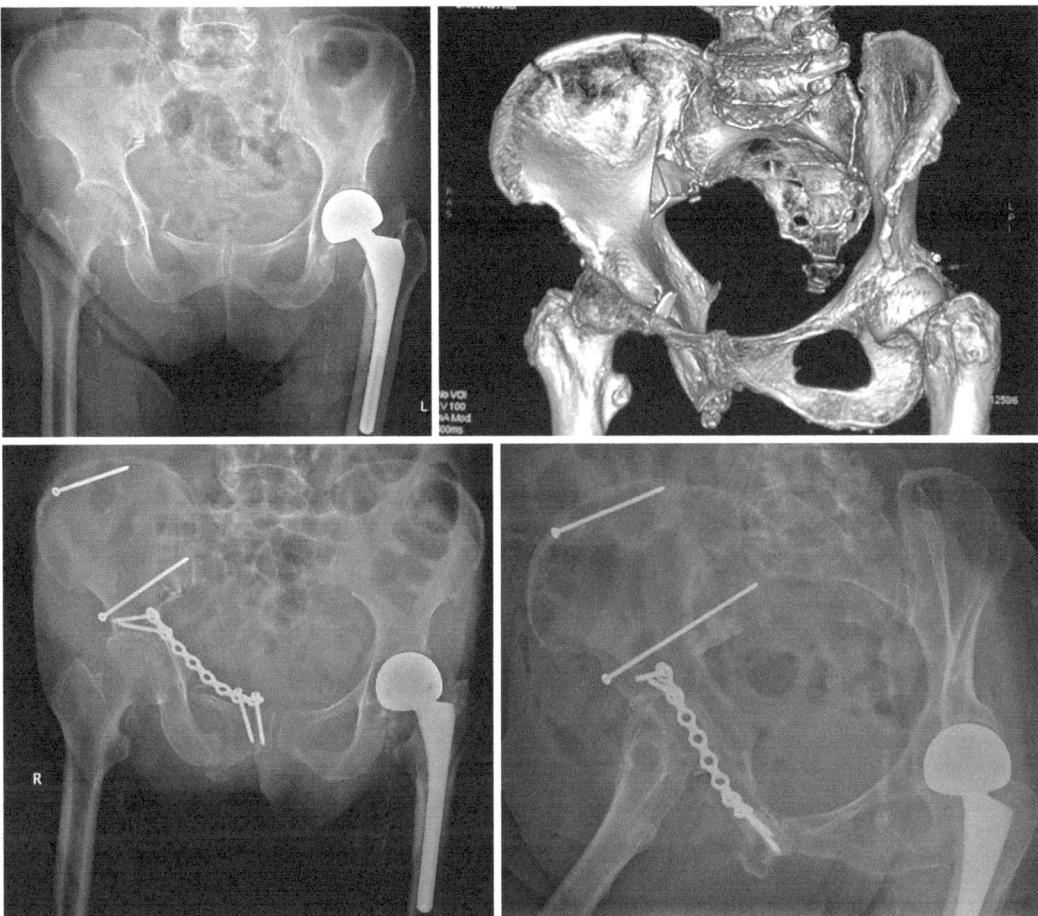

Fig. 7.11 An 87-year-old lady presented with fractures on right ilium and right pubic rami (type IIIa). As there was severe pain from fracture instability, surgery was performed. The ilium was stabilized with an iliac crest screw and a supra-acetabular screw from anterior to posterior. Plate fixation via a modified Stoppa approach was performed for the anterior injury

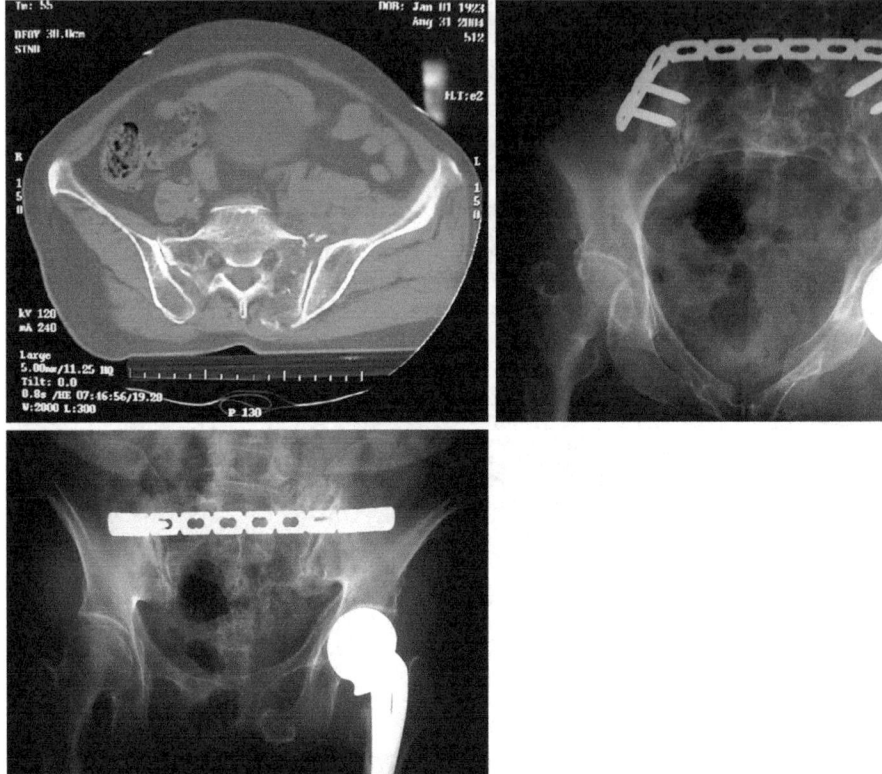

Fig. 7.12 An 83-year-old patient with a type IIIc fracture. In view of her advanced osteoporosis, a more stable fixation with posterior bridge plating was chosen. This was performed in a minimally invasive manner with the patient in prone position. An 4.5/5 mm locked compression plate was manually bent and angular stable screws were inserted through the ilium into the lateral mass of the sacrum. The patient was mobilized with weight bearing

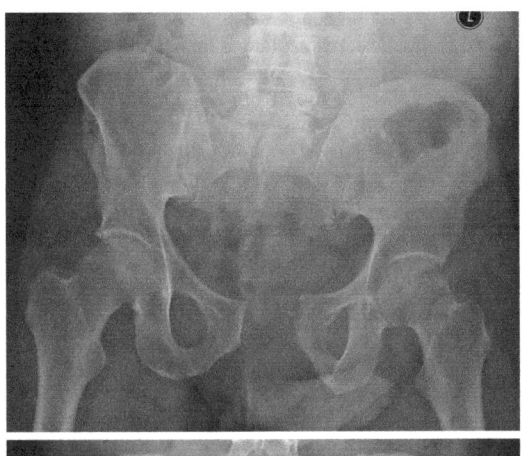
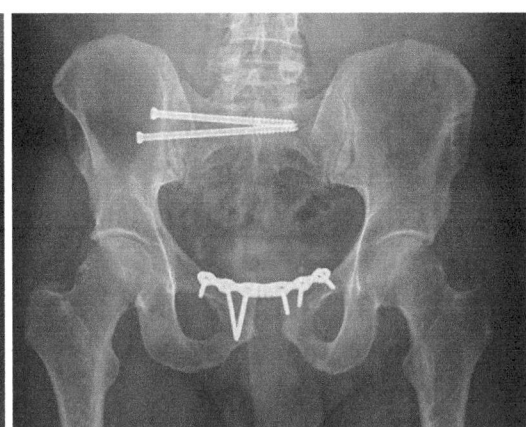
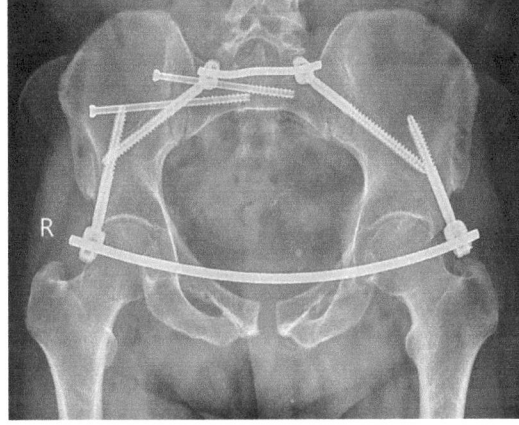

Fig. 7.13 A patient with FFP IV/Tiles type C anterior and posterior pelvic ring injury who developed intraabdominal sepsis followed by infection and loosening of the primary fixation. To avoid contamination of the surgical site, the INFIX was used re-stabilize the anterior pelvic ring while an interconnected S2AI screw is used to supplement the posterior ring. The patient is allowed to mobilize immediately following fixation

7.7 Conclusion

FFPs are a commonly encountered type of fragility fracture. The understanding of the pathoanatomy helps identifying subgroups of patients with instability who may suffer from prolonged pain and significant functional compromise. The primary management of these patients is nonoperative treatment and adequate pain control. Subgroups of patients with more severe injuries can be treated with minimally invasive fixation and mobilized safely with significantly less pain. Management of osteoporosis also plays in critical role in the prevention of secondary fractures.

References

1. Andrich S, Haastert B, Neuhaus E, Neidert K, Arend W, Ohmann C, et al. Epidemiology of pelvic fractures in Germany: considerably high incidence rates among older people. PLoS One. 2015;10(9):e0139078.
2. Loggers SAI, Joosse P, Jan PK. Outcome of pubic rami fractures with or without concomitant involvement of the posterior ring in elderly patients. Eur J Trauma Emerg Surg. 2019;45(6):1021–9.
3. Lau TW, Leung F. Occult posterior pelvic ring fractures in elderly patients with osteoporotic pubic rami fractures. J Orthop Surg (Hong Kong). 2010;18(2):153–7.
4. Rommens PM, Hofmann A. Comprehensive classification of fragility fractures of the pelvic ring: recommendations for surgical treatment. Injury. 2013;44(12):1733–44.

5. Scheyerer MJ, Osterhoff G, Wehrle S, Wanner GA, Simmen HP, Werner CM. Detection of posterior pelvic injuries in fractures of the pubic rami. Injury. 2012;43(8):1326–9.

6. Soles GL, Ferguson TA. Fragility fractures of the pelvis. Curr Rev Musculoskelet Med. 2012;5(3):222–8.

7. O'Connor TJ, Cole PA. Pelvic insufficiency fractures. Geriatr Orthop Surg Rehabil. 2014;5(4):178–90.

8. Steinitz D, Guy P, Passariello A, Reindl R, Harvey EJ. All superior pubic ramus fractures are not created equal. Can J Surg. 2004;47(6):422–5.

9. Young JW, Burgess AR, Brumback RJ, Poka A. Pelvic fractures: value of plain radiography in early assessment and management. Radiology. 1986;160(2):445–51.

10. Tile M, Helfet DL, Kellam JF, Vrahas M. Fractures of the pelvis and acetabulum. Baltimore: Williams & Wilkins; 1995.

11. Rommens PM. Paradigm shift in geriatric fracture treatment. Eur J Trauma Emerg Surg. 2019;45(2):181–9.

12. Avilucea FR, Archdeacon MT, Collinge CA, Sciadini M, Sagi HC, Mir HR. Fixation strategy using sequential intraoperative examination under anesthesia for unstable lateral compression pelvic ring injuries reliably predicts union with minimal displacement. J Bone Joint Surg Am. 2018;100(17):1503–8.

13. Schmerwitz IU, Jungebluth P, Lehmann W, Hockertz TJ. Minimally invasive posterior locked compression plate osteosynthesis shows excellent results in elderly patients with fragility fractures of the pelvis. Eur J Trauma Emerg Surg. 2021;47(1):37–45.

14. Chaus GW, Weaver MJ. Anterior subcutaneous internal fixation of the pelvis: placement of the INFIX. Oper Tech Orthop. 2015;25(4):262–9.

15. Fang C, Alabdulrahman H, Pape HC. Complications after percutaneous internal fixator for anterior pelvic ring injuries. Int Orthop. 2017;41(9):1785–90.

16. Mahmood B, Pasternack J, Razi A, Saleh A. Safety and efficacy of percutaneous sacroplasty for treatment of sacral insufficiency fractures: a systematic review. J Spine Surg. 2019;5(3):365–71.

17. Collinge CA, Crist BD. Combined percutaneous iliosacral screw fixation with sacroplasty using resorbable calcium phosphate cement for osteoporotic pelvic fractures requiring surgery. J Orthop Trauma. 2016;30(6):e217–22.

Management of Femoral Neck and Per-Trochanteric Fractures Including New Technology

8

Dennis King Hang Yee

8.1 Introduction

Neck of femur fracture and trochanteric fractures are the most frequent and typical major injuries in fragility fracture patients. The goal of treatment is to allow early mobilization and weight bearing as tolerated to reduce the risk of complications associated with immobility. Most elderly hip fracture patients are not able to comply with partial or non- weight bearing walking.

8.2 Classification and Decision Making

8.2.1 Neck of Femur Fracture

The intracapsular portion of the femoral neck has no periosteum. Hence, fractures need to heal by endosteal healing [1]. Neck of femur fractures were traditionally classified by Garden classification (Fig. 8.1), Type I and II are nondisplaced or minimal displaced fractures and type III and IV are displaced fractures [2]. A truly nondisplaced or valgus impacted fracture could be treated with internal fixation. Displaced frac-

tures should be treated with arthroplasty, as internal fixation leads to a high risk of reoperation (approximately 23%) and lower health-related quality of life [3, 4].

A major limitation of the Garden classification system is that it solely relies on the AP radiograph. This is important as impacted fracture with retroversion (apex anterior or posterior tilt) >20° on lateral view had been correlated with a higher risk of fixation failure [5–7]. However, despite its limitations, Garden classification is still the most widely used system for describing femoral neck fractures [8].

Pauwel proposed a biomechanical classification, grouping fractures based on the inclination of the fracture line with reference to the horizon [9] (Fig. 8.2). A higher Pauwel type denotes increasing angle of inclination and the force transitions from being compressive to shearing [10]. However, its clinical usage is limited by difficulties in accurate assessment of fracture line inclination in preoperative radiographs [11], and changes in appearance of the fracture line inclination based on rotation of the leg [2].

8.2.2 Trochanteric Fracture

The gluteal musculature abducts the proximal main fragment after trochanteric fracture, pulling the fracture into varus deformity. If the lesser tro-

D. K. H. Yee (✉)
Department of Orthopaedics and Traumatology,
Queen Mary Hospital, The University of Hong Kong,
Pokfulam, Hong Kong
e-mail: yeedns@ortho.hku.hk

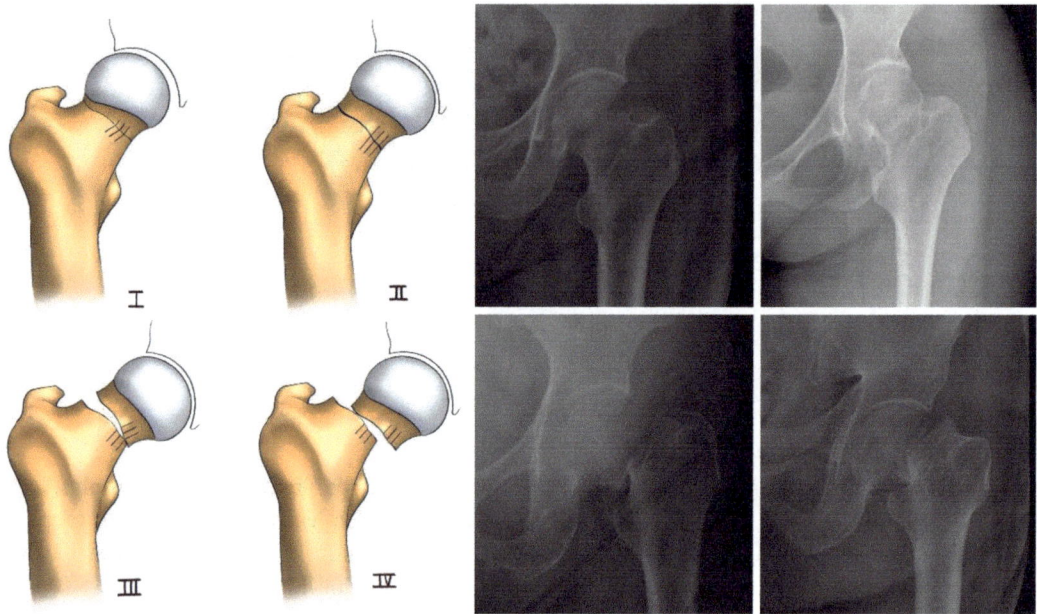

Fig. 8.1 Diagrams and corresponding radiographs of Garden classifications I–IV

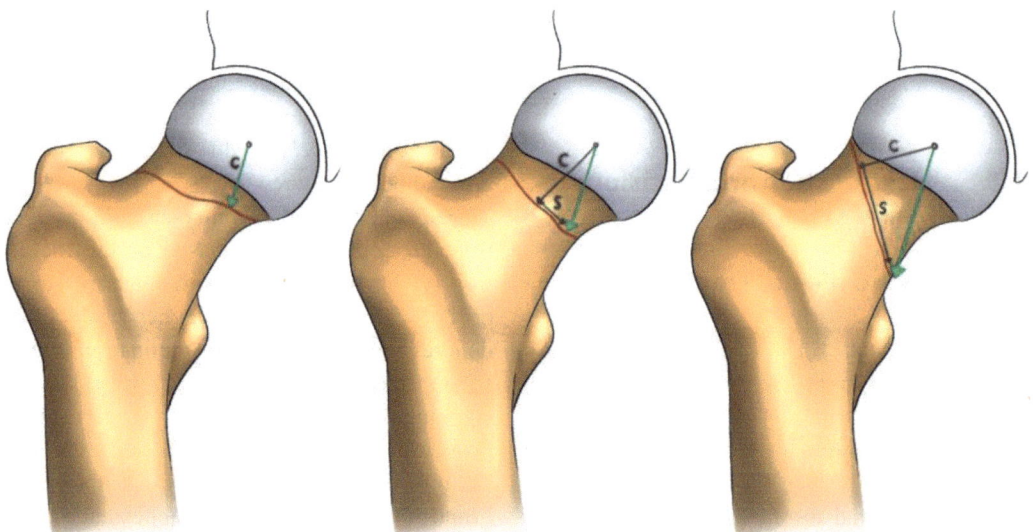

Fig. 8.2 Pauwel's classification Type I, II, and III. The inclination of the fracture line from the horizontal line determines the ratio between compressive and shearing forces. C: compression force across the fracture. S: shear force across the fracture. Type 1, up to 30°; Type 2, 30–50°; Type 3, more than 50°

chanter (iliopsoas) is connected to the head–neck fragment, flexion and external rotation of the fragment results. The shaft is usually adducted and external rotated because of the adductor and hamstring muscles pull [1]. On a traction table, gravity may cause posterior translation of the distal main fragment.

Classification and choice of implants are based on the stability of the fracture. Unstable fractures are characterised by the presence of

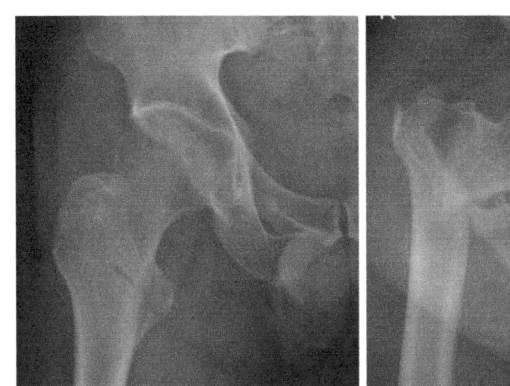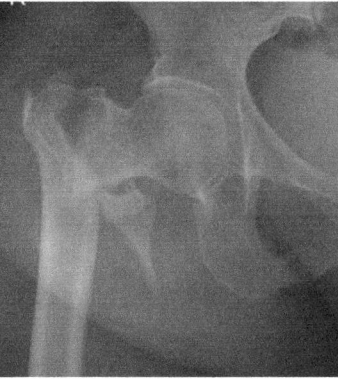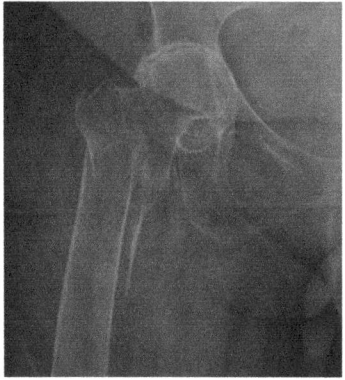

Fig. 8.3 Examples of AO/OTA classification of proximal femur fractures A1, A2, and A3 (right to left)

significant posteromedial fragments, reverse obliquity patterns, or subtrochanteric extension.

The AO/OTA Fracture and Dislocation Classification is recommended for trochanteric and subtrochanteric fractures [12] (Fig. 8.3). Intertrochanteric fractures are classified as extracapsular fractures of the proximal femur region.

A1. A1 fractures are simple two fragment fractures with the fracture line running through the greater trochanter. Closed reduction is routinely achieved on traction table with traction and internal rotation.

A2. Fractures with incompetent lateral wall (≤20.5 mm) or large lesser trochanteric fragments remain unstable after reduction and are classified as A2 fractures. These fractures tend towards more varus displacement. The medial column may collapse and the lesser trochanter may be pulled by the iliopsoas, causing it to migrate proximally. A2 fractures are considered unstable and the use of cephalomedullary nail is generally recommended for fixation [13].

A3. Fractures with lateral starting points beneath the greater trochanter, and a main fracture line running between the greater and lesser trochanter in a horizontal and reversed fashion are classified as A3.

8.3 Management of Undisplaced/Impacted Neck of Femur Fracture

8.3.1 Reduction Versus In Situ Fixation

Previous studies showed that femoral neck shortening is associated with worse hip function [14], the role of reduction prior to fixation of valgus impacted neck of femur fracture has been called into question. Mahajan described a technique with trans-fixation wire that stabilizes the head so that the distal fragment can be easily and gently manipulated in a controlled manner [15]. A similar technique was introduced by Noda et al. specifically for valgus impacted neck of femur fracture, using a trans-acetabular pin [16]. However, clinical outcomes including patient reported outcome score, incidence of non-union or avascular necrosis were not reported by the authors.

Yamamoto studied the outcomes of closed reduction of retroversion in patients with preoperative posterior tilt of ≥20° [17]. Defining sufficient close reduction as posterior tilt ≤5°, they found that secondary operation rate was lower in the sufficient reduction group (5/34 cases) than in the insufficient reduction group (3/6 cases) (Odds ratio = 5.8).

Author's preference: The author does not advocate intraoperative reduction manoeuvres

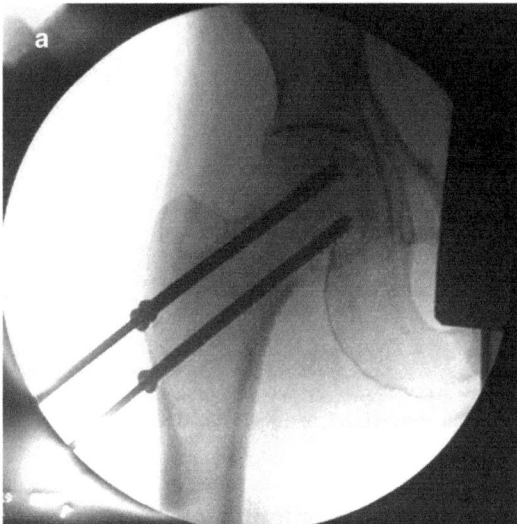
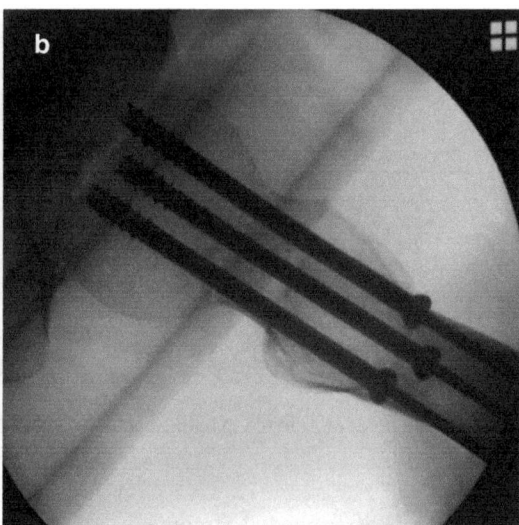
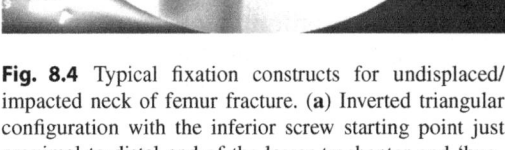

Fig. 8.4 Typical fixation constructs for undisplaced/impacted neck of femur fracture. (**a**) Inverted triangular configuration with the inferior screw starting point just proximal to distal end of the lesser trochanter and 'hugging' the medial femoral neck cortex. The superior screws are maximally spaced to increase the construct stiffness. (**b**) The posterior screw supports the posterior femoral neck cortex to resist retroversion deformity

due to the lack of high-quality supporting evidence. Intraoperative screening with the patient on the traction table is important especially in the detection of excessive retroversion. If retroversion is more than 20°, conversion to hemiarthroplasty is recommended.

8.3.2 Cannulated Screw Fixation Constructs

There is no consensus on the optimal device for fixation of intracapsular fractures in osteoporotic patients. In a biomechanical study, dynamic hip screw plus anti-rotation screw constructs were shown to have comparable axial stiffness to three cannulated screw fixation. However, the former were superior in terms of cycles until 15 mm leg shortening, and also cycles until 15 mm femoral neck shortening [18], albeit such benefits are not demonstrated in clinical studies. A meta-analysis on internal fixation implants for intracapsular proximal femoral fractures in adults revealed no major differences between implants in patient survival or complications [19]. Fracture fixation in the operative management of hip fractures (FAITH) showed similar reoperation rate within 24 months between those treated with sliding hip screw and cancellous screws [20]. However, avascular necrosis was more prevalent in the sliding hip screw group.

In an evaluation of mechanical outcomes comparing different configurations of cannulated compression screws for fixation of Pauwels type III femoral neck fracture, inverted triangular configurations showed the best mechanical advantage, while being less likely to cutout [21].

The starting point on the lateral diaphyseal cortex for the inferior screw should be just above the inferior border of the lesser trochanter. This decreases the possibility of iatrogenic subtrochanteric fracture due to stress riser effect and achieves a high screw placement angle.

Screws should be spaced out maximally to increase construct stiffness [22].

1. The inferior screw should be placed close to the medial cortical bone of the femoral neck to resist inferior displacement of the femoral head (Fig. 8.4). The screw has two supporting points (inferior femoral neck cortex and lateral diaphyseal cortex), preventing cantilever failure of the construct (Figs. 8.5 and 8.6).

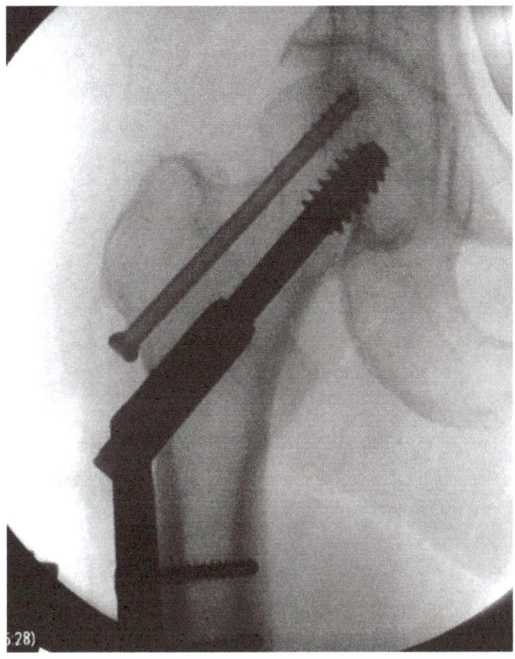

Fig. 8.5 Pauwel 3 fractures are fixed with dynamic hip screw plus anti-rotation screw. Anti-rotation guide pins should be used. The femoral head screw should be over-turned then back to correct the rotational displacement created by the strong torque exerted during screw insertion

2. The posterior superior screw should be placed close to the posterior cortex of the femoral neck to minimize retroversion of the femoral head (Figs. 8.4 and 8.6).

Increased resistance when advancing the 2.8 mm or 3.2 mm guide wire across the femoral neck should alert the surgeon of the possibility of an "in-out-in" screw. Hoffmann et al. placed the posterior and cranial screw of the inverted triangle configuration under fluoroscopy guidance using standard technique in ten cadavers. A 70% incidence of cortical breach for cranial posterior screw was noted despite appearing radiographically contained [23] (Fig. 8.7).

The anterior cortex is typically non-comminuted as it is at the tension side of the fracture. The author prefers to use partially threaded screws, tightening the anterior superior screw first to prevent increase of the deformity.

The ideal fixation method should also minimise femoral neck shortening. Weil et al. found

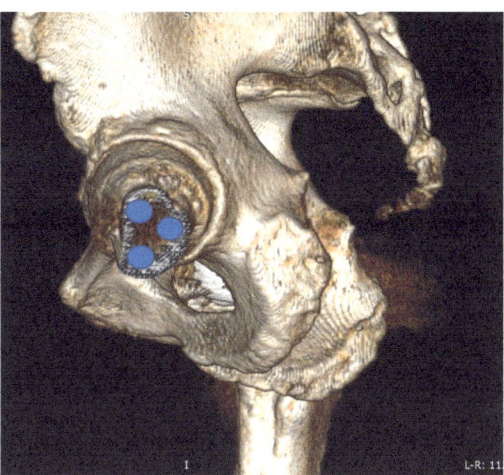

Fig. 8.6 Cross sectional cut over femoral neck is shown. Screws should be spaced out in an inverted triangle configuration

femoral neck shortening occurred in 56% of their patients, with severe shortening in 22% of patients. While femoral neck shortening did not significantly correlate with fracture type, quality of reduction, age, or neck shaft angle, there was a negative correlation between patient self-reported outcome score (SF-12) results and overall femoral neck shortening [14].

Author's preference: Dynamic hip screw plus anti-rotation screw are used for Pauwel 3 fractures in order to counteract the strong shearing force (Fig. 8.5). Three cannulated screws construct is used for Pauwel 1 and 2 neck of femur fractures (Fig. 8.4a, b).

8.3.3 Femoral Neck System

The femoral neck system (DePuy Synthes, Zuchwil, Switzerland) is a minimally invasive implant that combines the advantages of angular stability of the dynamic hip screw with the minimal invasive surgical technique of cannulated screws. Biomechanical testing showed superior mean axial stiffness compared with DHS-screw and DHS-blade [18].

Insertion of the femoral neck system implant does not require "screwing in" the bolt, which eliminates the risk of fracture rotation (Fig. 8.8).

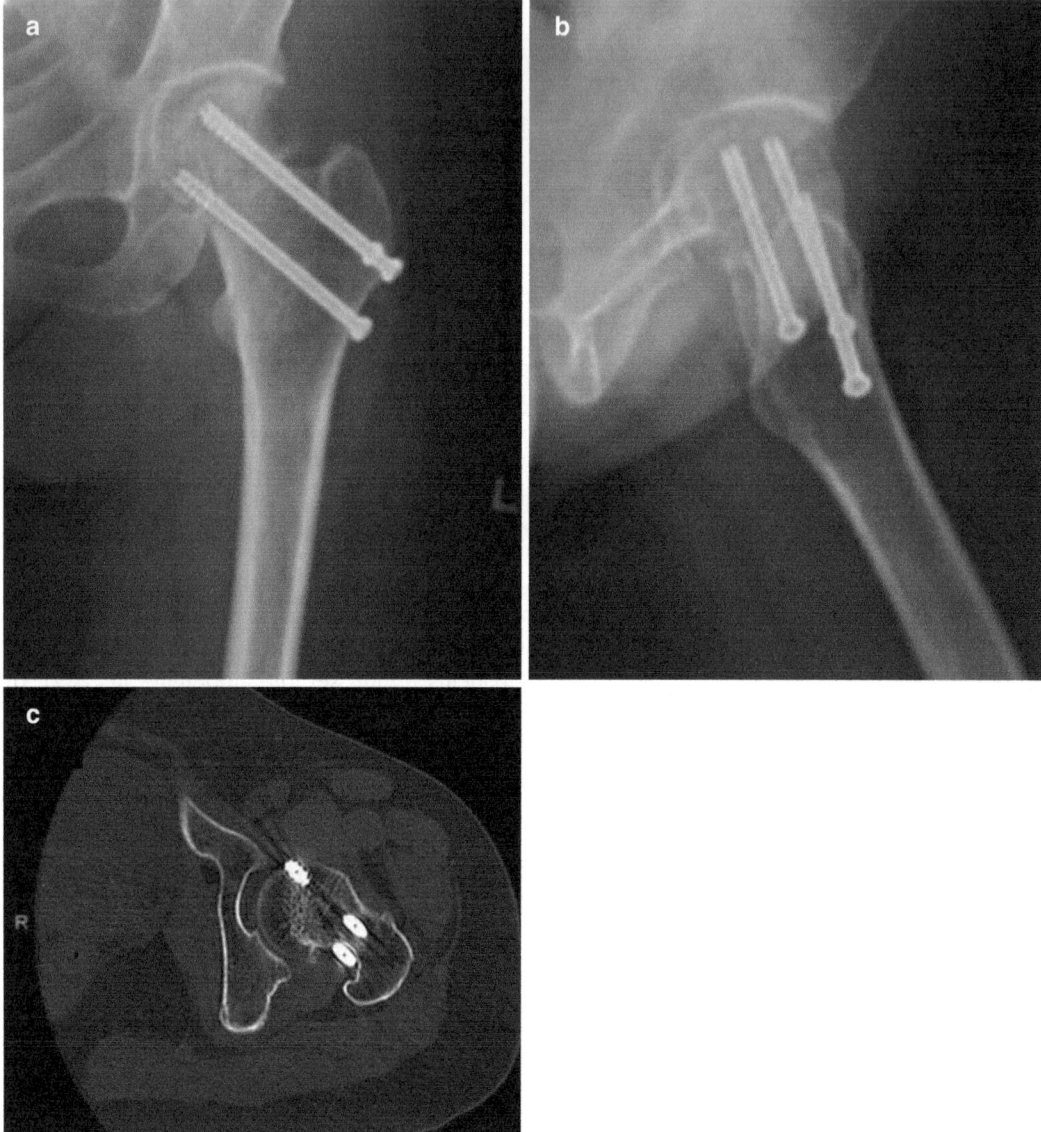

Fig. 8.7 (**a** and **b**) Three cannulated screws inserted in inverted triangular configuration for valgus impacted neck of femur fracture. No apparent cortical breach noted on AP and lateral radiograph. (**c**) Computed tomography scan of the same patient showed posterior superior screw violated posterior femoral neck cortex, and anterior superior screw was too long with risk of acetabular cartilage erosion

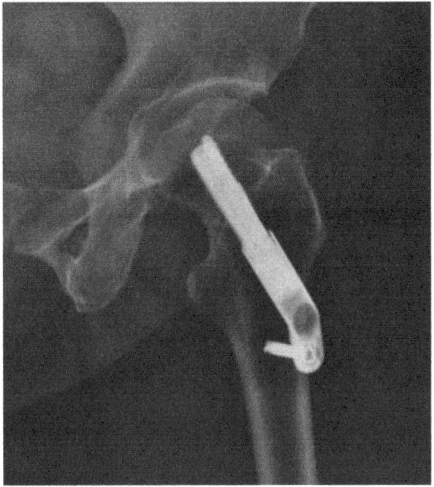

Fig. 8.8 Femoral neck system for valgus impacted neck of femur fracture. It is important to position the locking screw at the centre of the bone. The distal locking screw should be inserted after insertion of the bolt but before the anti-rotation screw, allowing rotation of the plate to ensure proper positioning of the distal locking screw

8.4 Management of Displaced Neck of Femur Fracture

Displaced femoral neck fractures in geriatric patients are best treated by arthroplasty, as internal fixation has a high reoperation rate for nonunion, malunion, shortening, and avascular necrosis [3, 4, 24].

8.4.1 Approach

Surgical approaches for hemiarthroplasty/total hip arthroplasty can be divided into three categories: posterior approaches, lateral approaches, and anterior approaches [25–27].

A meta-analysis involving all studies on hemiarthroplasty for neck of femur fracture which compared outcomes by approach [27] found that a posterior approach was associated with a higher risk of dislocation when compare with lateral approaches (OR = 2.90; 95%CI: 1.63 to 5.14; $P < 0.0003$) or anterior approaches (OR = 2.61; 95%CI: 1.26 to 5.43; $P < 0.01$).

8.4.2 Total Hip Replacement Vs. Hemiarthroplasty

The Hip Fracture Evaluation with Alternatives of Total Hip Arthroplasty versus Hemi-Arthroplasty (HEALTH) trial [28] compared both methods in a randomized controlled trial involving 1495 patients older than 50 years old who had a displaced neck of femur fracture. After randomizing patients to receive either hemiarthroplasty or total hip arthroplasty, they found no statistically significant difference between the two groups with regard to secondary hip procedure within 24 months of follow-up. Furthermore, total hip arthroplasty provided clinically unimportant improvements over hemiarthroplasty in function and quality of life over 24 months.

Two other randomized controlled trials comparing hemiarthroplasty and total hip replacement with modern implants have reported long term data (7–12 years) [29, 30]. Tol et al. [29] demonstrated that there was no difference in functional outcomes at 12 years post-operatively. Avery et al. [30] showed there was a lower mortality and a trend towards superior function in patients with total hip replacement. However, three hips had dislocated in the total hip replacement group versus none in the hemiarthroplasty group.

The National Institute for Health and Care Excellence (NICE) guidelines recommend total hip replacement for displaced neck of femur fracture in those who can ambulate outdoors with the use of no more than a stick, are not cognitively impaired, and are medically fit for anaesthesia [31].

8.4.3 Cemented Vs. Cementless Prosthesis

Tanzer et al. [32] compared the best three cemented and the best three cementless femoral stems using data from the Australian Orthopaedic Association National Joint Replacement Registry. Cementless femoral stem fixation was associated with a higher early rate of revision in patients older than 75 years; however, there was no difference between the two groups after 3 months.

Veldman et al. [33] conducted a systematic review and meta-analysis of current generation hip stems comparing cementless and cemented hemiarthroplasty for displaced neck of femur fracture, including 950 patients over a total of five randomized controlled trials. They found that although operating times were significantly shorter for cementless stems, such implants were associated with more complications versus cemented stems; especially implant-related complications such as periprosthetic fractures, aseptic loosening, and dislocation.

It is known that cardiorespiratory and hemodynamic reactions secondary to cement implantation syndrome may occur during cementation, and in some patients this can be fatal [34]. Meta-analysis of large, national registries studied the risk of death within 48 h of hip hemiarthroplasty between patients treated with cemented and cementless implants. Compared with the cementless group, mortality was increased in the cemented group. For every 183 patients treated

with a cemented implant, one death would be expected compared with the cementless [34].

In conclusion, cemented hemiarthroplasty was associated with an increased risk of perioperative death compared with cementless fixation. However, there was an increased risk of other complications and revision surgeries associated with cementless fixation for geriatric neck of femur fracture population. The surgeon needs to consider both the risk of perioperative death and the potential of longer-term complications.

8.5 Management of Trochanteric Fracture

8.5.1 Cephalomedullary Nail Versus Extramedullary Fixation

Several comparative studies compare outcome parametes of intramedullary fixation versus extramedullary fixation.

In a study utilizing postoperative day 1 serum creatinine phosphokinase levels as a biochemical marker to assess muscle damage and inflammation, dynamic hip screws were found to result in greater soft tissue damage compared with fractures stabilized by proximal femoral nail [34]. However, Saudan et al. reported no differences in complications, rate of reoperations, and mobility score between patients treated with either technique in AO/OTA 31-A1 and A2 pertrochanteric fractures [35].

Leung et al. noted similar postoperative mobility and hip function when comparing Gamma nails with dynamic hip screws for pertrochanteric fracture [36]. This finding was also concurred by Radford et al., with a lower rate of wound complications in nail group. However, a high incidence of femoral shaft peri-implant fracture was noted in the Gamma nail group [37].

In further literature, it has been proposed to use dynamic hip screw only in stable fractures (AO/OTA 31-A1 to A2.1). Cephalomedullary nails should be the preferred treatment option for other more unstable fractures [1, 38].

8.5.2 Long Nail Versus Short Nail

In a prospective randomized controlled trial comparing short and long cephalomedullary nails for pertrochanteric hip fractures with up to 3 cm of subtrochanteric fracture line extension, patients treated with short nails had significantly shorter operative times and lower estimated blood loss. Functional outcomes and rates of peri-implant fracture and lag screw cut-out were comparable between the two groups [39].

8.5.3 Tip Apex Distance

To calculate tip apex distance, the distance between the tip of the femoral neck screw and the subchondral border of the femoral head is measured in AP and lateral view and summated (Fig. 8.9). For patients treated with dynamic hip screw, studies have shown that tip apex distance below 25 mm results in significantly less screw cut-out [40].

The value of tip-apex distance has been questioned for constructs fixed with cephalomedullary nails. A cadaveric study showed positioning of lag screw inferior in the head and neck was at least as biomechanically stable as centre–centre positioning, even for larger tip-apex distances (>25 mm) [41]. For clinical studies, Caruso reported one of the largest cohorts ($n = 571$) in which tip-apex distance was found to be a highly significant predictor of screw cut-out with cut-offs of 30.7 mm [42]. A significantly higher risk of screw cut-out was correlated with lag-screw positioning in the upper part of the femoral head in the anteroposterior radiological view, posterior in the latero-lateral radiological view, and in the Cleveland peripheral zones [42].

Cephalomedullary nails with helical blade likely behave differently compared with cephalomedullary nails with lag screw. Cut-out risk has been reported to be bimodally distributed for such devices, with increased risk in tip-apex distance of less than 20 mm or more than 30 mm [43].

8.5.4 Operative Techniques in Cephalomedullary Nail

8.5.4.1 Positioning

The patient is placed supine on a traction table with C-arm on opposite side of the table. The

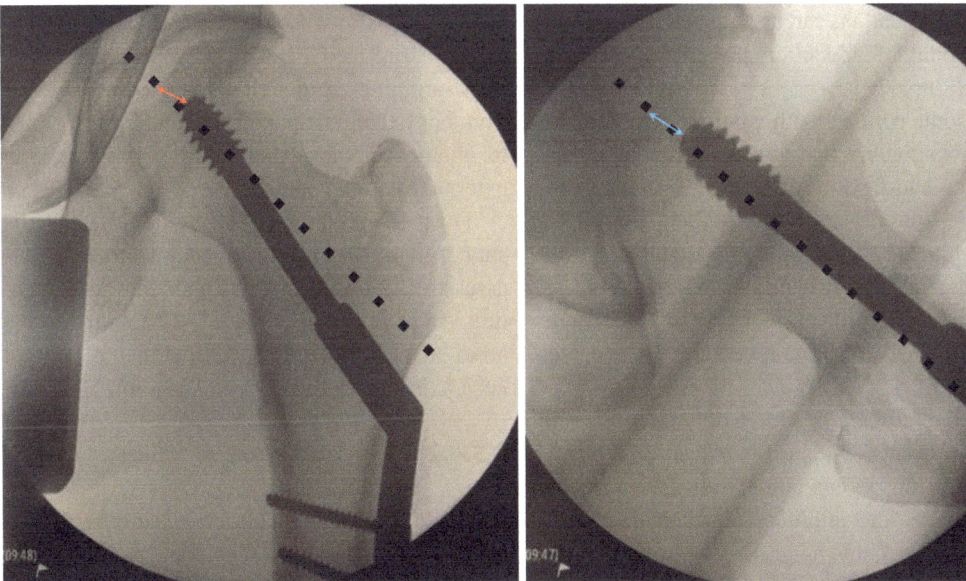

Fig. 8.9 Calculation of the Tip Apex Distance. Red arrow: Xap. Blue arrow: Xlat. Tip Apex Distance = Xap + Xlat

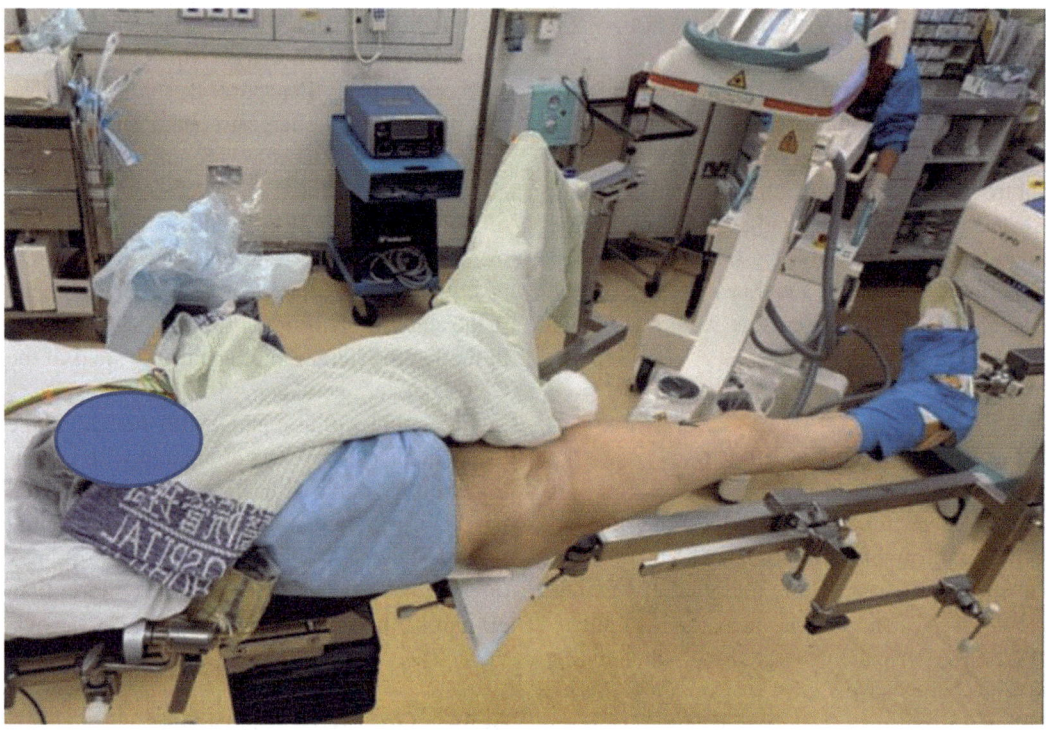

Fig. 8.10 Traction table and hemilithotomy position of the patient

contralateral leg is held in abducted, flexed, externally rotated position (hemilithotomy position) to allow good access for the C-arm to obtain AP and lateral image (Fig. 8.10). The tension of the adductor tendons can be palpated to gauge the safe amount of abduction possible in patients with stiff hip.

For some patients with significant hip arthrosis and contracture that does not allow adequate abduction and flexion for C-arm passage, extension of the contralateral hip and flexion of the injured hip can be attempted for quality intraoperative lateral images, using a small rolled towel bump under the ipsilateral torso to roll the patient away from the surgeon about 15 degrees (Fig. 8.11).

The injured side is addicted to facilitate nail insertion. A lateral support is placed on the ipsilateral rib to prevent lateral translation of the body towards the injured side when traction is applied, which could neutralize the hip adduction necessary for nail entry (Fig. 8.11).

Some surgeons also choose to position patients laterally to assist with fracture reduction [44].

It is important to be able to obtain good X-rays in orthogonal planes. A straight vertical C-arm gives a true AP view of the hip only when the hip is internal rotated 10–15°, hence the position of the C-arm must be individualized to the hip position. For example, the C-arm should roll forward to obtain AP view when the hip is reduced in external rotation position.

The true lateral view of the femur in which the shaft is in line with the head–neck segment allows assessment of the sagittal alignment of the fracture. The C-arm should be at 45° relative to the torso so that it is perpendicular to the femoral neck axis and "parallel" with hip joint.

8.5.4.2 Reduction and Entry Site Preparation

In patients with unstable fracture patterns, the use of a traction table may accentuate sagittal plane deformity, namely, posterior translation of distal

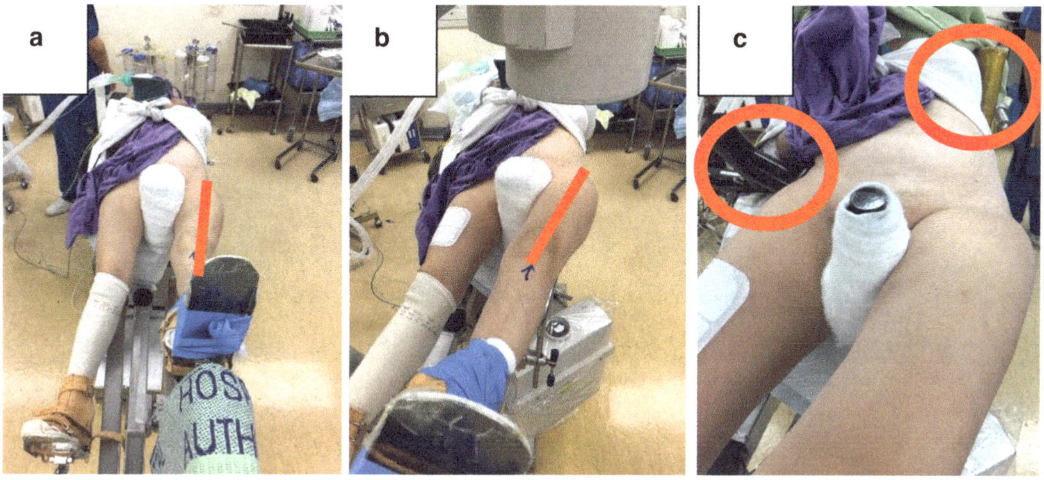

Fig. 8.11 Patient positioning on the traction table. (**a, b**) Adduction of injured hip allows passage of cephalomedullary nail. (**c**) Lateral support put at ipsilateral rib counteracts the lateral translation force on the torso when the injured limb is under traction. Coupled with contralateral pelvic support, this maintains the adduction posture of the injured hip

segment and apex posterior angulation [45]. In such cases, thigh support can be added to the traction table to elevate the distal fragment (Fig. 8.12).

In patients with fracture patterns that failed closed reduction, percutaneous reduction techniques represent the first step of escalation. Percutaneously inserted curved artery forceps placed anteriorly over the proximal fragment can correct head–neck fragment flexion and maintain it during reaming (Fig. 8.13). Most of the time this can be performed through the anticipated blade insertion wound.

8.5.4.3 Reaming

Almost all current cephalomedullary nails accommodate for trochanteric entry site by having a proximal lateral bend [1]. The recommended nail entry point is the tip of the greater trochanter or just medial to it on anteroposterior fluoroscopy [46]. An over lateral starting point leads to varus malreduction. In patients with fracture line involving the tip of the greater trochanter, the thin bone bridge lateral to the tip may break during reaming, resulting in lateralization of the nail entry [47]. Special care must be taken

during reaming to ensure a channel is reamed through the bone instead of simply displacing the fracture. This can be achieved by applying firm pressure on the greater trochanter during reaming with a mallet [48]. The reamer needs to be pushed medially during reaming to ensure adequate medial reaming of the relatively hard bone at the base of the neck. Otherwise, it may result in medialization and varus displacement of the proximal head fragment (Fig. 8.14). A slightly medial entry point could also help to minimise these problems.

Reaming of the femoral canal is usually not necessary except in patients who cannot accept the nail with the smallest diameter. Forceful entry may result in iatrogenic femur fracture. Cephalomedullary nails should be inserted with manual force only. Anterior endosteal impingement should be suspected in difficult nail insertion situation.

The lateral end of the blade should be outside the lateral cortex to avoid blockage of the gliding mechanism [49] (Fig. 8.15).

Before distal static locking bolt is inserted, traction should be released to eliminate any existing fracture gaps.

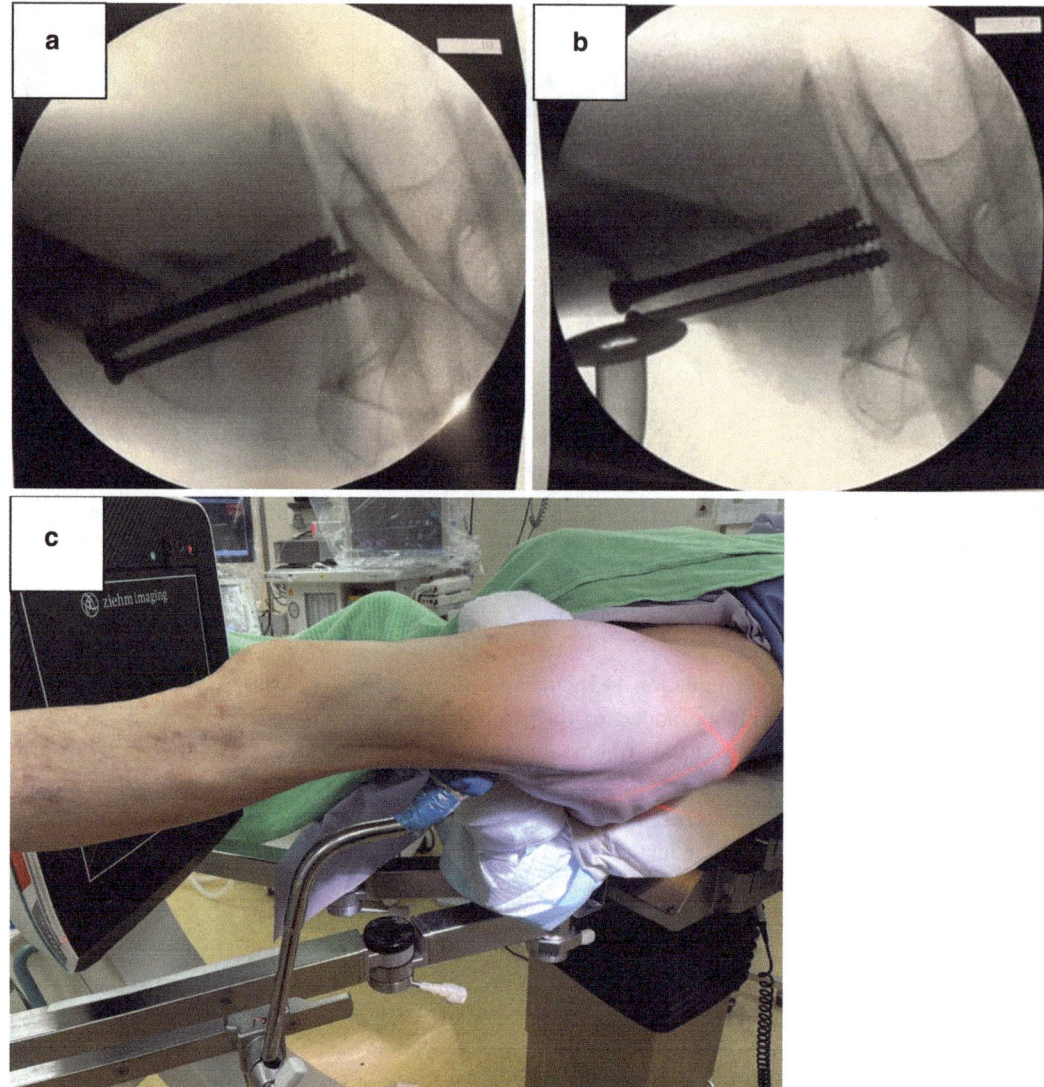

Fig. 8.12 (a–c) Patient with peri-implant fracture after previous cannulated screw fixation for neck of femur fracture. Posterior sagging of the femur shaft was noted after the patient was put on the traction table. Posterior thigh support was added to translate the femoral shaft anteriorly. Image intensifier confirmed restoration of the anterior cortex line

8.5.4.4 Tips: Rotational Alignment in Intertrochanteric Fracture

The typical rotational deformity in intertrochanteric fracture is internal rotation of the proximal fragment and external rotation of the distal fragment due to the pull of the iliopsoas (Remarks: iliopsoas act as an external rotator of the distal fragment in intertrochanteric fracture, but in intact bone it is an internal rotator).

Both AP and lateral view can help the surgeon to assess the rotational profile intraoperatively (Fig. 8.16a, b). The amount of internal rotation can differ in each case depending on the fracture pattern. Less commonly, when iliopsoas insertion

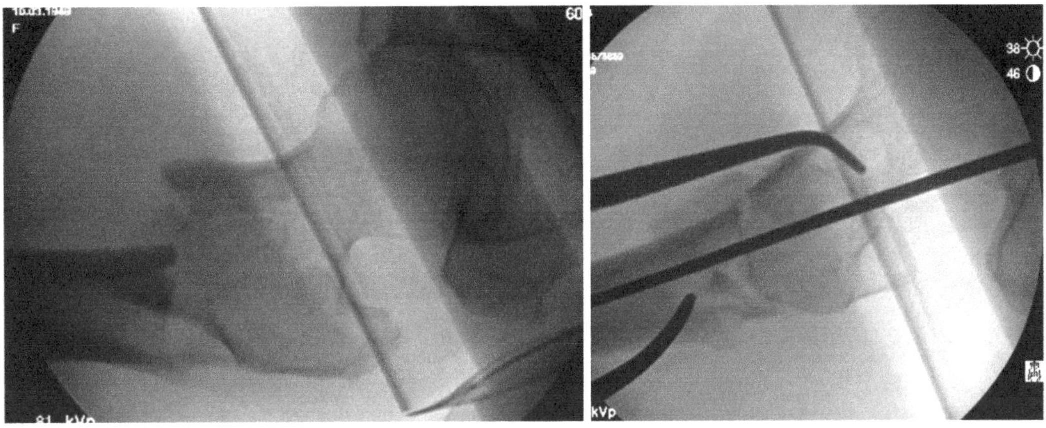

Fig. 8.13 Intraoperative C arm image of a patient with A3 TOF. Percutaneous long artery forceps were introduced from the lateral wound, which would be used for blade entry, to correct the flexion deformity. Another pair of artery forceps was introduced distally to correct the posterior sagging of the femoral shaft

is attached to the proximal fragment, external rotation of the distal fragment may be required for reduction (Fig. 8.17).

8.5.5   Cement Augmentation

Hip fractures have devastating health impacts on the elderly. Failed fixation leads to poor functional outcomes and high mortality rates [50–52] and can still occur even if immediate postoperative radiographs satisfy traditional criterion.

PMMA-augmented implants have been shown to produce higher failure loads and reduced cutout events for conventional hip screws and sliding hip screws [53, 54]. Biomechanical studies comparing cement augmentation and blade fixation in the cephalomedullary device demonstrated improved rotational stability, pull-out and cut-out resistance for cement-augmented Proximal Femoral Nail-Antirotation (PFNA, Depuy Synthes, Paoli, PA) in foam models and human cadaveric bones [54–56]. A randomized controlled study on cement augmentation in PFNA showed six patients were complicated by mechanical failure in the non-augmented group, versus none in the augmented group. However, this result was unable to reach statistical significance [57]. In a retrospective cohort involving 110 patients with TFN-Advanced Proximal Femoral Nailing System (TFNA, DePuy Synthes, Paoli, PA), 63 patients had cement augmentation and 47 patients did not have cement augmentation. There was a significantly lower rate of fixation failure in the group with cement augmentation [58] (Fig. 8.18).

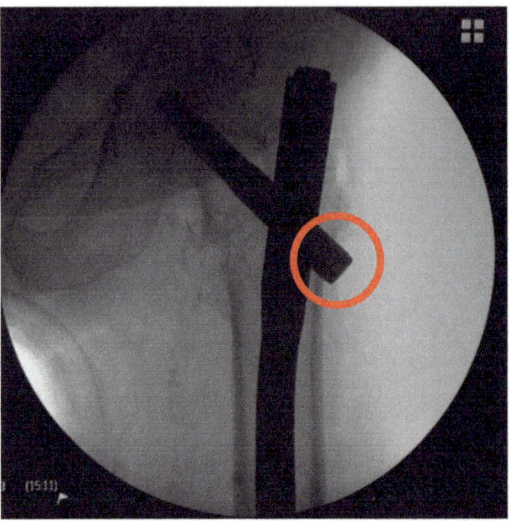

Fig. 8.15 The lateral end of the blade must be outside the cortex to avoid blockage of the gliding hole

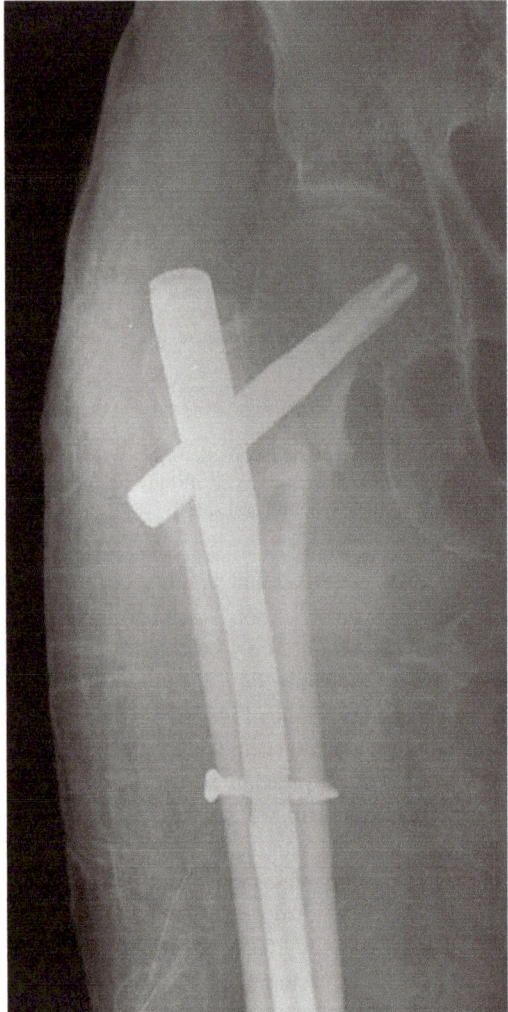

Fig. 8.14 Medial translation of the head–neck fragment was evident on this postoperative X-ray. The likely reason is inadequate entry site bone preparation due to reamer entry through the fracture site displacing the fracture

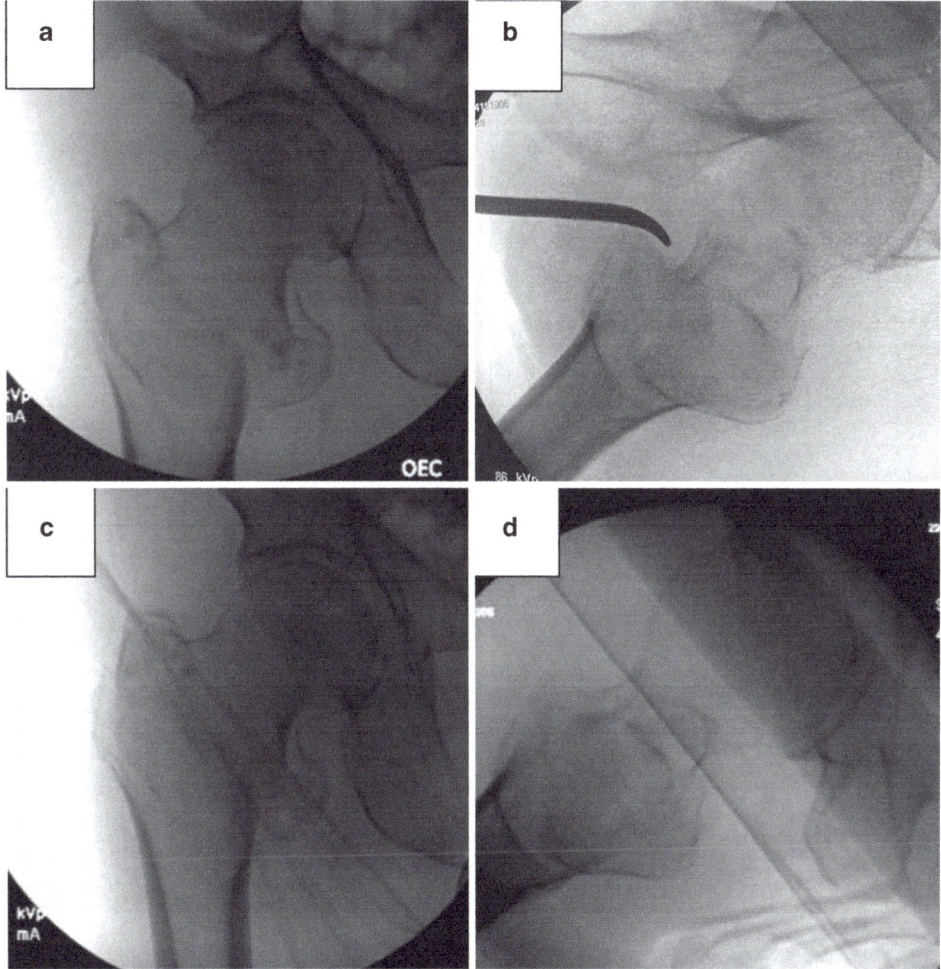

Fig. 8.16 (**a** and **b**) Alignment of medial cortex on AP view and anterior cortex on lateral view indicates correct rotational profile

Fig. 8.17 (**a**) Part of the lesser trochanter (iliopsoas) is attached with the proximal fragment. In this patient, when the distal fragment was in internal rotation, there was a rotational mismatch as evidenced by the disruption of the medial cortex line. (**b**) Lateral view of the same patient showed anterior cortex line disruption (**c**) External rotation of the distal fragment restores medial cortex line. (**d**) Lateral view shows anterior cortex line restored with external rotation of the distal fragment

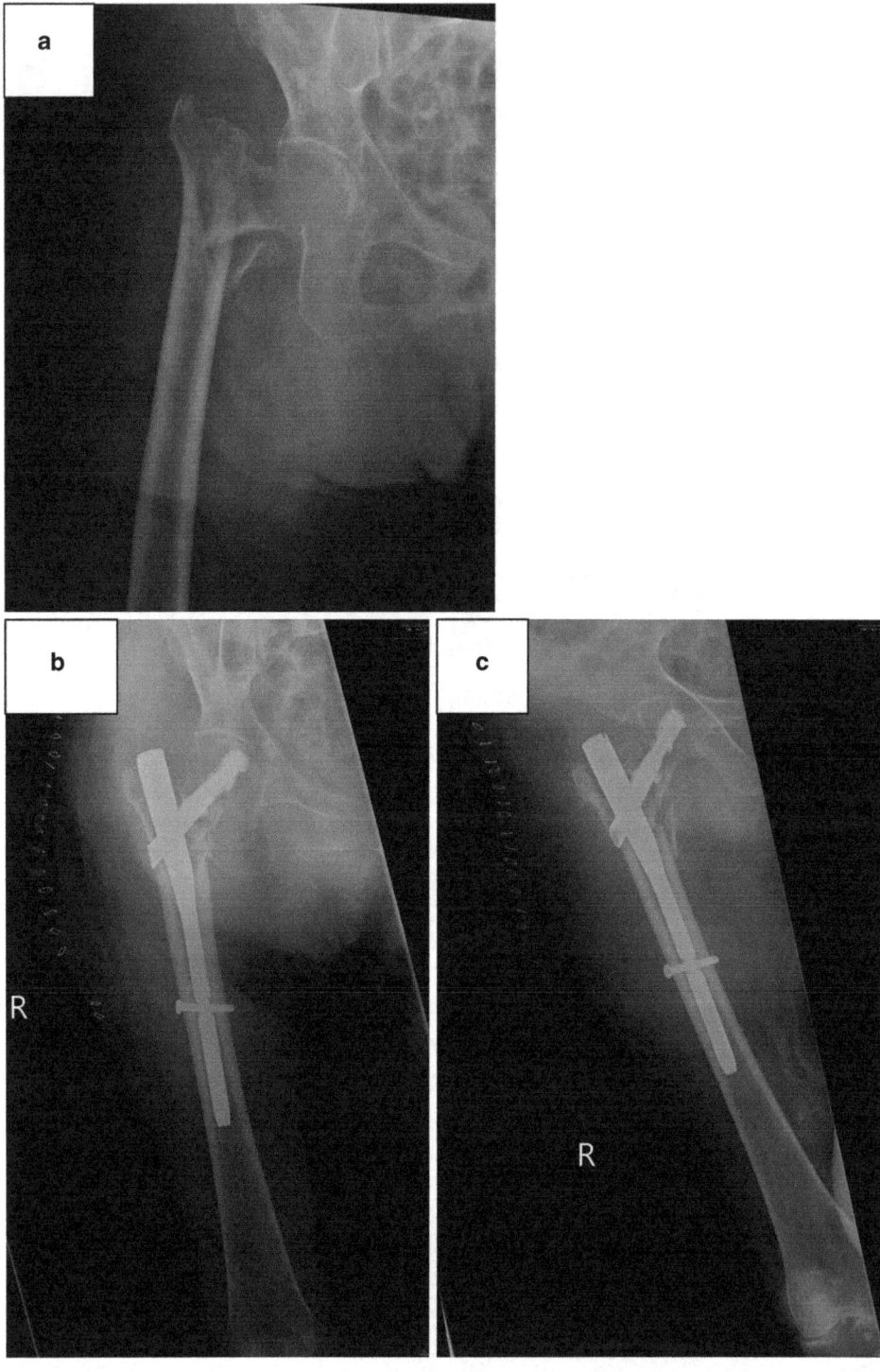

Fig. 8.18 A 96-year-old patient fell 3 months ago with intertrochanteric fracture. She was advised conservative treatment in another hospital due to her age and comorbidities and became bedbound since the injury. She presented 3 months later with persistent hip pain and decided for surgical fixation. (**a**) X-ray showing subacute intertrochanteric fracture with varus deformity and shortening. (**b**, **c**) Open reduction and fixation with TFNA and cement augmentation. The fracture healed at 6 months

8.6 Specific Complications

8.6.1 Cut-Out/Cut-Through

Cut-out is defined as perforation of the femoral neck screw/blade through the femoral head with varus or rotational collapse of the head–neck fragment. Cut-through is defined as medial perforation of the blade through the femoral head without loss of reduction of the head–neck fragment [59] (Fig. 8.19).

Cut-through is a unique complication of blade devices. Three mechanisms had been proposed: jamming of the sliding mechanism, sharp end of the blade allowing cutting into the femoral head, and Z-effect. Z-effect describes the central migration of neck–head device in relation to the nail during loading [60].

Good fracture reduction and implant placement are important to prevent cut-out/cut-through complications [60]. The quality of reduction can be judged by criteria set by

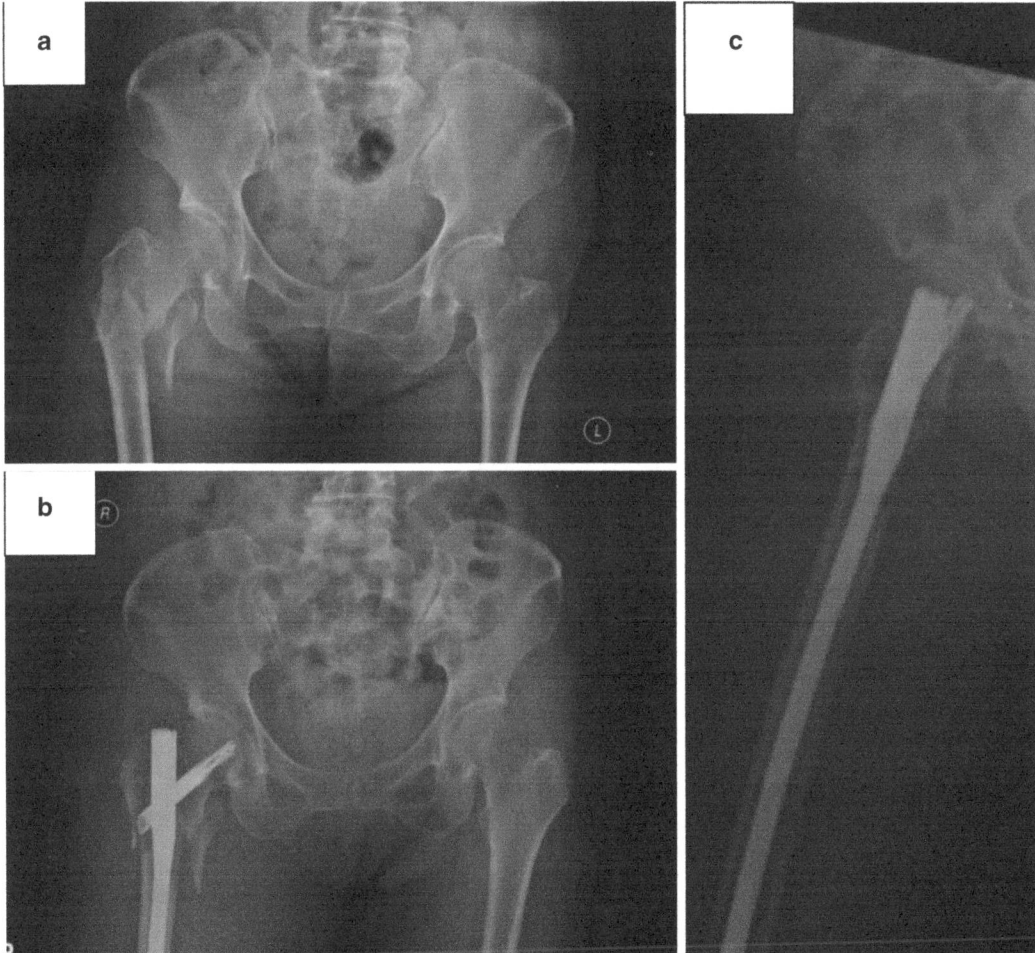

Fig. 8.19 TFNA blade cut-through and revised with cemented TFNA. (**a**) A3 TOF fracture in an 86-year-old gentleman after fall injury. (**b**) AP view of postoperative radiograph showing fracture fixation with long TFNA with satisfactory reduction and implant position. (**c**) Lateral view of postoperative radiograph. (**d**) AP view X-ray at 2 months postop showed blade cut-through. (**e**) Lateral X-ray at 2 months. (**f**) Sagittal cut computed tomography showed rotation of the fracture around the blade. (**g**) Revision fixation with cemented TFNA. The blade was positioned in the anterior femoral head to avoid the old track. X-ray taken at 5 months postop showed fracture union. (**h**) Lateral radiograph at 5 months

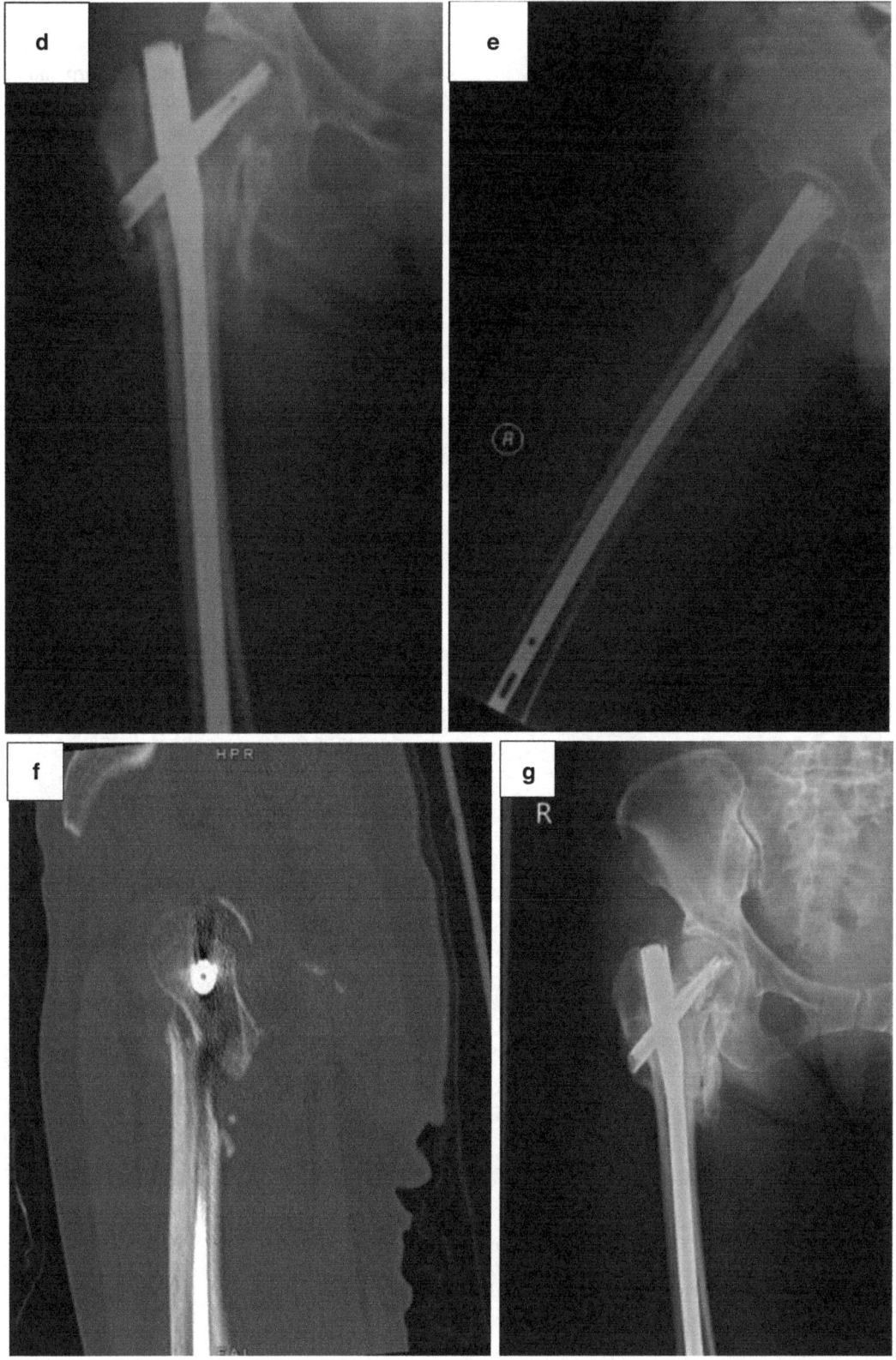

Fig. 8.19 (continued)

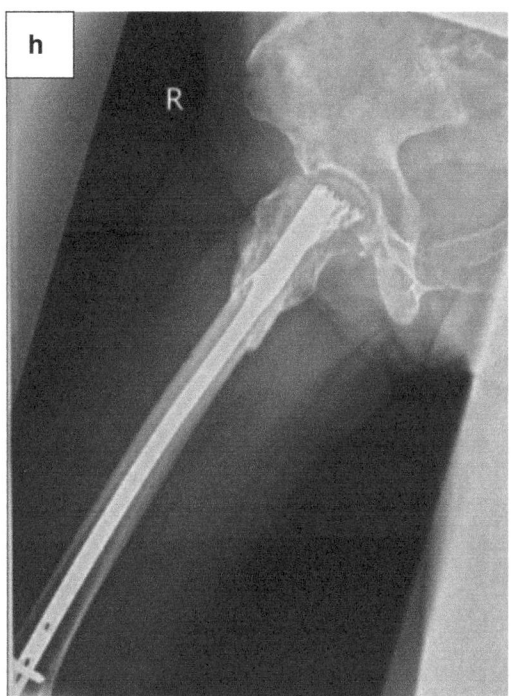

Fig. 8.19 (continued)

Baumgaertner [61]. Good reduction is defined as a normal or slight valgus alignment on the anteroposterior radiograph with less than 20 degrees of angulation on the lateral radiograph, and no more than 4 mm of displacement of any fragment. For a reduction to be considered acceptable, it has to meet the criteria of a good reduction with respect to either angulation or displacement, but not both. A poor reduction meets neither criteria .

8.6.2 Cephalomedullary Nail Infection

The incidence of infection in intertrochanteric fracture treated with cephalomedullary nailing is around 1.1–3.2% [62]. The general principles of fracture-related infection apply, which entails early operative debridement with antimicrobial therapy and retention of implant until fracture union in early infection [63]. In severely compromised host or fulminant infection (especially with infection in intramedullary canal), removal of the cephalomedullary nail for thorough debridement and insertion of antibiotic loaded cement spacer is. Deep infection can have delayed presentations (Fig. 8.20).

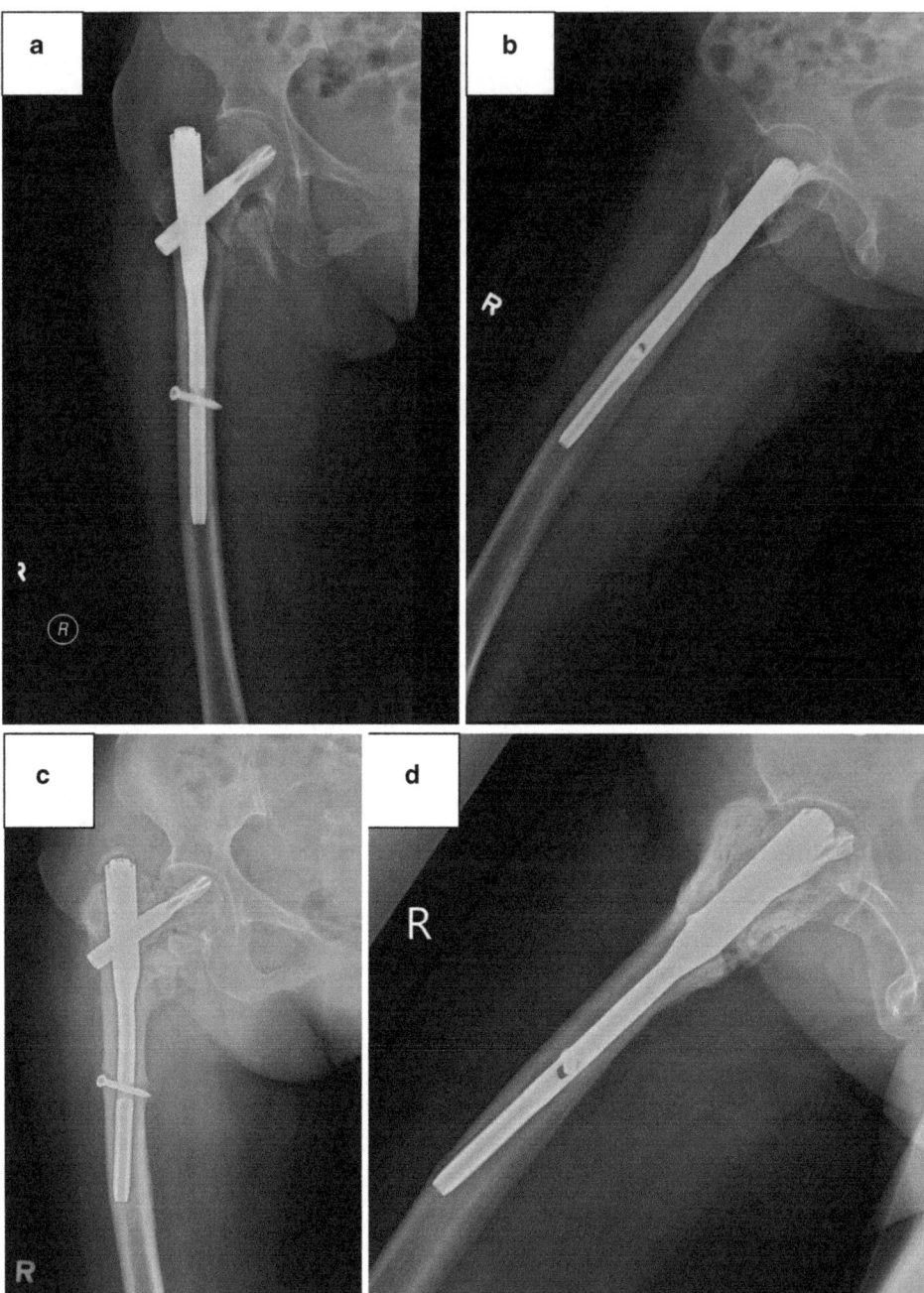

Fig. 8.20 Deep infection following cephalomedullary nail fixation of trochanteric fracture. (**a**, **b**) Postoperative X-ray showing satisfactory reduction and implant position. (**c**, **d**) X-ray taken 1.5 years postop showing hypertrophic non-union with migration of blade position within the femoral head, halo around the distal locking bolt and around the nail with erosion of endosteal cortex. (**e**, **f**) Contrast CT confirmed nonunion and rim enhancing collection around the proximal femur. Ultrasound guided aspiration of the collection grew methicillin resistant staphylococcus aureus. (**g**) Removal of implant and debridement of the intramedullary canal with reamer irrigator aspirator (DePuy Synthes, Zuchwil, Switzerland). Antibiotic loaded cement rod was inserted. Clearance of infection was confirmed by normalization of inflammatory markers (white cell count, erythrocyte sedimentation rate and C reactive protein), negative culture from ultrasound guided aspiration and low increased FDG uptake (SUVmax 2.8–3.7) in PET-CT scan. (**h**) Long TFNA with cement augmentation was performed 2 months after the last debridement surgery. X-ray at 1 year postop after TFNA insertion showed fracture union

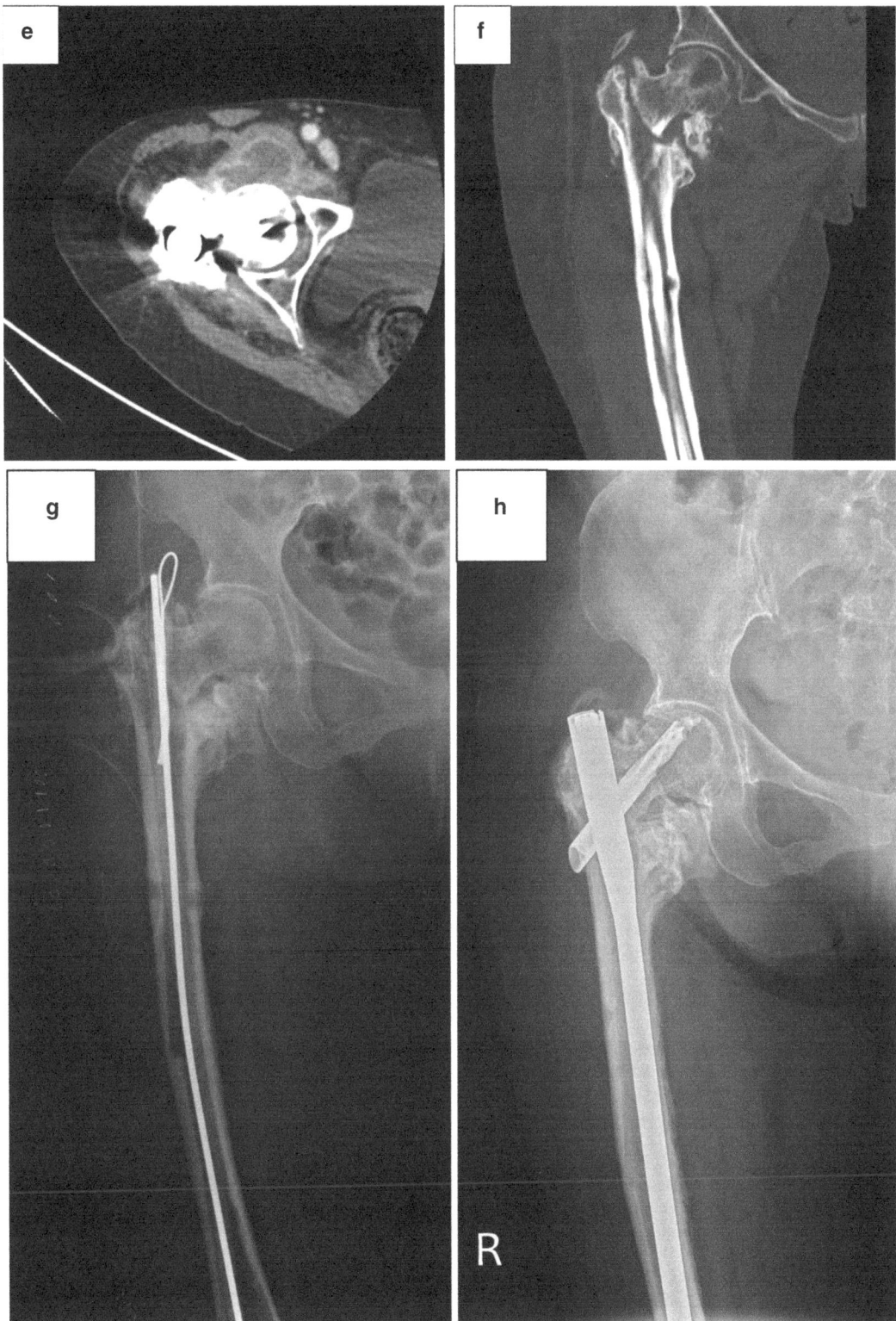

Fig. 8.20 (continued)

8.7   Summary and Conclusion

Proximal femur fractures frequently occur in fragility fracture patients. Suboptimal management could lead to disastrous outcomes. Attention to details aids in preventing complications. New technologies such as cement augmentation can help to reduce complications in osteoporotic bones.

References

1. Braun BJ, Pohlemann T. Proximal femur fractures. In: Egol KA, Leucht P, editors. An evidence-based approach to evaluation and management. Cham: Springer; 2018.
2. Garden R. Low-angle fixation in fractures of the femoral neck. J Bone Joint Surg. 1961;43-B(4):647.
3. Gjertsen JE, et al. Internal screw fixation compared with bipolar hemiarthroplasty for treatment of displaced femoral neck fractures in elderly patients. J Bone Joint Surg Am. 2010;92(3):619–28.
4. Hedbeck CJ, et al. Internal fixation versus cemented hemiarthroplasty for displaced femoral neck fractures in patients with severe cognitive dysfunction: a randomized controlled trial. J Orthop Trauma. 2013;27(12):690–5.
5. Palm H, et al. A new measurement for posterior tilt predicts reoperation in undisplaced femoral neck fractures: 113 consecutive patients treated by internal fixation and followed for 1 year. Acta Orthop. 2009;80(3):303–7.
6. Dolatowski FC, et al. Preoperative posterior tilt of at least 20 degrees increased the risk of fixation failure in Garden-I and -II femoral neck fractures. Acta Orthop. 2016;87(3):252–6.
7. Okike K, et al. Not all Garden-I and II femoral neck fractures in the elderly should be fixed: effect of posterior tilt on rates of subsequent arthroplasty. J Bone Joint Surg Am. 2019;101(20):1852–9.
8. Zlowodzki M, et al. Perception of Garden's classification for femoral neck fractures: an international survey of 298 orthopaedic trauma surgeons. Arch Orthop Trauma Surg. 2005;125(7):503–5.
9. Pauwels F. Der schenkelhalsbruch, ein mechanisches problem : grundlagen des heilungsvorganges, prognose und kausale therapie. Zeitschrift für orthopädische Chirurgie, Bd. 63. Beilageheft, 1935.
10. Bartonicek J. Pauwels' classification of femoral neck fractures: correct interpretation of the original. J Orthop Trauma. 2001;15(5):358–60.
11. Linton P. Types of displacement in fractures of the femoral neck and observations on impaction of fractures. J Bone Joint Surg Br. 1949;31B(2):184–9.
12. Meinberg EG, et al. Fracture and dislocation classification Compendium-2018. J Orthop Trauma. 2018;32(Suppl 1):S1–S170.
13. Falkensammer ML, Benninger E, Meier C. Reduction techniques for trochantericand subtrochanteric fractures of the femur: a practical guide. Acta Chir Orthop Traumatol Cech. 2016;83(5):300–10.
14. Weil YA, et al. Femoral neck shortening and varus collapse after navigated fixation of intracapsular femoral neck fractures. J Orthop Trauma. 2012;26(1):19–23.
15. Mahajan RH, Kumar S, Mishra B. Technique for gentle accurate reproducible closed reduction of intracapsular fracture of neck of femur. Injury. 2017;48(3):789–90.
16. Noda M, et al. Innovative technique of minimally invasive closed reduction for impacted femoral neck fractures (MICRIF). J Orthop Surg (Hong Kong). 2019;27(1):2309499019832418.
17. Yamamoto T, Kobayashi Y, Nonomiya H. Undisplaced femoral neck fractures need a closed reduction before internal fixation. Eur J Orthop Surg Traumatol. 2019;29(1):73–8.
18. Stoffel K, et al. Biomechanical evaluation of the femoral neck system in unstable Pauwels III femoral neck fractures: a comparison with the dynamic hip screw and cannulated screws. J Orthop Trauma. 2017;31(3):131–7.
19. Parker MJ, Stockton G. Internal fixation implants for intracapsular proximal femoral fractures in adults. Cochrane Database Syst Rev. 2001;4:CD001467.
20. Fixation Using Alternative Implants for the Treatment of Hip Fractures Investigators. Fracture fixation in the operative management of hip fractures (FAITH): an international, multicentre, randomised controlled trial. Lancet. 2017;389(10078):1519–27.
21. Li J, et al. Optimum configuration of cannulated compression screws for the fixation of unstable femoral neck Fractures: finite element analysis evaluation. Biomed Res Int. 2018;2018:1271762.
22. Gurusamy K, Parker MJ, Rowlands TK. The complications of displaced intracapsular fractures of the hip: the effect of screw positioning and angulation on fracture healing. J Bone Joint Surg Br. 2005;87(5):632–4.
23. Hoffmann JC, et al. Is the cranial and posterior screw of the "inverted triangle" configuration for femoral neck Fractures safe? J Orthop Trauma. 2019;33(7):331–4.
24. Waaler Bjornelv GM, et al. Hemiarthroplasty compared to internal fixation with percutaneous cannulated screws as treatment of displaced femoral neck fractures in the elderly: cost-utility analysis performed alongside a randomized, controlled trial. Osteoporos Int. 2012;23(6):1711–9.
25. Parker MJ, Pervez H. Surgical approaches for inserting hemiarthroplasty of the hip. Cochrane Database Syst Rev. 2002;3:CD001707.
26. Kunkel ST, et al. A systematic review and meta-analysis of the direct anterior approach for hemiar-

throplasty for femoral neck fracture. Eur J Orthop Surg Traumatol. 2018;28(2):217–32.

27. van der Sijp MPL, et al. Surgical approaches and hemiarthroplasty outcomes for femoral neck fractures: a meta-analysis. J Arthroplasty. 2018;33(5):1617–1627e9.

28. Investigators H, et al. Total hip arthroplasty or hemiarthroplasty for hip fracture. N Engl J Med. 2019;381(23):2199–208.

29. Tol MC, et al. Hemiarthroplasty or total hip arthroplasty for the treatment of a displaced intracapsular fracture in active elderly patients: 12-year follow-up of randomised trial. Bone Joint J. 2017;99-B(2):250–4.

30. Avery PP, et al. Total hip replacement and hemiarthroplasty in mobile, independent patients with a displaced intracapsular fracture of the femoral neck: a seven- to ten-year follow-up report of a prospective randomised controlled trial. J Bone Joint Surg Br. 2011;93(8):1045–8.

31. Excellence, N.I.f.H.a.C.E.I.f.H.a.C. Addendum to clinical guideline 124, hip fracture: management. NICE: London; 2017.

32. Tanzer M, et al. Is cemented or Cementless femoral stem fixation more durable in patients older than 75 years of age? A comparison of the best-performing stems. Clin Orthop Relat Res. 2018;476(7):1428–37.

33. Veldman HD, et al. Cemented versus cementless hemiarthroplasty for a displaced fracture of the femoral neck: a systematic review and meta-analysis of current generation hip stems. Bone Joint J. 2017;99-B(4):421–31.

34. Dahl OE, Pripp AH. Does the risk of death within 48 hours of hip hemiarthroplasty differ between patients treated with cemented and cementless implants? A meta-analysis of large, National Registries. Clin Orthop Relat Res. 2021;480:343.

35. Saudan M, et al. Pertrochanteric fractures: is there an advantage to an intramedullary nail?: a randomized, prospective study of 206 patients comparing the dynamic hip screw and proximal femoral nail. J Orthop Trauma. 2002;16(6):386–93.

36. Leung KS, et al. Gamma nails and dynamic hip screws for peritrochanteric fractures. A randomised prospective study in elderly patients. J Bone Joint Surg Br. 1992;74(3):345–51.

37. Radford PJ, Needoff M, Webb JK. A prospective randomised comparison of the dynamic hip screw and the gamma locking nail. J Bone Joint Surg Br. 1993;75(5):789–93.

38. Neuerburg C, Kammerlander C, Kates SL. In: Blauth M, Nicholas JA, editors. Trochanteric and subtrochanteric femur, in osteoporotic fracture care. New York: Thieme; 2018.

39. Shannon SF, et al. Short versus long cephalomedullary nails for pertrochanteric hip fractures: a randomized prospective study. J Orthop Trauma. 2019;33(10):480–6.

40. Baumgaertner MR, Solberg BD. Awareness of tip-apex distance reduces failure of fixation of trochanteric fractures of the hip. J Bone Joint Surg Br. 1997;79(6):969–71.

41. Kane P, et al. Is tip apex distance as important as we think? A biomechanical study examining optimal lag screw placement. Clin Orthop Relat Res. 2014;472(8):2492–8.

42. Caruso G, et al. A six-year retrospective analysis of cut-out risk predictors in cephalomedullary nailing for pertrochanteric fractures: can the tip-apex distance (TAD) still be considered the best parameter? Bone Joint Res. 2017;6(8):481–8.

43. Nikoloski AN, Osbrough AL, Yates PJ. Should the tip-apex distance (TAD) rule be modified for the proximal femoral nail antirotation (PFNA)? A retrospective study. J Orthop Surg Res. 2013;8:35.

44. Sonmez MM, et al. Strategies for proximal femoral nailing of unstable intertrochanteric fractures: lateral decubitus position or traction table. J Am Acad Orthop Surg. 2017;25(3):e37–44.

45. Henley MB, Gardner MF, Gardner MJ. Harborview illustrated tips and tricks in fracture surgery. Philadelphia: Lippincott Williams & Wilkins (LWW); 2018.

46. Ostrum RF, Marcantonio A, Marburger R. A critical analysis of the eccentric starting point for trochanteric intramedullary femoral nailing. J Orthop Trauma. 2005;19(10):681–6.

47. Siddiqui YS, Khan AQ, Asif N, Khan MJ, Sherwani MKA. Modes of failure of proximal femoral nail (PFN) in unstable trochanteric fractures. MOJ Orthop Rheumatol. 2019;11(1):7–16.

48. Lindskog DM, Baumgaertner MR. Unstable intertrochanteric hip fractures in the elderly. J Am Acad Orthop Surg. 2004;12(3):179–90.

49. Cheung JP, Chan CF. Cutout of proximal femoral nail antirotation resulting from blocking of the gliding mechanism during fracture collapse. J Orthop Trauma. 2011;25(6):e51–5.

50. Davis TR, et al. Intertrochanteric femoral fractures. Mechanical failure after internal fixation. J Bone Joint Surg Br. 1990;72(1):26–31.

51. Mainds CC, Newman RJ. Implant failures in patients with proximal fractures of the femur treated with a sliding screw device. Injury. 1989;20(2):98–100.

52. Parker MJ. Valgus reduction of trochanteric fractures. Injury. 1993;24(5):313–6.

53. Muhr G, Tscherne H, Thomas R. Comminuted trochanteric femoral fractures in geriatric patients: the results of 231 cases treated with internal fixation and acrylic cement. Clin Orthop Relat Res. 1979;138:41–4.

54. Stoffel KK, et al. A new technique for cement augmentation of the sliding hip screw in proximal femur fractures. Clin Biomech (Bristol, Avon). 2008;23(1):45–51.

55. Sermon A, et al. Biomechanical evaluation of bone-cement augmented proximal femoral nail antirotation blades in a polyurethane foam model with low density. Clin Biomech (Bristol, Avon). 2012;27(1):71–6.

56. Sermon A, et al. Potential of polymethylmethacrylate cement-augmented helical proximal femoral nail anti-rotation blades to improve implant stability—a biomechanical investigation in human cadaveric femoral heads. J Trauma Acute Care Surg. 2012;72(2):E54–9.

57. Kammerlander C, et al. Cement augmentation of the proximal femoral nail antirotation (PFNA)—a multicentre randomized controlled trial. Injury. 2018;49(8):1436–44.

58. Yee DKH, et al. Cementation: for better or worse? Interim results of a multi-centre cohort study using a fenestrated spiral blade cephalomedullary device for pertrochanteric fractures in the elderly. Arch Orthop Trauma Surg. 2020;140(12):1957–64.

59. Brunner A, et al. What is the optimal salvage procedure for cut-out after surgical fixation of trochanteric fractures with the PFNA or TFN?: a multicentre study. Injury. 2016;47(2):432–8.

60. Frei H-C, et al. Central head perforation, or "Cut Through," caused by the helical blade of the proximal femoral nail antirotation. J Orthop Trauma. 2012;26(8):e102–7.

61. Baumgaertner MR, et al. The value of the tip-apex distance in predicting failure of fixation of peritrochanteric fractures of the hip. JBJS. 1995;77(7):1058–64.

62. Mavrogenis AF, et al. Complications after hip nailing for fractures. Orthopedics. 2016;39(1):e108–16.

63. Metsemakers WJ, et al. General treatment principles for fracture-related infection: recommendations from an international expert group. Arch Orthop Trauma Surg. 2020;140(8):1013–27.

Terence Cheuk Ting Pun and Frankie Leung

9.1 Introduction

Subtrochanteric femur fracture is a subset of the proximal femur fracture with a major fracture line across the area between the lesser trochanter and the junction of the proximal and middle thirds of the femoral shaft. It accounts for 5–22% of all proximal femur fracture cases [1, 2]. Although the principles of intramedullary nailing are similarly applied, subtrochanteric femur fracture differs from intertrochanteric and femoral shaft fracture from both anatomical and surgical perspectives. This is a unique meta-diaphyseal fracture in which surgical outcome is heavily dependent on the quality of reduction. Successful intramedullary fixation requires both a high-quality fracture reduction and an accurate entry point. Significant complications and poor clinical outcomes can be anticipated if either step is not properly executed. In the past decade, there has been an increasing trend on the incidence of atypical femoral fractures associated with bisphosphonates [3]. Healing problems after fixation have often been reported [4, 5].

9.2 Characteristic of Subtrochanteric Region of Femur

Several anatomical and biomechanical characteristics of subtrochanteric segment make it a technically demanding condition to treat once a fracture occurs. These include the femoral bowing, eccentric loading of body weight onto femur, and tension-band effect of the iliotibial band and vastus lateralis. Hence, the subtrochanteric segment is subject to the largest asymmetric difference in stress in two opposite directions in a single long bone. The medial and posteromedial cortices are under massive compressive force, whereas the lateral cortex experiences high tensile force. Bone naturally heals under compression. But since the lateral cortex is under great tension, it is important to reduce the fracture leaving no lateral cortical gaps and no varus mal-alignment.

The subtrochanteric segment is mainly composed of cortical bone. It has a slower turnover rate as compared to cancellous bone in the intertrochanteric segment. On the other hand, anatomical studies have shown that the vascularity of the subtrochanteric region does not differ from other metaphyseal segment of long bone. Hence, the fracture will heal uneventfully if strong and stable fixation can maintain the fracture reduction until healing occurs.

T. C. T. Pun (✉) · F. Leung
Department of Orthopaedics and Traumatology,
Queen Mary Hospital, The University of Hong Kong,
Pokfulam, Hong Kong
e-mail: klleunga@hku.hk

© The Author(s), under exclusive license to Springer Nature Singapore Pte Ltd. 2024
F. Leung, T. W. Lau (eds.), *Surgery for Osteoporotic Fractures*,
https://doi.org/10.1007/978-981-99-9696-4_9

The subtrochanteric segment is subjected to multiple strong deforming forces related to the muscles that insert on the proximal femur. Deforming forces created by the hip abductors, external rotators, and the iliopsoas muscles result in a characteristic varus, externally rotated, and flexed deformity of the proximal fragment. Meanwhile, the pull of the adductors causes shortening and medialization of the distal fragment. Gravity leads to sagging of the distal fragment with patient in a supine position. Neutralization of all forces is needed to achieve a good reduction before definitive fixation.

9.3 Types of Subtrochanteric Fracture

Classification systems help to describe subtrochanteric femur fracture with different morphology and complexity, assist in selecting the method of reduction and mode of fixation, and provide prognostic information. In the AO classification, subtrochanteric fracture is classified under diaphyseal femur (32) rather than proximal femur (31) and it is denoted by 0.1 at the end. It takes into account of the energy of trauma (A, simple; B, wedge; or C, complex) and the mechanism (1, spiral; 2, oblique or bending; or 3, transverse).

Practically, subtrochanteric fractures present in a bi-modal distribution. Comminuted fractures occur in young patients involved in high-energy injuries such as motor vehicle collisions. Oblique and spiral fractures occur in elderly patients after low-energy injuries such as ground-level falls (Fig. 9.1). These patients have underlying osteoporosis, multiple co-morbidities, and limited physiological reserve. Early surgery with multidisciplinary team involvement, secondary fall prevention as well as bone health management are essential components of care.

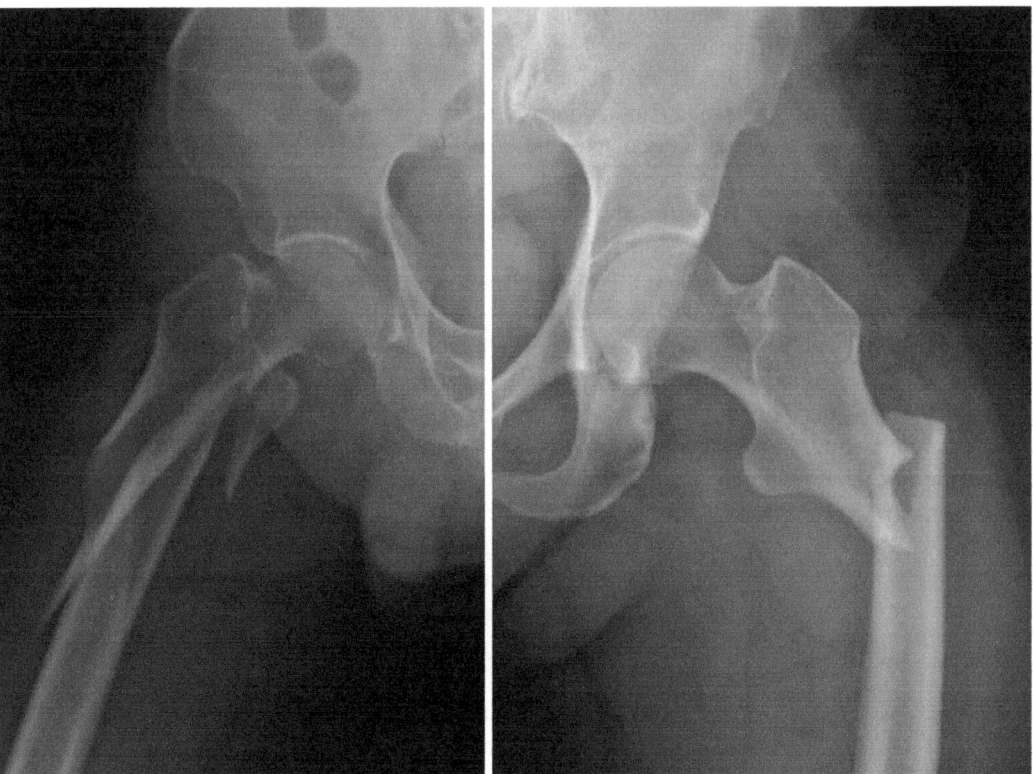

Fig. 9.1 Subtrochanteric fracture with normal healing potential following low-energy trauma (left) and atypical subtrochanteric fracture (right)

9.3.1 Atypical Femoral Fracture

Atypical femoral fracture is a low energy subtrochanteric or femoral shaft fracture in older patients taking long-term bisphosphonates or other anti-resorptive medication. They may have prodromal symptom of thigh pain. Atypical fracture is slower to heal, more intolerant to malreduction, and has a higher rate of fixation failure compared to subtrochanteric fractures with normal bone turnover (Fig. 9.2).

The presence of a more varus femorotibial angle, a more prominent lateral femoral bow, and an increased varus neck-shaft angle increase the tensile load on the lateral femoral cortex. These are the unfavorable femoral geometry that increases the risk of atypical femoral fracture. Diaphyseal atypical femoral fractures tend to be associated with a larger lateral bowing angle and a larger standing femorotibial angle, whereas subtrochanteric atypical femoral fractures are associated with a smaller femoral neck-shaft angle, i.e., a varus hip geometry.

Upon termination of bisphosphonate, the risk of atypical femoral fracture is reduced to approximately half at 3–15 months and 74–79% in the following years [6]. In patients without atypical femoral fractures, there is no consensus on discontinuation of anti-resorptive agents after several years of administration. They should

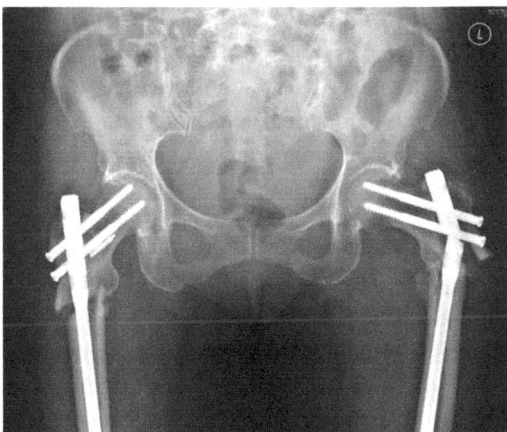

Fig. 9.2 Bilateral atypical subtrochanteric fracture developed into non-union and implant failure secondary to fracture mal-reduction

probably be continued in patients at high risk of fragility fractures. There may be a role of drug holiday after 3–5 years of treatment if the patients have mild to moderate, have low fracture risk (FRAX) score, and have no fragility fracture during the period of bisphosphonate use.

Cephalomedullary nailing is the preferred method of surgical fixation of both complete and incomplete atypical femur fracture. The fixation covers the full length of the femur and avoid stress concentration and re-fracture at the end of a plate fixation. Compared to standard subtrochanteric fractures, surgeon may encounter several difficulties when intra-medullary nailing is performed.

In atypical femoral fractures, the femoral canal is narrow with generalized cortical thickening. The narrowest diameter of the canal can be smaller than 9 mm. There is also significant anterolateral femoral bowing. Putting in a nail that does not fit the radius of curvature of the bone will straighten a curved bone at the fracture site, resulting in posteromedial fracture gaps, leg-length discrepancy or iatrogenic fractures. Nail may perforate the anterior cortex of the distal femur because of the eccentric nail position. Localized lateral endosteal thickening is present at the fracture site. The sclerotic beak deflects guidewire and reamers medially, promoting a varus mal-reduction. Any mal-reduction will impose prolonged stress on the implant, leading to fatigue failure. There is little room for error in reduction and surgical technique. Tips and tricks to tackle such problems will be described in the treatment section.

Other than fixation of complete fracture, the contralateral femur has to be screened because approximately 28% of patients have bilateral involvement [7]. In cases with normal X-ray radiographs on the contralateral side but there is still clinical suspicion or pain, computer tomography, magnetic resonance imaging or bone scan should be performed.

Incomplete fracture carries a risk of progression to a complete fracture as high as 28% within 6 months of diagnosis. Subtrochanteric location, functional pain, and a radiolucent line of more than 50% of the lateral cortex were identified as risk factors for progression to complete fracture [8]. Prophylactic treatment with cephalomedullary nailing is effective in preventing fracture progression and healing of fracture. However, nailing an incomplete fracture can be technically demanding. The "intact" but bowed femur will not give way to accommodate a nail with a mismatch in the radius of curvature.

Upon diagnosis of atypical femoral fracture, bisphosphonates or anti-resorptive agents should be discontinued. Dietary calcium and vitamin D status are assessed and adequate supplementation prescribed. In selected patients, teriparatide is prescribed to advance healing of atypical femoral fracture. Teriparatide is a recombinant form of parathyroid hormone that enhances bone healing in patients with delayed union or non-union.

9.3.2 Treatment of Subtrochanteric Femur Fracture

Cephalomedullary nail stands out to be the implant of choice in fixing these challenging fractures. The intramedullary devices have stronger biomechanical stiffness than extra-medullary implants, as they resist deforming forces with a shorter lever arm. Nails are by themselves load-sharing device, and the load-sharing effect is enhanced with adequate fracture reduction and fragment opposition. Allowing early weight bearing is particularly important for geriatric patients with limited upper limb power and cognition. Nails can span the whole femur length and can be inserted with less soft tissue dissection.

The standard implant is a long-reamed interlocking cephalomedullary nail. Trochanteric entry nail with a proximal valgus bend helps to prevent varus mal-alignment. Although it is designed for easier entry at the tip of greater trochanter, it is advisable to insert the nail medial to the tip or at the piriformis fossa in order to prevent varus mal-alignment. While short nails can span across the subtrochanteric segment of femur, subtrochanteric fracture is inherently unstable, long nails are the default option in fixation of subtrochanteric fracture. It also obviates the risk of peri-implant fracture at the tip of a short nail.

All long nails have a defined radii of curvature and they may not match patients' femoral bowing. In these special cases, one may need to alter the insertion technique, use an opposite side nail or a straight nail.

9.3.3 Pre-Operative Planning

Plain radiograph of the entire fractured femur is obtained for pre-existing deformities, retained hardware and distal stemmed prosthesis that could impede intramedullary nailing. Contralateral femur is imaged to serve as a template for neck shaft angulation, medullary diameter, anterior and lateral bowing, limb length and rotational profile. This is particularly valuable in comminuted fracture with limited cortical read to judge reduction. Contralateral femur is screened for incomplete fractures in cases of atypical femoral fracture.

Surgeons select the type of operating table and the way to position the patient according to patient body habitus and surgeon preference. Depending on the fracture pattern, surgical instruments for reduction include femoral distractor, 5.0 mm Schanz pin, large reduction forceps, collinear clamp, bone hook, long hemostatic forceps, flexible wires, and small reduction plates.

9.4 Goals of Fracture Reduction

The reduction goals in subtrochanteric fracture are restoration of length, axis, and rotation. Varus or flexion mal-reduction is poorly tolerated. Another reduction goal is restoration of medial cortical support. Lack of cortical support may result from mal-reduction, medial comminution, or a displaced medial wedge fragment. Medial cortical buttress after reduction supports the implant and counteract the bending forces and varus torque during postoperative mobilization. Intramedullary nail acts more like a load-sharing device in the presence of medial cortical support, and more like a load-bearing device in the absence of medial cortical support. Length is of less importance in geriatric fracture and fracture impaction is beneficial for stability of construct and healing (Fig. 9.3).

9.4.1 Reduction Techniques

9.4.1.1 Traction Table Setup

Often the proximal fragment will not be reduced by excessive distraction, which worsens the deformity and makes further percutaneous or mini-open reduction difficult. Rotational adjustment of the distal fragment by the footplate will not be accurate until the proximal fragment is brought out of flexion. Intra-operative adjustment of rotation is needed. Support of distal fragment with a post helps to correct the posterior translation (Fig. 9.4).

9.4.1.2 Percutaneous Extra-Focal Techniques

Nailing unreduced subtrochanteric fracture has a high failure rate. Meta-diaphyseal fracture will not reduce by itself with reaming nor nailing. The entry point created in an unreduced proximal fragment is likely to be suboptimal. Manipulation of the proximal fragment using a nail is likely to remove metaphyseal bone and the entry hole will be enlarged in an undesirable direction.

A simple yet effective method of reducing subtrochanteric fracture is the use of long hemostatic forceps. Through a percutaneous incision, the forceps are introduced from posterolateral to anteromedial, and rest on the anteromedial sur-

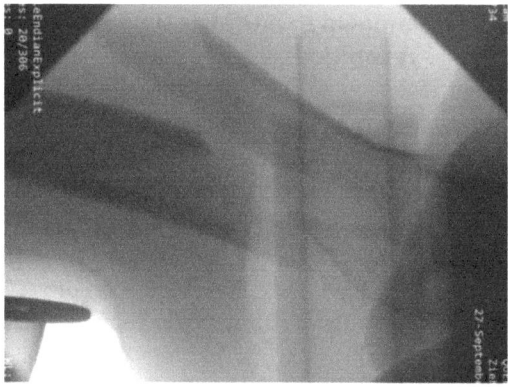

Fig. 9.4 A post is positioned under the distal fragment to correct the posterior sagging

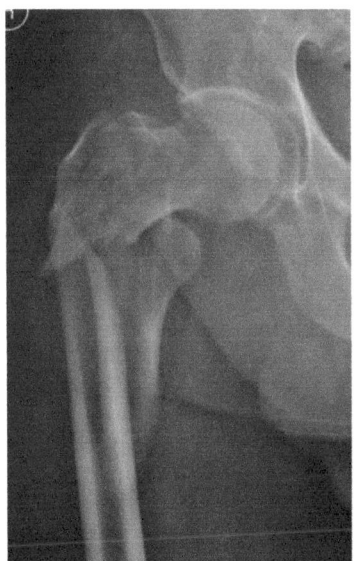
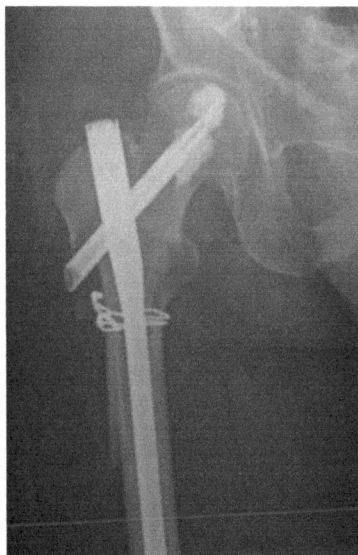
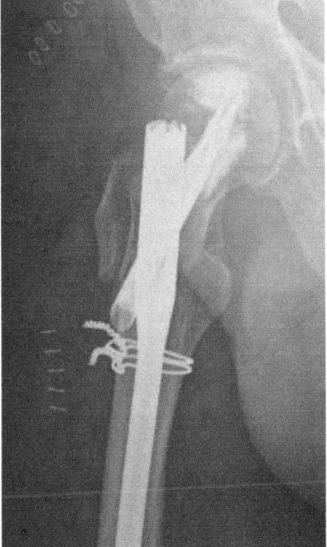

Fig. 9.3 The goal of reduction is to restore the neck-shaft angle or over-reduce it to a slight valgus position. There should be no sagittal plane deformity. In comminuted fractures, placement of cerclage wiring around large medial wedge fragment helps to restore medial cortical support. It supports the implant to counteract varus torque during post-operative mobilization. A positive cortical buttress, defined as the medial cortex of head-neck fragment being superomedial to the medial cortex of the shaft, also helps to prevent varus collapse

face of the proximal fragment. By lifting the forceps handle upward, the flexion, abduction, and external rotational deformities of the proximal fragment are corrected. A narrow Hohmann retractor can also serve the same purpose.

Direct manipulation of the individual bone fragment can be achieved with ball-tipped pusher or Schanz pin and bone hook respectively. These tools remain in the wounds until proximal locking is completed.

9.4.1.3 Mini-Open Intra-Focal Techniques

When reduction is not satisfactory after closed reduction or percutaneous methods, one should have a low threshold to carry out a limited open reduction. Current evidence supports the mechanical advantages of preventing varus malalignment and restoration of the medial cortical support over the disadvantages of open dissection. A well-aligned fracture via limited open reduction is always preferable to a closed malreduction in subtrochanteric fractures. This is particularly true for atypical femoral fractures. Our own study showed that a good reduction with both <4 mm maximal cortical displacement and <10° angulation can improve the operative outcome of atypical femoral fractures [9].

For short oblique or transverse fractures, a vastus lateralis split through a limited incision

can be used. The vastus lateralis should be elevated for longer exposure in long oblique and spiral fractures. The periosteum should be maintained at all times.

Reduction forceps or clamps are introduced parallel to the skin incision with their prongs closed. They are turned perpendicular to the fracture plane and their prongs are opened gently to span the fracture site. Pointed or serrated jaw-bone reduction forceps or Verbrugge bone holding clamp can be applied for fractures primarily in the coronal plane. Collinear clamp or Verbrugge bone holding clamp can be applied for fractures primarily in the sagittal plane. The reduction quality can be assessed by palpation and fluoroscopy (Fig. 9.5).

In oblique and spiral fractures, cerclage wires can be applied percutaneously through specially designed wire passers (Figs. 9.6 and 9.7). The passer prongs should be applied close to bone to avoid trapping neurovascular structures. In osteoporotic bone, excessive tightening should be avoided to prevent iatrogenic fracture.

9.4.1.4 Implant Assisted Reduction

One of the most common methods of correcting deformity during nailing is the poller screw technique. It works in meta-diaphyseal fracture by narrowing the canal diameter and directing the nail to a desired position. Poller screw can be left

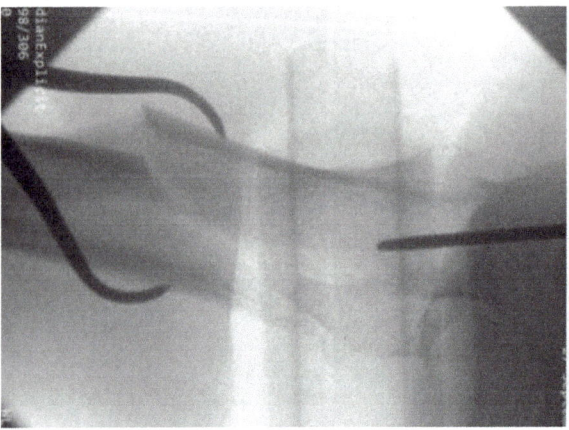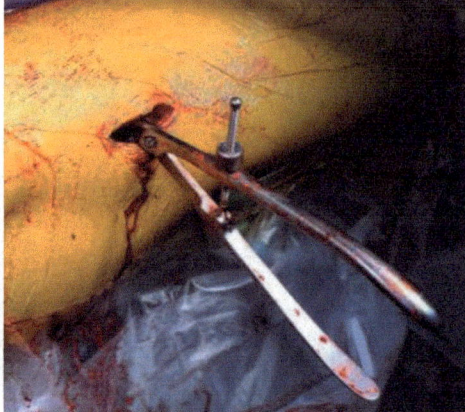

Fig. 9.5 Pointed reduction forceps or collinear clamp can be applied through the limited incision

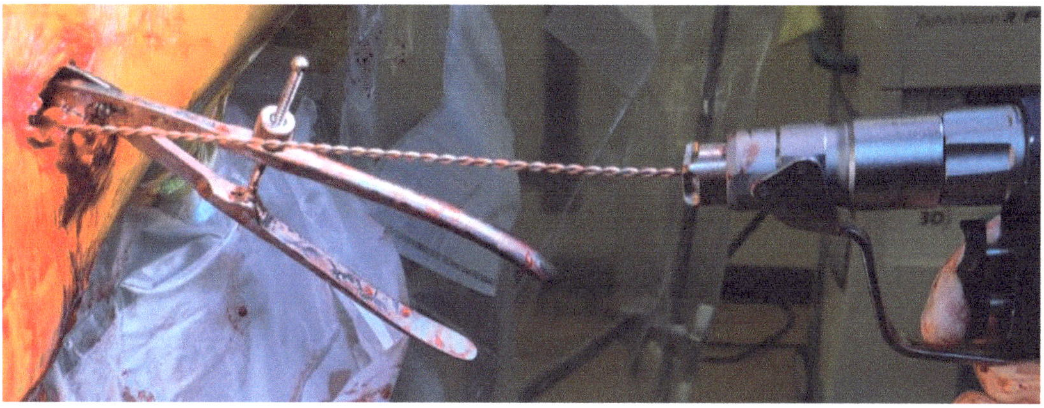

Fig. 9.6 After provisional reduction of fracture with reduction forceps, a cerclage wire is placed and tensioned

in place for additional stability. Alternatively a thick blocking pin can serve the same purpose and can be inserted and removed easily.

When deciding on the position of the poller screw or pin, a simple guideline is to place it at site where the reaming guide rod should not pass through (Figs. 9.8 and 9.9). For example, to prevent a varus deformity, an anterior-to-posterior poller screw is inserted in the proximal fragment, medial to the path of the nail, close to the fracture site where there is no comminution. It ensures a more lateral reaming path along the lateral cortex. In case of atypical fractures, poller screw also helps to divert the reamer to remove the endosteal beak of the lateral cortex, thus prevent varus mal-reduction after nail insertion.

To correct or prevent a flexion deformity, a lateral-to-medial poller screw is placed in the proximal fragment, posterior to the nail path, near the fracture site where there is no comminution. It ensures a reaming path along the anterior cortex.

As the degree of fracture comminution increases, it is often difficult to obtain and maintain a satisfactory reduction for intramedullary nailing with percutaneous techniques. Moreover, the use of reduction clamps and cerclage may not be feasible in transverse or highly comminuted fracture pattern. A short 3.5 mm plate with monocortical screws can also be used to temporarily stabilize the fracture for subsequent nailing. The plate is contoured in slight valgus and applied to the lateral cortex. This technique of provisional plating with limited soft tissue stripping can provide excellent reduction.

9.4.1.5 Importance of Entry Point

Most nails require a trochanteric entry point. However, medialization of the entry hole can lead to slight valgus alignment, which is desirable in subtrochanteric fractures. The key in obtaining the correct entry site is provisional fracture reduction because the site is concealed if the proximal fragment remains displaced (Fig. 9.10).

Before putting in a guide wire through the entry point, an AP view of the proximal fragment should be scrutinized that it has been brought out of external rotation. When the proximal fragment is in neutral rotation, the lesser trochanter profile is obscured, the femoral neck is elongated and not overlapping with the greater trochanter (Fig. 9.11).

Sometimes a correct entry site is difficult to obtain in the usual manner such as in patient with morbid obesity, in revision cases where an incorrect nail entry site was used, and in atypical femoral fractures with varus alignment. Open takedown of lateral endosteal beak with a rasp further helps in reduction in atypical femoral fracture. Moreover, an inside-out technique can also be used for retrograde reaming of the proximal fragment (Fig. 9.12).

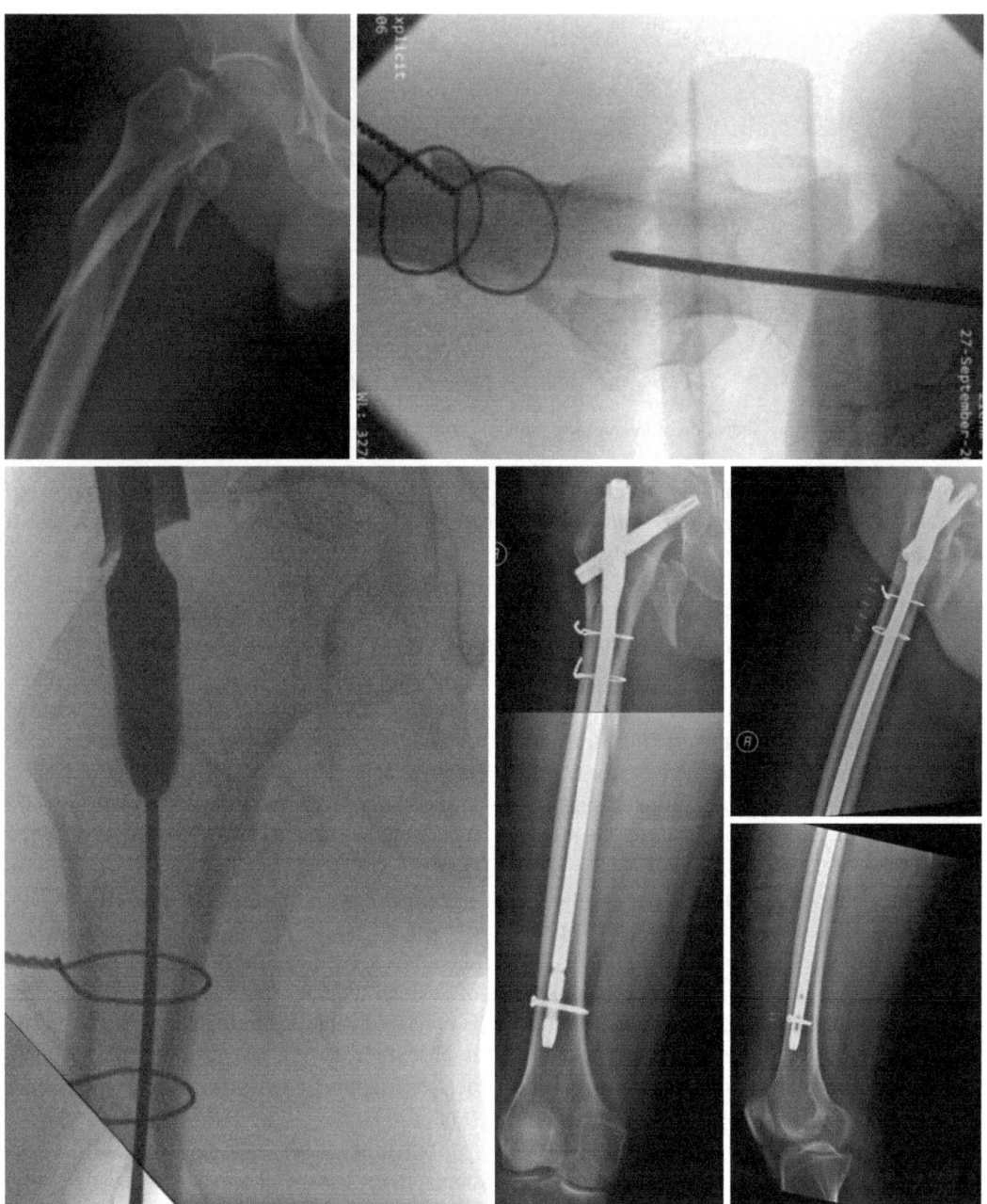

Fig. 9.7 Example of cerclage wire-assisted cephalomedullary nailing in a long spiral subtrochanteric fracture

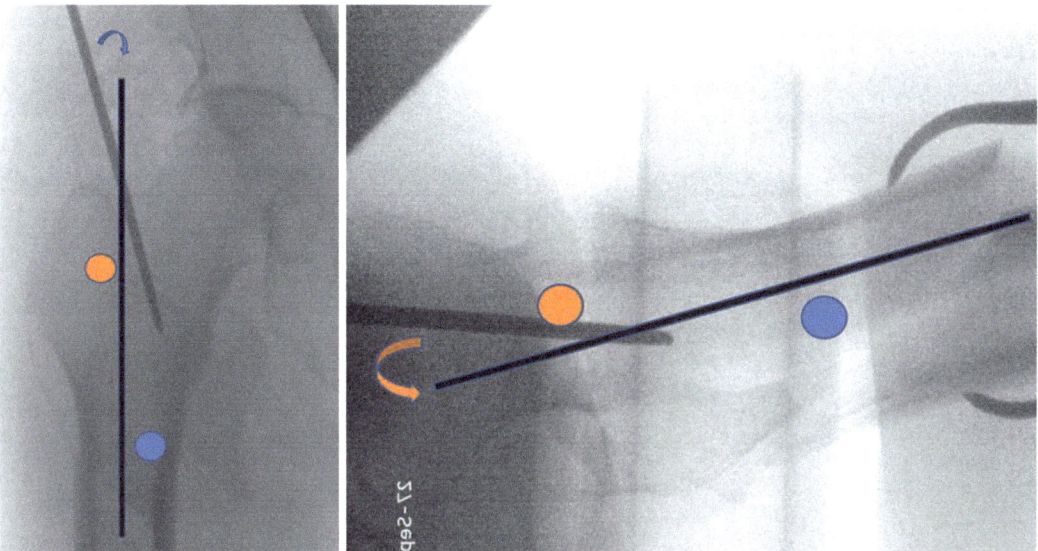

Fig. 9.8 Poller screw or blocking pin placement in subtrochanteric fracture. Blue dots denote the sites of placement to correct varus (coronal) and flexion (sagittal) deformity. Orange dots denote the sites of placement to divert reamer and nail to go through the proper entry site

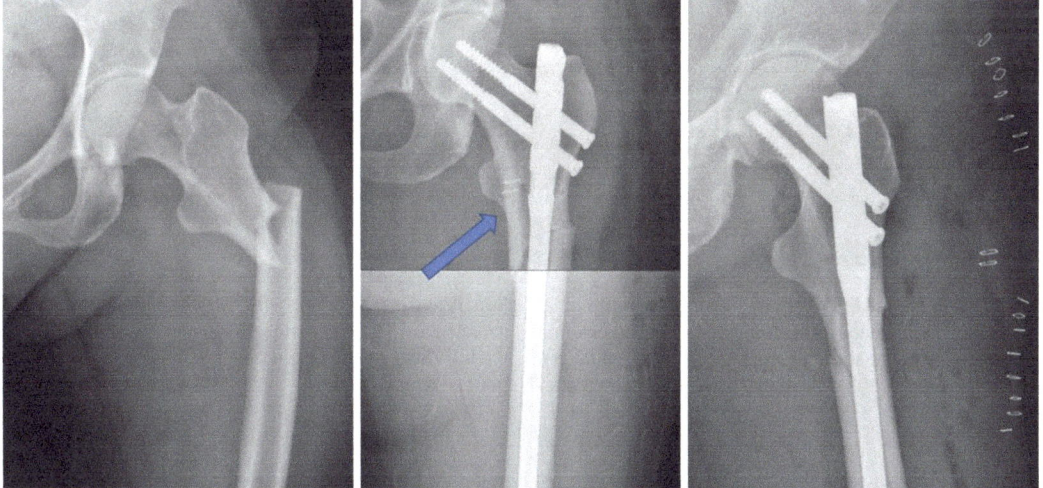

Fig. 9.9 Reduction of atypical subtrochanteric femur fracture is facilitated by placement of an anterior-to-posterior blocking pin medial to the nail in the proximal fragment. The pin also diverts the reamer to remove the endosteal beak

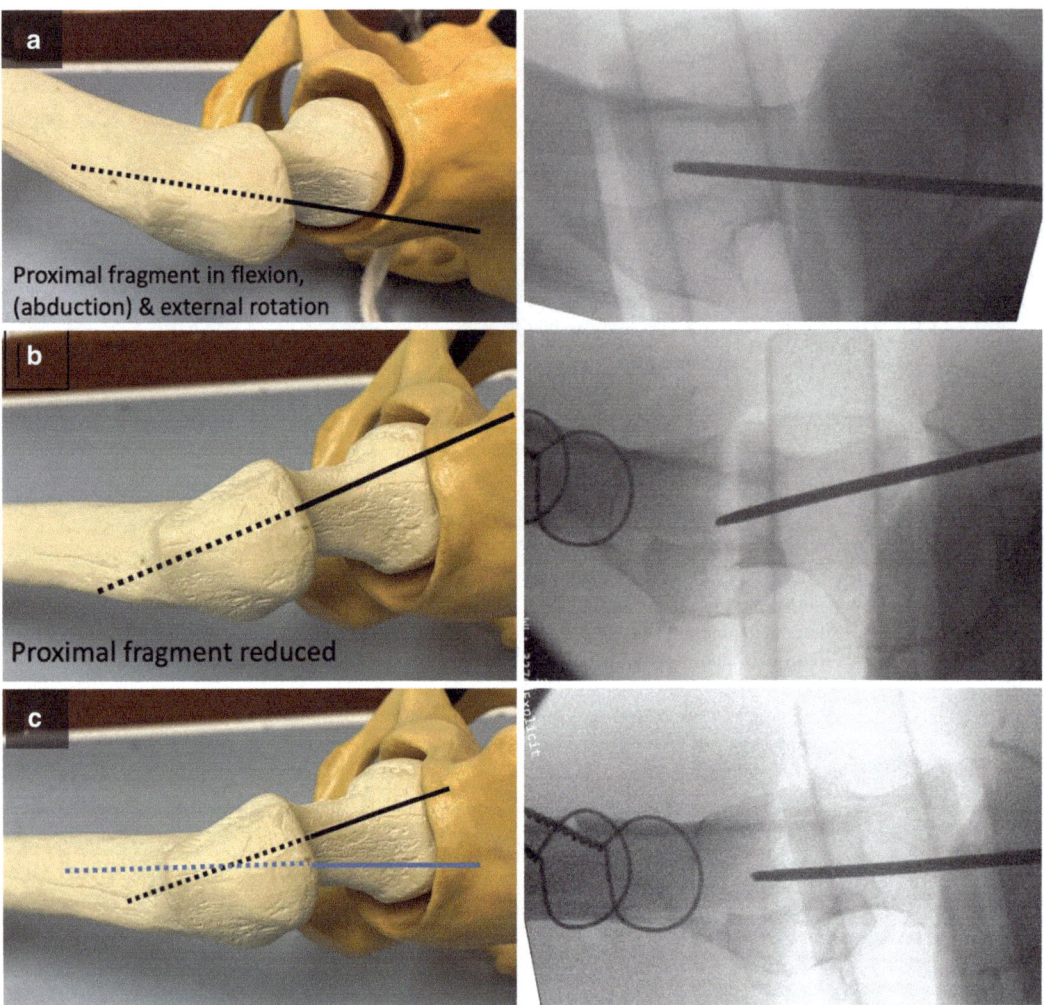

Fig. 9.10 Bone model (**a**) shows an unreduced proximal fragment that remained in flexion, abduction and external rotation. The entry site and trajectory of the guide pin (black line) appeared satisfactory. (**b**) With fracture reduc-tion, the erroneous guide wire entry site and trajectory are revealed. (**c**) The entry site was too anteriorly situated and the trajectory pointed posteriorly. A new guide wire (blue line) is then re-inserted

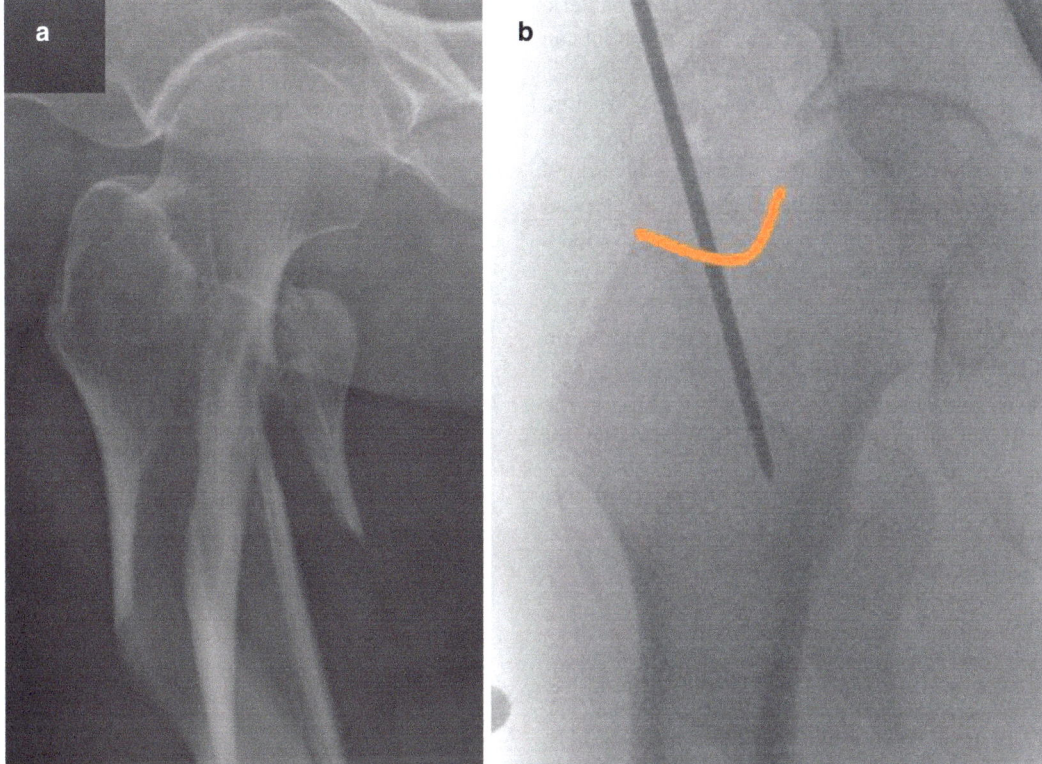

Fig. 9.11 (**a**) The femoral neck is obscured by the greater trochanter when the proximal fragment is externally rotated. (**b**) The femoral neck is elongated and not over-lapping with the greater trochanter when the proximal fragment is in neutral rotation. Insertion of guide wire when the curved contour (orange line) is seen

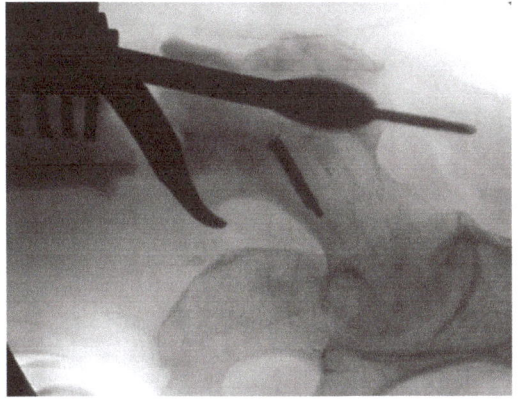

Fig. 9.12 Retrograde reaming in revision nailing of an atypical fracture

9.5 Outcome

After the surgery, elderly patients should start mobilization as soon as possible, usually on the first postoperative day. Weight bearing walking is allowed, and a daily physiotherapy program is initiated to achieve early ambulation.

The quality of fracture reduction is proven to be the most important factor in bone union and time to union. Failure to restore the anatomical neck-shaft angle leaving post-operative gaps at anterior and lateral fracture site are significantly associated with delayed union or non-union [9].

Intramedullary nailing of subtrochanteric femur fracture with normal healing potential can yield excellent results. Higher rate of failure is observed in atypical subtrochanteric fracture with union rate around 70% [5]. The healing time of standard subtrochanteric fracture is around 4.3 months [10]. The healing time of atypical subtrochanteric femur fracture was observed at a mean of 10.7 months.

Subtrochanteric fractures in elderly patients significantly affect their short and long-term quality of life. Although hip pain is often not severe, there will likely be a deterioration in the walking ability and functioning in activities of daily living.

References

1. Mattisson L, Bojan A, Enocson A. Epidemiology, treatment and mortality of trochanteric and subtrochanteric hip fractures: data from the Swedish fracture register. BMC Musculoskelet Disord. 2018;19(1):369.
2. Ekstrom W, Nemeth G, Samnegard E, Dalen N, Tidermark J. Quality of life after a subtrochanteric fracture a prospective cohort study on 87 elderly patients. Injury. 2009;40(4):371–6.
3. Leung F, Lau T-W, To M, Luk KD-K, Kung AWC. Atypical femoral diaphyseal and subtrochanteric fractures and their association with bisphosphonates. BMJ Case Rep. 2009;2009:bcr1020081073-bcr.
4. Luo Q, Fang C, Shen W-Y, Lau T-W, Leung F. A lesson from the failure of intramedullary fixation of atypical subtrochanteric fractures: a report of two cases. JBJS Case Connect. 2013;3(1):e22.
5. Cho J-W, Oh C-W, Leung F, Park K-C, Wong MK, Kwek E, et al. Healing of atypical subtrochanteric femur fractures after Cephalomedullary nailing: which factors predict union? J Orthop Trauma. 2017;31(3):138–45.
6. Black DM, Geiger EJ, Eastell R, Vittinghoff E, Li BH, Ryan DS, et al. Atypical femur fracture risk versus fragility fracture prevention with bisphosphonates. N Engl J Med. 2020;383(8):743–53.
7. Meier RPH, Perneger TV, Stern R, Rizzoli R, Peter RE. Increasing occurrence of atypical femoral fractures associated with bisphosphonate use. Arch Intern Med. 2012;172(12):930–6.
8. Min B-W, Koo K-H, Park Y-S, Oh C-W, Lim S-J, Kim J-W, et al. Scoring system for identifying impending complete fractures in incomplete atypical femoral fractures. J Clin Endocrinol Metabol. 2017;102(2):545–50.
9. Lai YS, Chau JYM, Woo SB, Fang C, Lau TW, Leung F. A retrospective review on atypical femoral fracture: operative outcomes and the risk factors for failure. Geriatr Orthop Surg Rehabil. 2019;10:2151459319864736.
10. Barquet A, Francescoli L, Rienzi D, López L. Intertrochanteric-subtrochanteric fractures: treatment with the long gamma nail. J Orthop Trauma. 2000;14(5):324–8.

Distal Femur Fractures and Periprosthetic Fractures around Distal Femur

10

Tak Man Wong

10.1 Introduction

Distal femoral fractures make up 4–6% of all osteoporotic femoral fractures [1]. Such fractures are associated with high morbidity and mortality. Studies showed that the mortality of elderly patients after distal femur fractures after at 6 months and 1 year were 17% and 30%, respectively [2, 3]. Similar to geriatric hip fractures, early surgical intervention of osteoporotic distal femur fractures can reduce both mortality and morbidity [4, 5].

Most of the osteoporotic distal femur fractures are caused by low energy trauma such as fall on level ground. The fracture occurs mainly at metaphyseal region and sometimes it extends distally causing intra-articular fracture. The fracture is usually shortened, in varus and extended position because of the pull of quadriceps, adductors, and gastrocnemius.

Hoffa fracture is a subtype and occurs in the coronal plane. The incidence of Hoffa fracture is between 8.7% and 13% of distal femur fractures [6]. The incidence is much higher in elderly and was reported up to 44% of supracondylar-intercondylar fractures [7].

Periprosthetic fractures following total knee replacement (TKR) usually occur over distal femur and the incidence is between 0.3 and 2.5% of patients within 2–4 years after TKR [8, 9]. The risk factors for periprosthetic fractures over femur include anterior notching, osteoporosis, osteolysis, long-term steroid, revision TKR, and ankylosis of knee joint, etc. [10, 11].

10.2 Classification

The most popular classification of distal femur fractures is AO classification, which divides the fractures into extra-articular (type 33A), partial articular (type 33B), and complete articular (type 33C). For each type, it is further subdivided into subgroups according to the fracture pattern and complexity (Fig. 10.1).

For Hoffa fractures, the most commonly used one is Letenneur classification [12]. The classification divides Hoffa fractures into three types (Fig. 10.2). In type I, the fracture line runs parallel to posterior cortex. In type II, the fracture line is parallel to the base of posterior condyle but posterior to the lateral collateral ligament. Type II is further subdivided into IIa, IIb, and IIc, based on how posterior the fracture line is. Type IIc fracture has a higher risk of nonunion due to poorer blood supply resulting from minimal soft tissue attachment [13–15].

T. M. Wong (✉)
Department of Orthopaedics and Traumatology, Queen Mary Hospital, The University of Hong Kong, Pokfulam, Hong Kong
e-mail: wongtm@hku.hk

© The Author(s), under exclusive license to Springer Nature Singapore Pte Ltd. 2024
F. Leung, T. W. Lau (eds.), *Surgery for Osteoporotic Fractures*,
https://doi.org/10.1007/978-981-99-9696-4_10

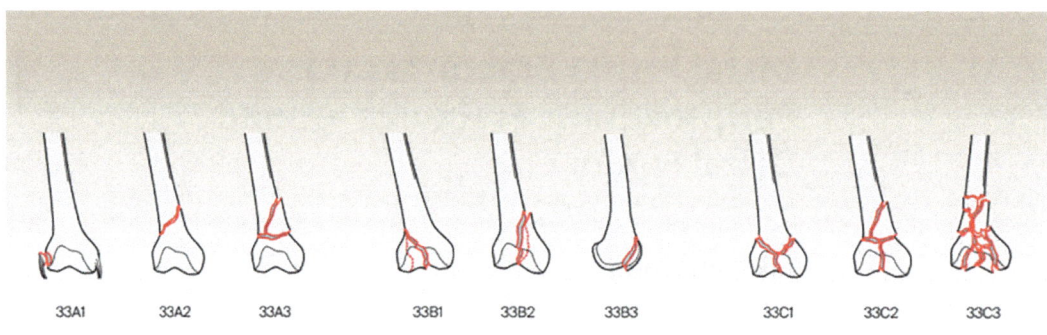

33 Distal end segment

33A   Extraarticular
33A1 Avulsion
33A2 Simple
33A3 Wedge or multifragmentary

33B   Partial articular
33B1 Lateral condyle, sagittal
33B2 Medial condyle, sagittal
33B3 Frontal/coronal

33C   Complete articular
33C1 Simple articular, simple metaphyseal
33C2 Simple articular, wedge or multifragmentary metaphyseal
33C3 Multifragmentary articular, simple, wedge or multifragmentary
         metaphyseal

Fig. 10.1 The AO classification of distal femur fractures. (*Copyright by AO Foundation, Switzerland. Source: AO Classification*, https://classification.aoeducation.org/)

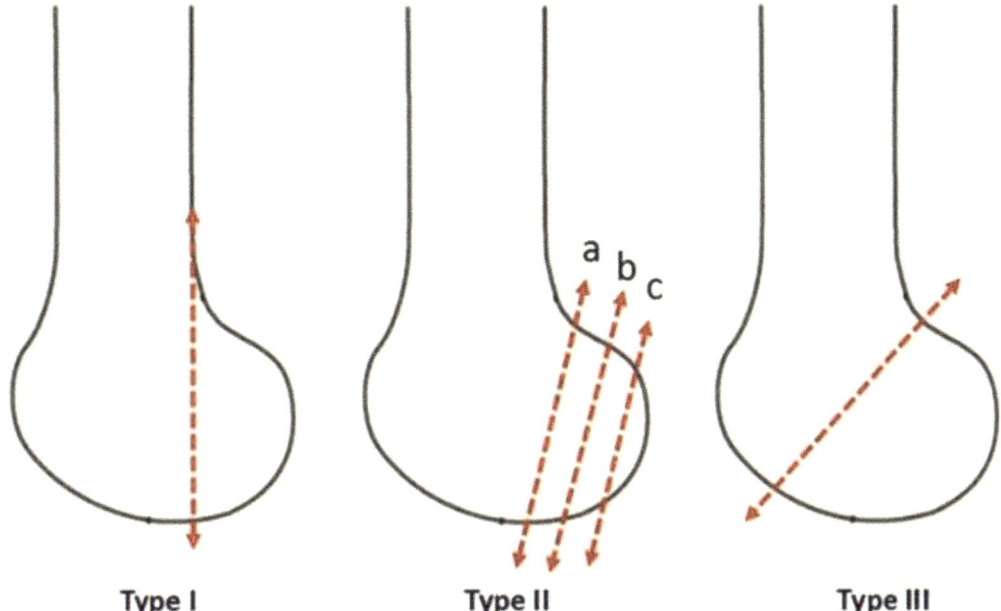

Fig. 10.2 Classification of Hoffa Fractures described by Letenneur. (*Reproduced from Letenneur J, Labour PE, Rogez JM, et al. Hoffa's fractures. Report of 20 cases [in French]. Ann Chir 1978; 32:213–9* [12]. *Elsevier Masson SAS. All rights reserved*)

In periprosthetic fractures following total knee arthroplasty, the most commonly used classification system is from Rorabeck and Taylor [10], which focuses on the fracture displacement and stability of prosthesis. Type I is non-displaced fracture with stable prosthesis. Type II is displaced fracture with stable prosthesis, while type III is displaced fracture with unstable prosthesis (Fig. 10.3).

I   II   III

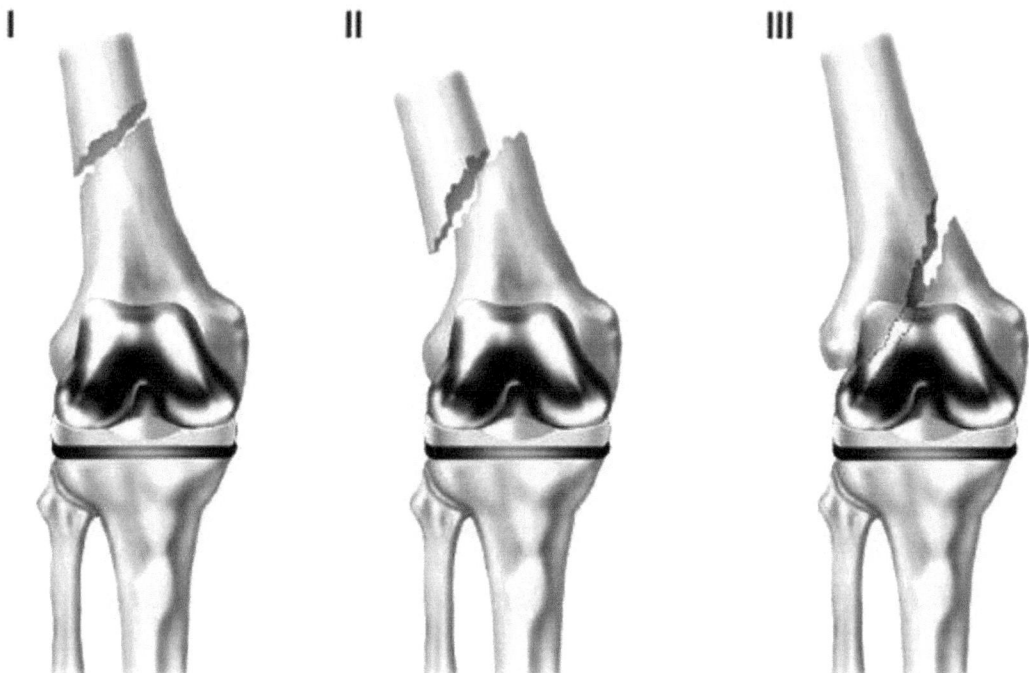

Fig. 10.3 Classification of periprosthetic fracture over distal femur described by Rorabeck and Taylor. (*Reprinted with permission from Copyright Clearance Center. Rorabeck CH, Taylor JW. Classification of periprosthetic* *fractures complicating total knee arthroplasty. Orthop Clin North Am. 1999 Apr;30 (2):209–14* [10]. *doi: 10.1016/s0030-5898(05)70075-4. PMID: 10196422*)

10.3 Management

For the management of distal femur fractures and periprosthetic fractures, surgical fixation is usually indicated for early mobilization and ambulation. Besides, surgical fixation can achieve immediate pain relief and better limb function. Occasionally, non-operative treatment can be used for undisplaced fractures or surgically unfit patients. Apart from high mortality as in proximal femur fractures, complications including nonunion (14%), joint stiffness (35%), post-traumatic osteoarthritis (50%) can occur. In case of periprosthetic fractures over distal femur, the nonunion rate is up to 42% if non-surgical management is adopted [16].

Before surgery, a CT Scan is necessary to delineate the fracture pattern and detect intra-articular involvement. In case of periprosthetic fractures, it is important to rule out aseptic loosening in which revision of total knee replacement is needed.

Historically, distal femur fractures were treated with fixed angled blade plates and non-locking condylar buttress plates. However, with recent advances in orthopedic implants such as locking plates, a more angular stable fixation can be achieved. Another effective method of fixation is retrograde intramedullary nailing. However, it is contraindicated if the TKR femoral component is either closed box (e.g., posterior stabilizing total knee system) or having a long stem. Moreover, it cannot be used in femur with proximal implant (e.g., hip arthroplasty or proximal femoral nail) or very distal femoral fractures [17].

10.3.1 Surgical Techniques in Plating

The goals of surgical treatment should be restoration of length, axis, and rotation and achieving relative stability. Precise reduction of each fragment is not necessary except for intra-articular fractures.

Generally speaking, a longer plate (13–14 hole) should be used in complex and comminuted fractures while a shorter plate (10-hole) could be considered in simple fractures [18]. For adequate fixation of proximal segment, the screws should be wide apart, and engaging 6–8 cortices.

The patient is placed in supine position on a radiolucent operating table. A rolled towel or pillow is put under the knee to correct the extension deformity caused by gastrocnemius (Fig. 10.4).

The surgical approach depends on fracture complexity. For intra-articular fractures, anterolateral parapatellar approach (Fig. 10.5) should be adopted. To reduce intra-articular fragments, large peri-articular reduction clamps can be used. The fragments are reduced anatomically, followed by the insertion of cancellous lag screws at subchondral region to achieve absolute stability and to allow lateral plating over free zone (Figs. 10.6 and 10.7).

For extra-articular fractures, a lateral incision starting from joint line and extend proximally is used. Simple oblique or spiral fractures can be reduced temporarily by reduction forceps (Fig. 10.8a, b) or cerclage wires (Fig. 10.9a–c).

After reduction, a locking plate is inserted through submuscular tunnel between vastus lateralis and periosteum. The plate is fixed temporarily with k-wires. Correct plate placement and

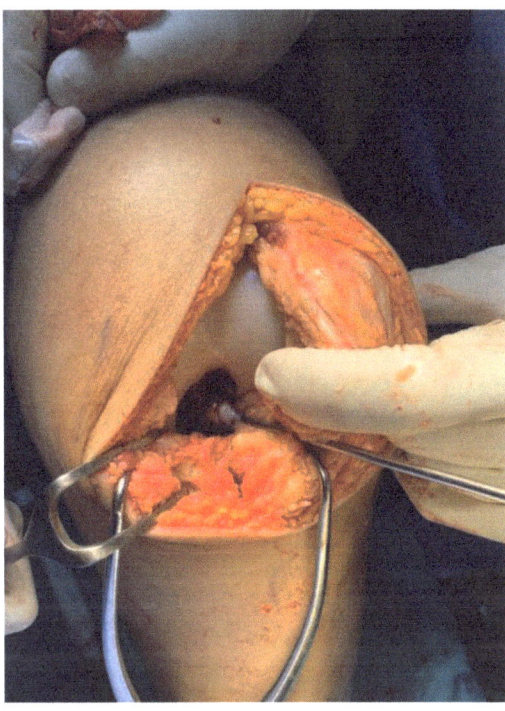

Fig. 10.5 Parapatellar approach to expose the intra-articular fracture

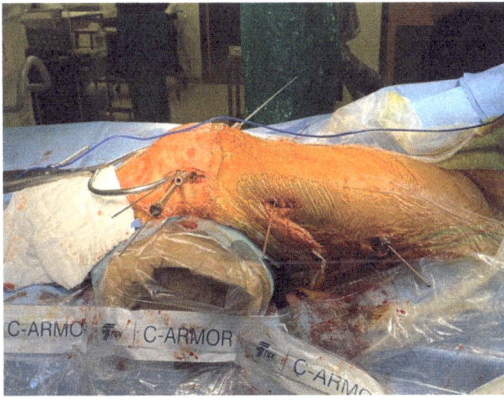

Fig. 10.4 Surgical limb is placed on a support to facilitate reduction of distal fragment

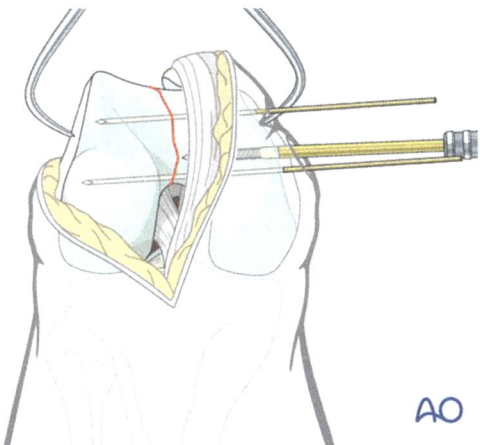

Fig. 10.6 Intra-articular fracture is temporarily reduced by reduction clip and k-wires. (*Copyright by AO Foundation, Switzerland. Source: AO Surgery Reference*, https://surgeryreference.aofoundation.org)

fracture alignment should be confirmed before definitive fixation.

In case of medial supracondylar bone loss, distal transcondylar fractures, medial Hoffa fractures or periprosthetic distal femur fractures, dual plating is advisable to provide a more stable fixation (Fig. 10.10a, b) [19]. Since there is no specific pre-contoured plate for medial side, either a 3.5 or 4.5 mm locking compression plate can be used.

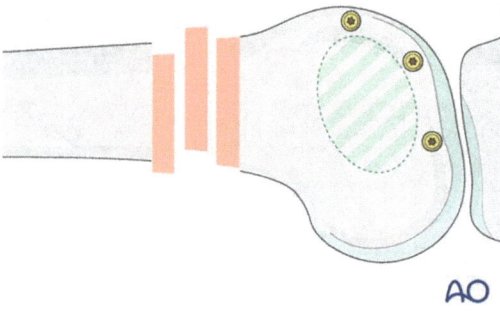

Fig. 10.7 Lag screws are placed subchrondrally. (*Copyright by AO Foundation, Switzerland. Source: AO Surgery Reference*, https://surgeryreference.aofoundation. org)

10.3.2 Surgical Techniques in Intramedullary Nailing

Retrograde nailing is indicated in extra-articular, periprosthetic, and simple intra-articular fractures (33 C1 or C2). The advantages of nailing include smaller wound and preservation of soft tissues and blood supply.

The patient is also placed in supine position on a radiolucent operating table. Medial parapatellar approach is commonly used for nail entry. In case of intra-articular fracture, it should be reduced and fixed before nail insertion. The intra-articular compression screws should be placed over subchondral region to prevent blocking of nail. To reduce the metaphysis, manual traction, femoral distractor, bone hook, or reduction clamp can be used. A guide pin is inserted above the intercondylar notch while preventing injuries of cruciate ligaments. In coronal plane, the guide pin should be inserted in the middle of the intercondylar notch. In sagittal plane, it should be just above the Blumensaat's line. Since the medullary canal is wider in elderly patients, there is a higher chance of fracture malalignment following nail

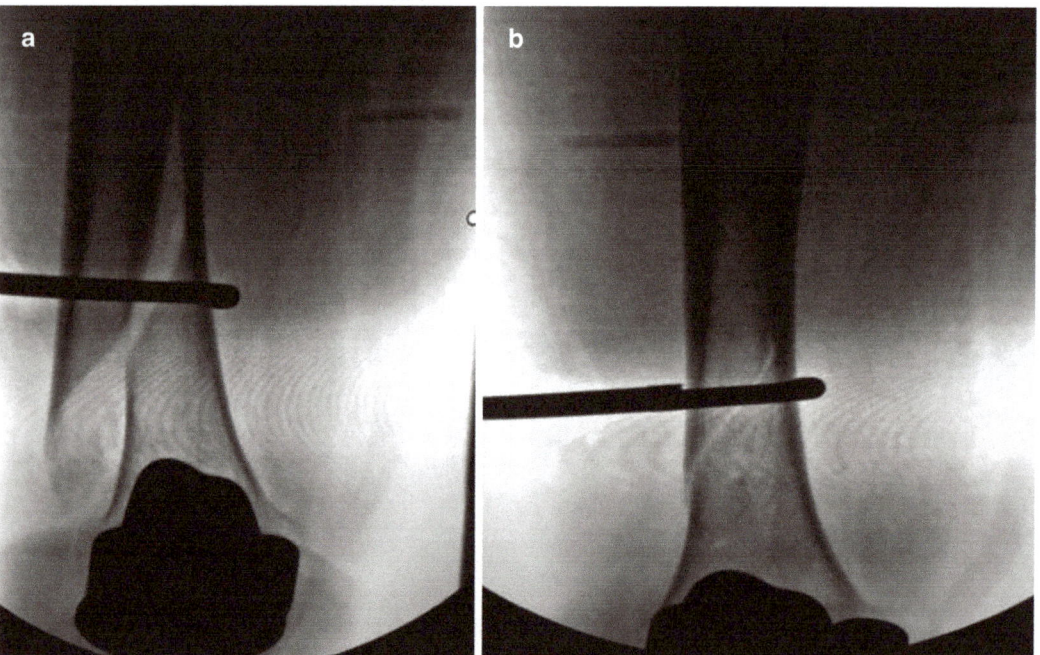

Fig. 10.8 (**a, b**) Distal femur fracture is temporarily reduced with colinear clamp

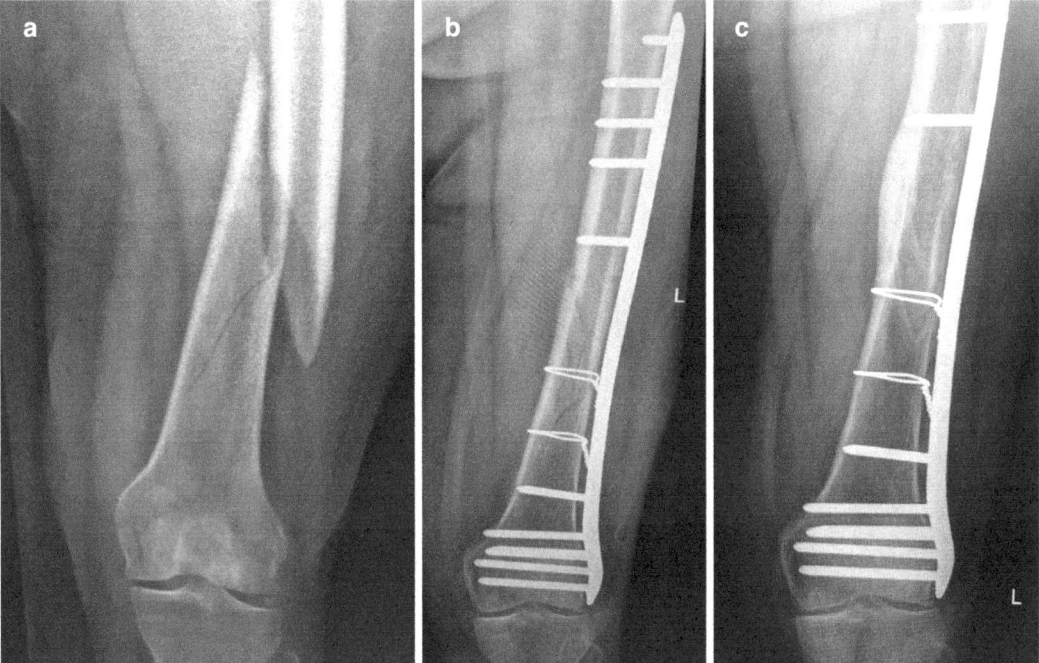

Fig. 10.9 (**a**) Long spiral distal femur fracture. (**b**) The fracture was fixed with cerclage wires and distal femur locking plate. (**c**) The fracture completely healed with good callus at 6 months after surgery

insertion. Before reaming, poller screws or blocking pins placed opposite to the direction of displacement could help to improve the fracture alignment (Fig. 10.11).

During reaming, it should be concentric and slow in speed to avoid damage of cortex and prevent fat extrusion which may result in pulmonary embolism. After reaming, the nail is inserted under traction, which should be advanced gently to avoid inadvertent propagation of fracture line or even iatrogenic fracture especially osteoporotic bones. Alignment is checked again before locking of the nail. It is preferable to perform distal locking via distal aiming device before proximal locking. A spiral blade is recommended for distal locking in extra-articular fracture to improve stability by increasing surface area. Proximal locking is performed by freehand and usually one dynamic screw. Finally, end cap is inserted to prevent any bone ingrowth into the nail and bleeding from medullary cavity.

For nailing of periprosthetic distal femur fractures, it is necessary to check if it is closed box or small open box [20, 21]. During insertion of guide pin, it is better to do an arthrotomy to have a better visualization to avoid the starting point posterior to blumensaat's line, which may damage the posterior cruciate ligament and also causes valgus and extension deformities [22]. Besides, direct visualization through arthrotomy can avoid damage of insert during nail insertion. The length of nail should be long enough to the level of lesser trochanter.

10.3.3 Surgical Techniques in Hoffa Fracture

The aim of surgery for Hoffa fracture is anatomical reduction with rigid fixation.

For surgical approach, it depends on the fracture pattern and complexity. A lateral or lateral parapatellar approach is used for lateral Hoffa while for medial fractures, a medial or medial parapatellar approach should be used. The knee is flexed for better exposure. Joystick technique

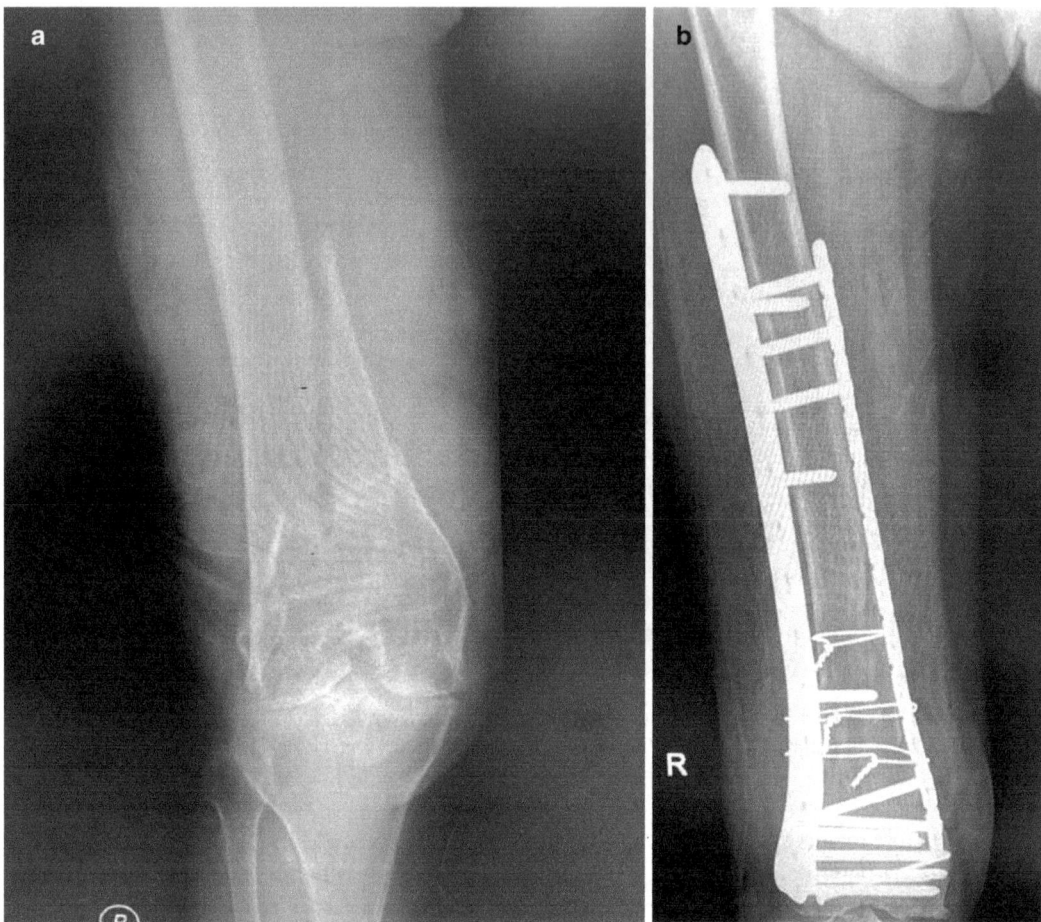

Fig. 10.10 (**a, b**) Comminuted distal femur fracture fixed by cerclage wires and dual plating. 4.5 mm locking compression plate used as buttress plate over medial side

is useful in controlling the small posterior fragment (Fig. 10.12). After reduction, two K-wires are inserted in anteroposterior direction to fix the fracture temporarily. Then two 3.5 mm cannulated screws are inserted in anteroposterior direction. Depending on the fragment size, larger screws can also be used. Both screws should be counter-sunk to avoid the screw heads above the articular surface.

In case of comminuted fractures or very osteoporotic bones, a plate should be added for further augmentation. A lateral or medial anti-glide plate has a greater anti-shearing strength and better structural support [23, 24]. A reverse contralateral proximal tibial plate can also be used for fixation (Figs. 10.13a, b and 10.14a, b) [25].

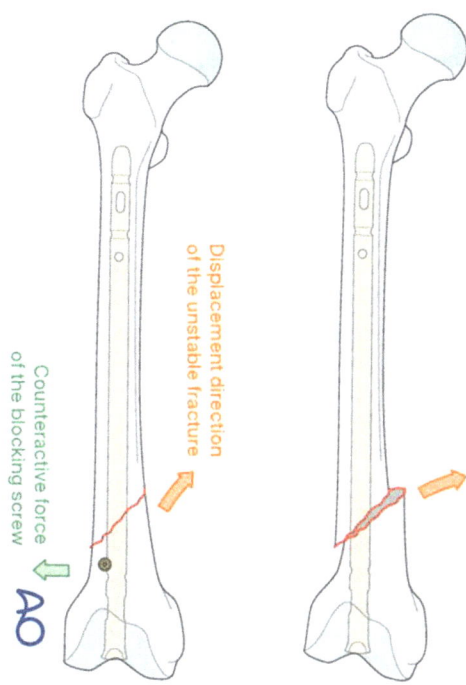

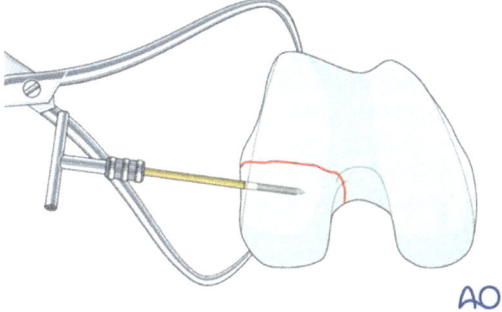

Fig. 10.12 A joystick technique is applied to hold the distal fragment and the fracture is temporarily reduced by pointed reduction. (*Copyright by AO Foundation, Switzerland. Source: AO Surgery Reference*, https://surgeryreference.aofoundation.org)

Fig. 10.11 Placement of poller screw opposite to the direction of displacement can counteract the force. (*Copyright by AO Foundation, Switzerland. Source: AO Surgery Reference*, https://surgeryreference.aofoundation.org)

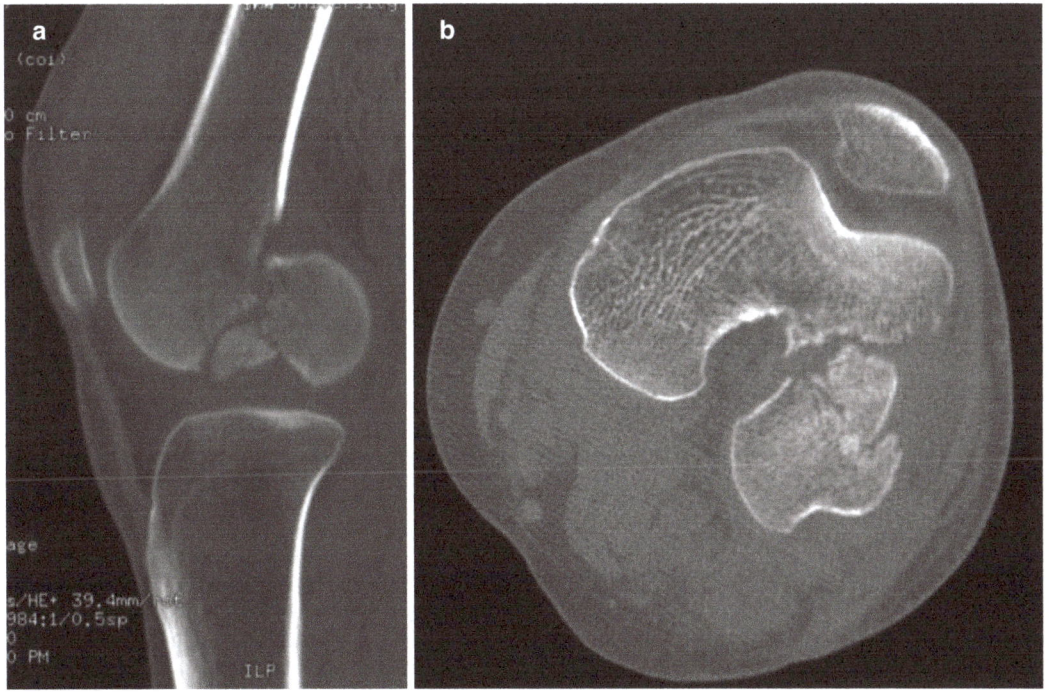

Fig. 10.13 (**a**, **b**) Showing lateral Hoffa fracture with comminution

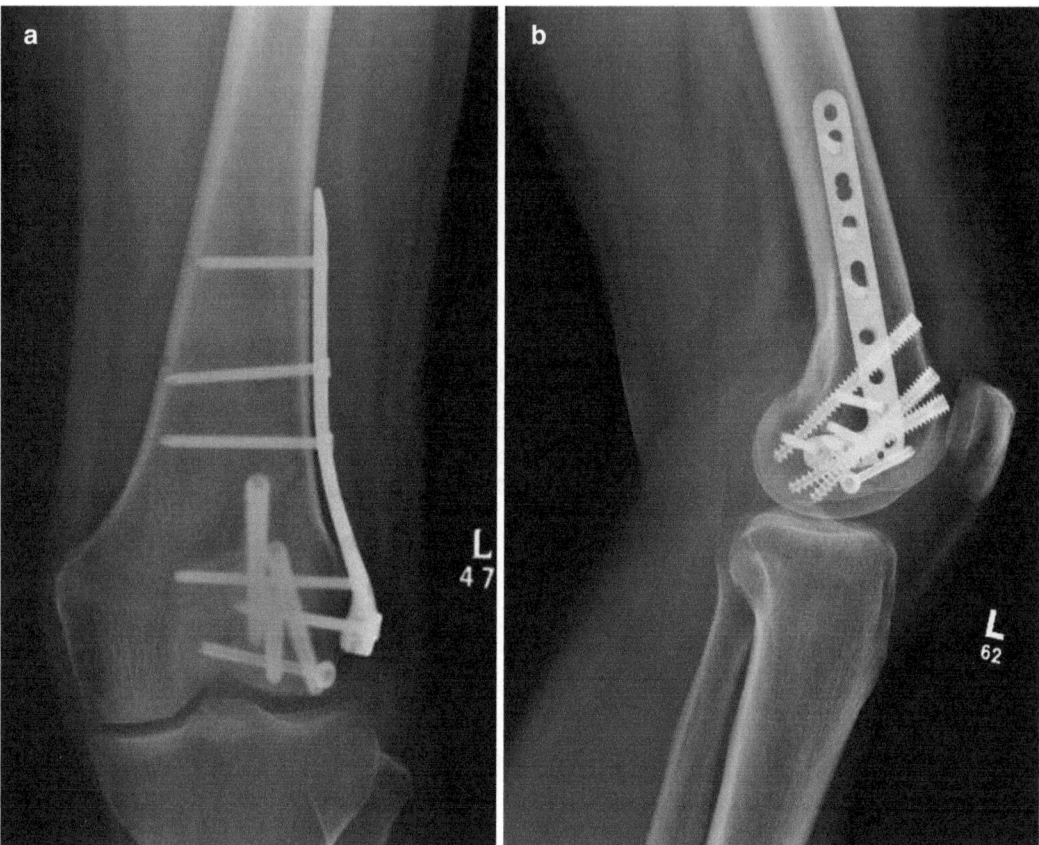

Fig. 10.14 (**a**, **b**) Showing the fracture fixed with headless screw and augmented with contralateral proximal tibial plate

10.4 Rehabilitation After Osteosynthesis of Distal Femur Fractures and Periprosthetic Fractures

After stable fixation, active and passive mobilization of affected knee should be started immediately. In general, early weight bearing should be started once the patient starts to recover the surgery, usually in a few days' time.

References

1. Myers P, Laboe P, Johnson KJ, Fredericks PD, Crichlow RJ, Maar DC, et al. Patient mortality in geriatric distal femur fractures. J Orthop Trauma. 2018;32(3):111–5.
2. Butt MS, Krikler SJ, Ali MS. Displaced fractures of the distal femur in elderly patients: operative versus non-operative treatment. J Bone Joint Surg Br. 1996;78:110–4.
3. Dunlop DG, Brenkel IJ. The supracondylar intramedullary nail elderly patients with distal femoral fractures. Injury. 1999;30:475–84.
4. Athar SM, Fazal MA, Hassan M, Ashwood N. Distal femoral fractures in the elderly: does early treatment with locking plates reduce mortality rates? Clin Res Open Access. 2017;3(1)
5. Ehlinger M, Ducrot G, Adam P, Bonnomet F. Distal femur fractures. Surgical techniques and a review of the literature. Orthop Traumatol Surg Res. 2013;99(3):3, 53–60.
6. Gavaskar AS, Tummala NC, Krishnamurthy M. Operative management Hoffa fractures—a prospective review of 18 patients. Injury. 2011;42:1495–8.
7. Hill BW, Cannada LK. Hoffa fragments in the geriatric distal femur fracture: myth or reality. Geriatr Orthop Surg Rehabil. 2017;8(4):252.
8. Figgie MP, Goldberg VM, Figgie HE 3rd, Sobel M. The results of treatment of supracondylar fracture above total knee arthroplasty. J Arthroplasty. 1990;5:267–76.

9. Rorabeck CH, Taylor JW. Periprosthetic fractures of the femur complicating total knee arthroplasty. Orthop Clin North Am. 1999;30:265–77.

10. Rorabeck CH, Taylor JW. Classification of periprosthetic fractures complicating total knee arthroplasty. Orthop Clin North Am. 1999;30:209–14.

11. Ha CW, Shon OJ, Lim SW, Park KH. Minimally invasive plate osteosynthesis for periprosthetic distal femoral fractures after total knee arthroplasty. Knee Surg Relat Res. 2014;26:27–32.

12. Letenneur J, Labour PE, Rogez JM, et al. Hoffa's fractures. Report of 20 cases [in French]. Ann Chir. 1978;32:213–9.

13. Jiang Y, Wang Z, Zhang D, Gu G. Twenty-seven-year nonunion of a Hoffa fracture in a 46-year-old patient. Chin J Traumatol. 2015;18:54–8.

14. McDonough PW, Bernstein RM. Nonunion of a Hoffa fracture in a child. J Orthop Trauma. 2000;14:519–21.

15. Ozturk A, Ozkan Y, Ozdemir RM. Nonunion of a Hoffa fracture in an adult. Chir Organi Mov. 2009;93:183–5.

16. Hoffmann MF, Jones CB, Sietsema DL, Koenig SJ, Tornetta P 3rd. Outcome of periprosthetic distal femoral fractures following knee arthroplasty. Injury. 2012;43:1084–9.

17. Giddie J, Sawalha S, Parker M. Retrograde nailing for distal femur fractures in the elderly. SICOT J. 2015;1:31.

18. Stoffel K, Dieter U, Stachowiak G, et al. Biomechanical testing of the LCP- how can stability in locked internal fixators be controlled? Injury. 2003;34(Suppl 2):B11–9.

19. Sain A, Sharma V, Farooque K, et al. Dual plating of the distal femur: indications and surgical techniques. Cureus. 2019;11(12):e6483. https://doi.org/10.7759/cureus.6483.

20. Lombardo DJ, Siljander MP, Sobh A, Moore DD, Karadsheh MS. Periprosthetic fractures about total knee arthroplasty. Musculoskelet Surg. 2020;104(2):135–43. https://doi.org/10.1007/s12306-019-00628-9.

21. Shah JK, Szukics P, Gianakos AL, Liporace FA, Yoon RS. Equivalent union rates between intramedullary nail and locked plate fixation for distal femur periprosthetic fractures—a systematic review. Injury. 2020;51(4):1062–8. https://doi.org/10.1016/j.injury.2020.02.043.

22. Service B, Kang W, Turnbull N, Langford J, Haidukewych G, Koval K. Influence if femoral component design on retrograde nail starting point. J Orthop Trauma. 2015;29:380–4.

23. Sun H, He QF, Huang YG, et al. Plate fixation for Letenneur type I Hoffa fracture: a biomechanical study. Injury. 2017;48:1492–8.

24. Singh AP, Dhammi IK, Vaishya R, et al. Nonunion of coronal shear fracture of femoral condyle. Chin J Traumatol. 2011;14:143–6.

25. Liu ZH, Wang T, Fang C, Wong TM, Lin LL, Wang X, Leung F. Reverse contralateral proximal tibial plating and cannulated screws fixation for Hoffa fracture: a case report. Trauma Case Rep. 2021;32:100443.

Proximal Tibial Fractures

11

Christian Fang

11.1 Introduction

Proximal tibial fractures consist of 8% of all fractures in the elderly. The mechanism of injury is commonly lower energy in simple falls while ambulatory patients with higher energy mechanisms in motor vehicle and cycling accidents are also common. High energy related soft tissue conditions are rarer yet challenging to handle. Because of osteoporosis and bone metabolic disorders, articular depression and sizable cancellous defects are common. Medical comorbidities and coexisting osteoarthritis impose unique management challenges. The recovery of elderly patients is critically affected by comorbidities. Mobilization regimens favour early weight bearing. Prolonged immobilization in the elderly is associated with deconditioning and medical complications such as pressure sores, chest and urinary tract infections, loss of muscle mass, and contractures and should be avoided.

The mechanism of injury is a combination of varus or valgus force combined with axial loading at various degrees of knee flexion. With knee extension, valgus, axial impaction, and hyperextension causes the larger anterior femoral condyles to impact on the anterior plateau, causing the typical anterolateral split depression pattern.

With knee flexion, rollback of the condyles means that the contact point is located more posteriorly, therefore posterior plateau depression and shear fracture occur. On the other hand, greater axial loading energy and weaker bone lead to increased probability of bicondylar involvement.

11.2 Initial Assessment

The initial assessment must take into consideration the patient as a whole. Detailed history taking and physical examination are mandatory and associated injuries are excluded. Comorbidities, the use of antiplatelets and anticoagulants will complicate treatment. Diabetes, malnutrition, and peripheral vascular diseases are common factors causing wound complications.

In addition to standard anteroposterior and lateral radiographs, a CT scan is invaluable in the initial assessment of proximal tibial fractures. Multiplanar and 3D reformatting of CT scans are modern methods which provide critical information concerning the fracture pattern and allow better decision-making. 3D printing is a modern technique valuable for intuitive assessment of complex articular fracture patterns.

The useful classifications of intraarticular proximal tibial fractures are the updated AO/OTA system and the Schatzker systems. The original Schatzker classification [1] is popular for tibial

C. Fang (✉)
Department of Orthopaedics and Traumatology,
Queen Mary Hospital, The University of Hong Kong,
Pokfulam, Hong Kong

plateau fractures based on 2D radiographs and is still widely used for communication and decision-making. The updated AO/OTA system adopted from Chang [2] considers the 3D fracture morphology under CT assessment and divides the proximal tibia is divided into four columns [3]: The anterolateral (AL), posterolateral (PL), anteromedial (AM) and posterolateral (PL). An updated 3D/CT-based Schatzker classification [4] (Fig. 11.1) with anterior (A) and posterior (P) modifiers was recently proposed. A drawback for the above classifications is that they only describe the fracture location and do not take into account the degree of fracture displacement and comminution which is a significant decision-making factor.

Anterolateral (AL) column split depression is the commonest pattern, occurring in more than half of elderly patients, followed by multi-column patterns involving the posterolateral (PL) column and posteromedial (PM) column. Poor prognostic features include fracture-dislocations, pre-existing osteoarthritis, and multiple column involvement (Fig. 11.2).

11.2.1 Non-Operative Treatment

Undisplaced fractures and minimally displaced fractures (<3 mm) with no significant deviation in the lower limb mechanical alignment can be managed nonoperatively in a well-padded long leg plaster cylinder and the patient can start protected weight bearing. Elderly patients are less tolerant to immobilization and pressure ulcers may occur at prominent areas of the knee such as the fibula head, the patella, tibial tuberosity, and the Gerdy's tubercle. On the other hand, patients with undisplaced but mechanically unstable patterns at the metaphysis may benefit from minimal invasive osteosynthesis and early mobilization.

11.2.2 Operative Treatment Planning

Proximal tibial fractures have a highly variable fracture patterns and multiple surgical approaches can be used. The objective is to anatomically restore the mechanical axis and provide sufficient mechanical stability for early mobilization. The

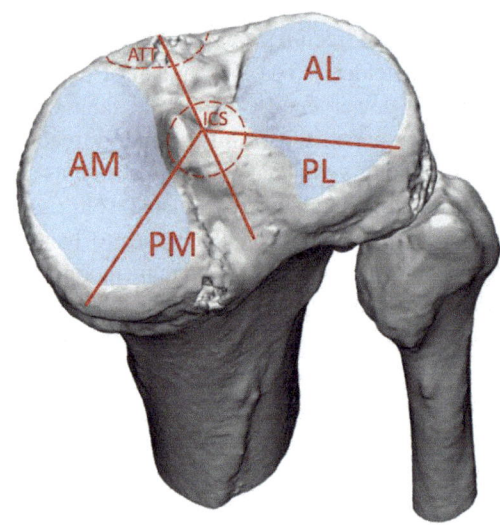

Fig. 11.2 Updated AO/OTA 4-column classification system with modifiers for four columns and two special zones. *AM* anteromedial, *PL* posteromedial, *AL* anterolateral, *PL* posterolateral, *ICS* intercondylar spine, *ATT* anterior tibial tuberosity

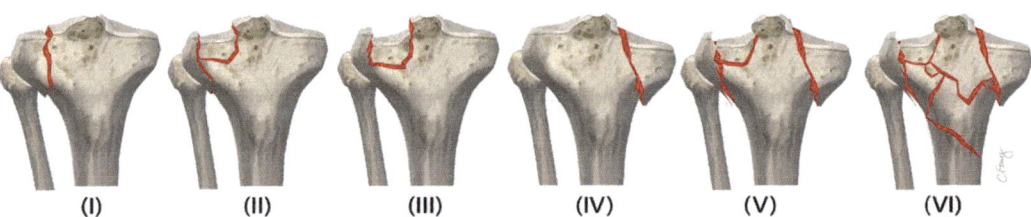

Fig. 11.1 [4] Schatzker classification of tibial plateau fracture types: I, lateral plateau split wedge; II, lateral plateau split wedge depression; III, lateral plateau pure depression; IV, medial plateau split wedge; V, bicondylar fracture with continuity between epiphysis and diaphysis; VI, bicondylar fracture with complete metaphyseal dissociation

treatment is more straightforward for extraarticular fractures. For intraarticular fractures, the main objective is to restore articular congruity, yet perfect restoration of the articular surface may not be possible in patients with severely comminuted articular depressions.

For geriatric patients with knee osteoarthritis, special considerations should be taken into account for the overall limb mechanical axis and articular surface status. Patients with pre-existing varus may well tolerate a depressed lateral plateau provided there are no significant steps or gaps. On the other hand, those with a non-reconstructable subchondral depression of the weight bearing medial side have good outcomes with immediate total knee arthroplasty (TKA).

11.2.3 Soft Tissue Handling

Higher energy trauma is associated with severe soft tissue problems in the proximal tibia. The thin tissue envelope is at risk of developing blisters and ulcerations. Compartment syndrome is common in high energy proximal tibial fractures. Patients who are on antiplatelet therapy and anticoagulants are at higher risk of significant subcutaneous ecchymosis. A high index of suspicion is necessary for its timely detection and decision for fasciotomy. Open fractures of the proximal tibia are managed in the same principle as younger adults although elderly patients are at a much higher risk of treatment failure and severe complications. Prophylactic antibiotics, early wound closure, and soft tissue coverage are effective means in preventing infections.

Wound complications are more common when incisions are placed over areas of poor soft tissue. Parallel surgical incisions should be placed at least 5–7 cm apart to avoid necrosis of the intermediate skin bridge. Haemorrhagic blisters and lesions with complete skin loss are absolute contraindications to the placement of implants underneath. Surgery may be delayed for up to 2 weeks for the swelling and soft tissue to improve. External fixators can be used for temporary maintenance of alignment and stability but have higher risk of loosening in osteoporotic

bone and are generally not well tolerated by the elderly as definitive treatment (Fig. 11.3).

11.2.4 Surgical Approaches

Various surgical approaches have been described for the proximal tibia. The principle of choosing the correct approach is to provide sufficient exposure for both reduction and placement of implants. Careful dissection with the preservation of blood supply to the soft tissue skin flap and periosteum of major bone fragments and avoidance of neurovascular damage is essential. Axial CT assessment of the fracture pattern is almost mandatory in determining the optimal surgical approach. Minimal invasive plate osteosynthesis (MIPO) technique with limited incisions should be used whenever a good reduction can be achieved by closed means. Arthroscopic assessment is applicable to specific fracture patterns which are minimally displaced and do not require extensive visualization for reduction. A list of common approaches are provided in the table below.

Choice of the surgical approach is dictated by the fracture pattern. The objective of the preoperative planning is to select the best approach which provides ease of access for fracture reduction and fixation and at the same time preserving biology to bone and soft tissue. Dual approaches are commonplace for multiple column fractures requiring bicondylar plate fixations. The first approach should be centred towards the most significantly displaced area and where direct fracture reduction and buttress plating can be applied. Periosteal stripping and detachment of the knee capsule is kept to a minimum so that devitalization of the main bone fragments is avoided.

The anterolateral (AL) sub-meniscal approach is the workhorse approach since the AL column is most commonly involved. The articular surface is approached via the sub-meniscal route following the most direct incision. However, the posterior or central articular surfaces may not be well seen in the anterolateral sub-meniscus approach. The thin Iliotibial band and capsular attachments to the Gerdy's tubercle should be preserved as the

Fig. 11.3 An 82-year-old female with Schatzker VI fracture presented with compromised soft tissues and blisters few days after admission. An external fixator and lateral plating was performed. Negative pressure dressing was applied to the wounds. With improved soft tissue conditions, completion of the fixation with medial plating using multiple small wounds was later performed

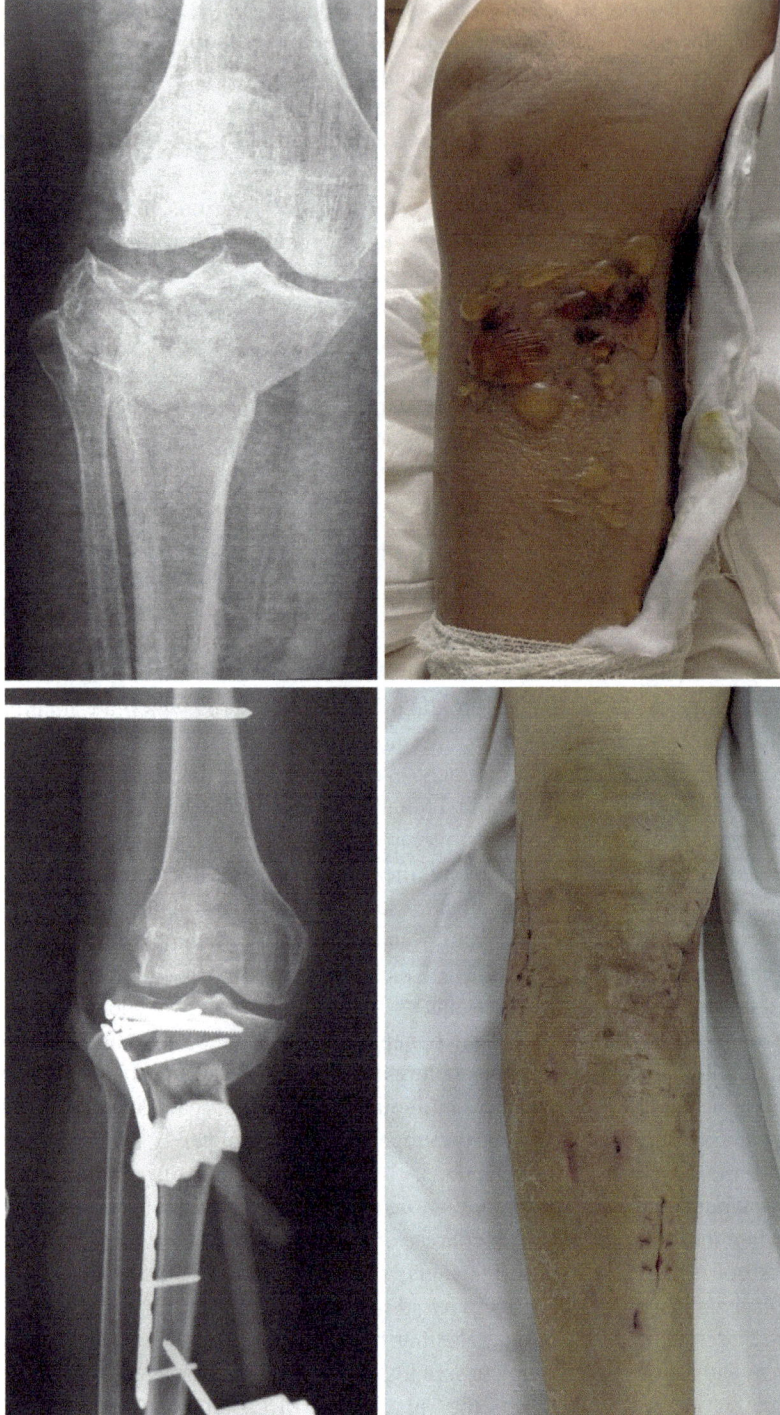

blood supply to the anterolateral fragment is maintained where the implant may be directly placed on. Moreover, detachment of this thin layer of soft tissue is often irreparable and does not help in reducing anterolateral implant prominence.

Posterolateral (PL) column depressed fractures are notoriously difficult to be approached. Improperly reduced PL fractures are associated with posterolateral subluxation of the knee and impaired long-term outcomes. The surgeon should be familiar with various approaches to the PL zone. The three useful techniques are the direct posterolateral approach behind the biceps femoris and common peroneal nerve [5], fibula neck osteotomy approach [6] and lateralized variation of the AL approach carried towards the posterolateral corner [7].

Variations of medial approaches are directed strategically to the injured AM and PM regions which require reduction and fixation efforts. The subcutaneous location of AM and PM regions has only thin, soft tissue coverage therefore incisions should be placed away from blisters and areas of doubtful skin viability. The pes anserinus tendons may interfere with medial plating and can be either tenotomized, plated on, or plated under which there are no clinical studies to demonstrate the effect of each different approach. A posteromedial approach [8] centred at the interval between the medial gastrocnemius medial hamstrings with the dissection carried subperiosteally under the soleus and popliteus muscles is useful for the reduction and buttressing of central posterior sheer fragments, without the need to expose the popliteal and tibial neurovascular structures.

Arthroscopic assisted reduction and fixation can minimize soft tissue trauma. This method is particularly valuable for assessment of articular splits and steps at the central or posterior plateau and for avulsion fractures of the cruciate ligaments which are not adequately assessed submeniscally. Additionally, the meniscus, the cruciate ligaments and the articular cartilage status can be accurately examined despite their role being less important in the elderly. In the author's experience, the continuous use of arthroscopy during fracture fixation is less practical as the equipment blocks articular reduction and interferes with fixation equipment and fluoroscopy. There is some risk of fluid extravasation and compartment syndrome with prolonged procedure. Hence, simple fractures with minimal comminution and a grossly intact articular rim are the best candidates for arthroscopic fixation [9] (Figs. 11.4, 11.5, 11.6, 11.7, 11.8, 11.9 and 11.10).

	Approach	Interval between	Indications	Pitfalls and dangers
Lateral	Anterolateral	Iliotibial band (ITB) and lateral joint capsule (sub-meniscal)	Anterolateral / lateral split and split depression	Complete detachment of soft tissue and devascularization of the lateral fragment. Wound breakdown in compromised skin.
	Direct lateral / para-LCL	ITB and lateral collateral ligament (LCL)	Posterolateral split and depression	Detachment of LCL with associated laxity, common peroneal nerve
	Fibula osteotomy	Common peroneal nerve and ITB (reflexion of biceps femoris and LCL)	Posterolateral metaphyseal buttressing plate and large depression	Common peroneal nerve and its branches. Anterior tibial artery. Posterolateral laxity with osteotomy non-union.
	Posterolateral	Common peroneal nerve and biceps femoris	Posterolateral split and depression	Common peroneal nerve, popliteal anterior tibial artery, and peroneal artery. LCL
Posterior	Direct Posterior	Neurovascular bundle and medial or lateral gastrocnemius head	Midline posterior shear and Posterior cruciate ligament (PCL) avulsions	Popliteal neurovascular bundle. Medial and lateral cutaneous sural nerves.
Medial	Posteromedial	Between medial head of gastrocnemius and soleus. Deep detachment of popliteus muscle insertion	Posteromedial / posterior split and depressions.	Saphenous nerve. Pes anserinus and medial gastrocnemius may need partial detachment
	Medial / anteromedial	Directly at Subcutaneous medial tibia	Anteromedial / medial tibial split and depressions	Saphenous nerve. Thin soft tissue envelope, wound breakdown in compromised skin.
Special	Parapatellar	Patella tendon and MCL	Large ACL intercondylar spine avulsion fractures	Skin bridge necrosis over anterior patella when too narrow
	Minimal invasive / percutaneous	Following anteromedial and anterolateral approaches	Various, closed reducible fractures or minimally displaced fractures	As above, depending on locations
	Arthroscopic	Standard anteromedial and anterolateral portals	ACL avulsions, simple and minimally displaced posterior column medial or lateral fractures	Difficulty in reduction of complex patterns, difficulty in visualizing anterior half of plateau

Fig. 11.4 Various surgical approaches to the tibial plateau

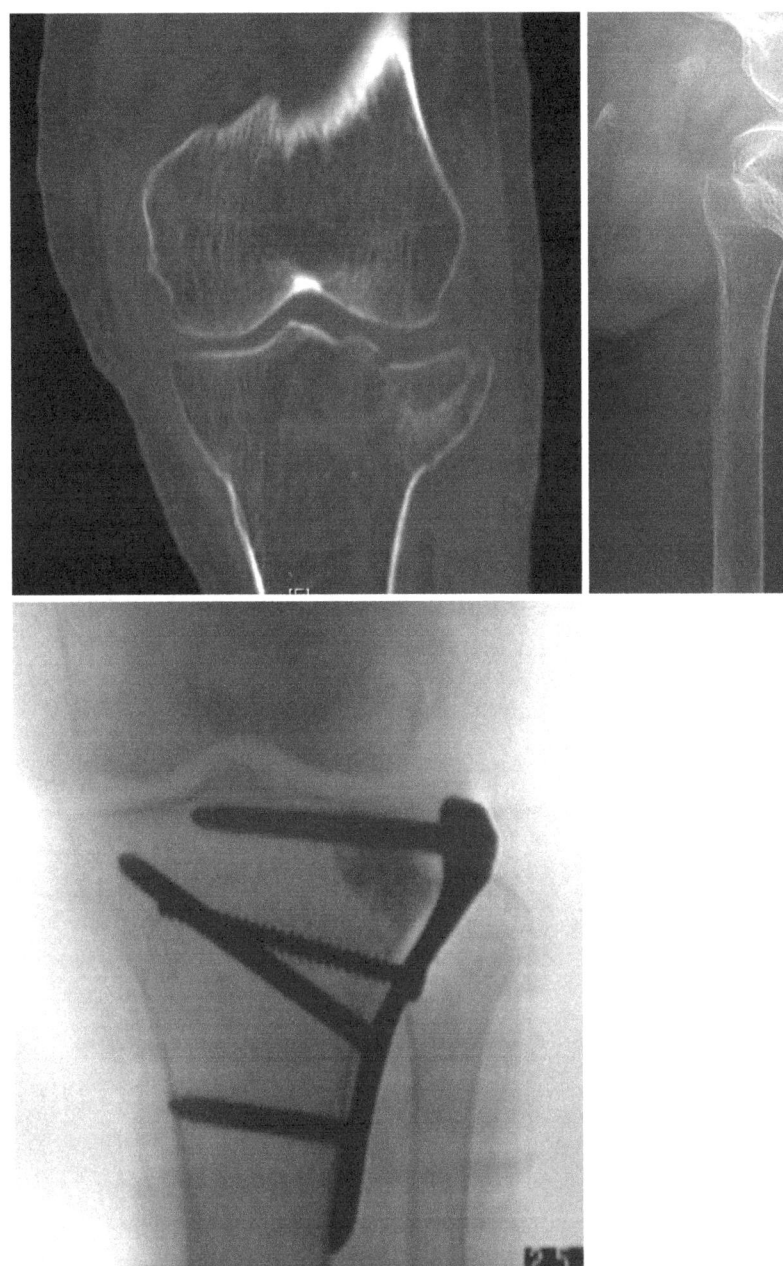

Fig. 11.5 A 100-year-old lady with internal fixation of a Schatzker II fracture. Tricalcium phosphate bone substitute is useful in providing intraoperative mechanical support to the depressed anterolateral fragment before subchondral placement of raft screws. Angle stable lateral buttressing plate provides sufficient stability for immediate postoperative weight bearing exercises

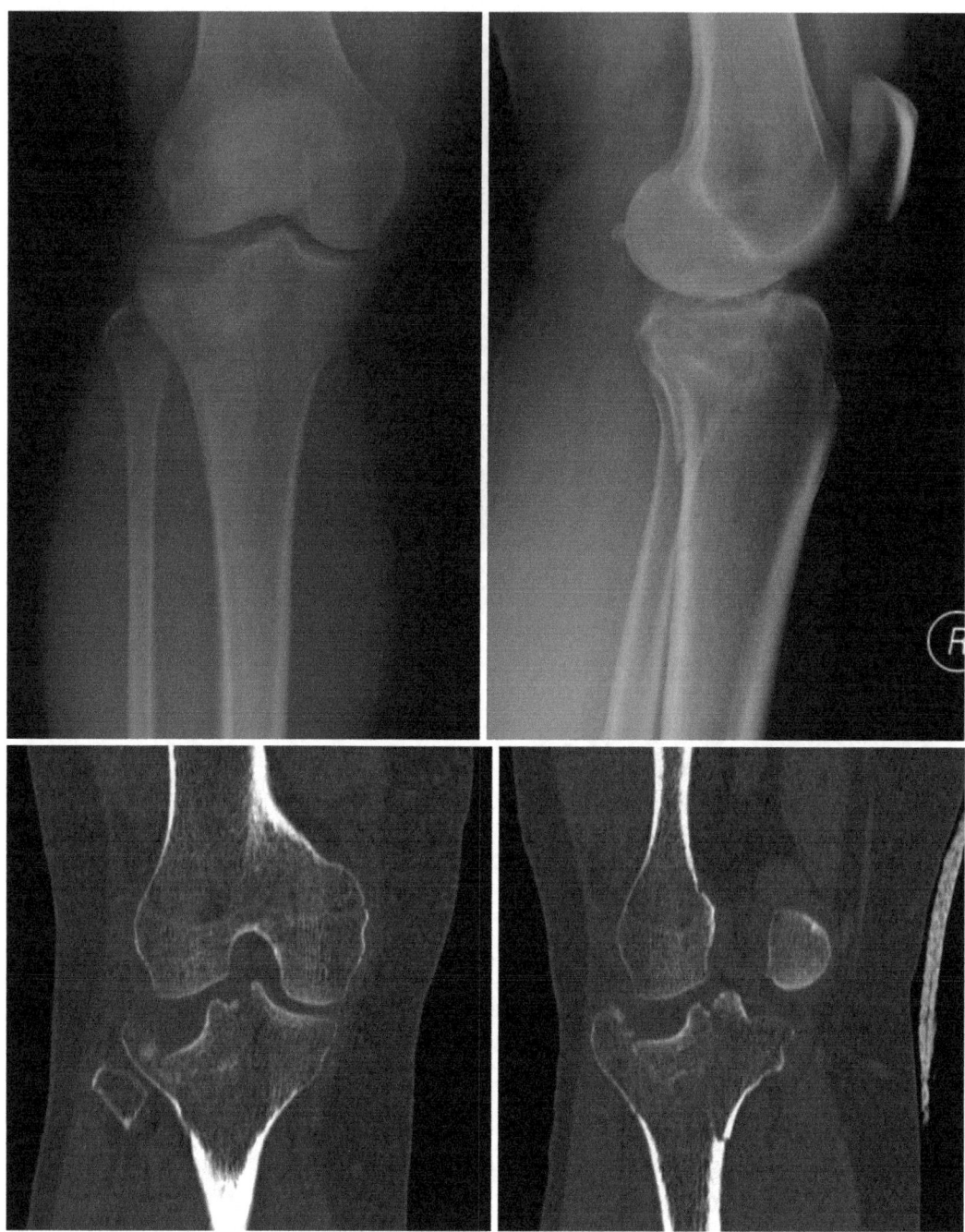

Fig. 11.6 A 77-year-old patient with Schatzker V fracture with posteromedial split and posterolateral depression. Detailed preoperative planning maximizing the use of CT data with multiplanar reformatting (MPR) and 3D reformatting plus the use of a 3D printed bone model to enhance tactile planning. Bicondylar plating is performed. Fixation is first carried out posteromedial with buttress plate. This is followed by direct lateral sub-meniscal incision and elevation of the sunken lateral posterior surface which is stabilized by raft screws and a locking plate. Postoperative weight bearing is encouraged. The patient is walking unaided and pain free at 3 months with no collapse of the fracture site

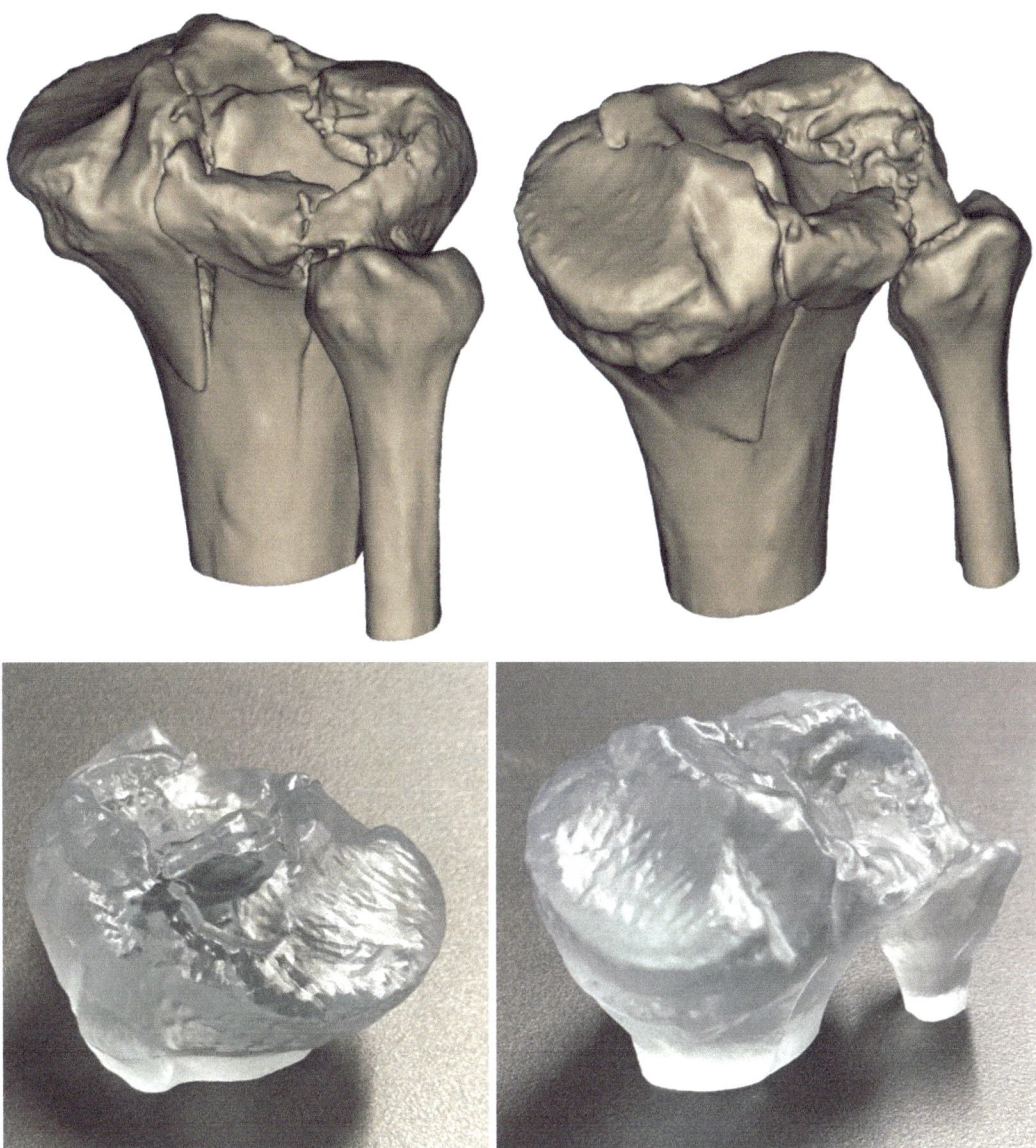

Fig. 11.6 (continued)

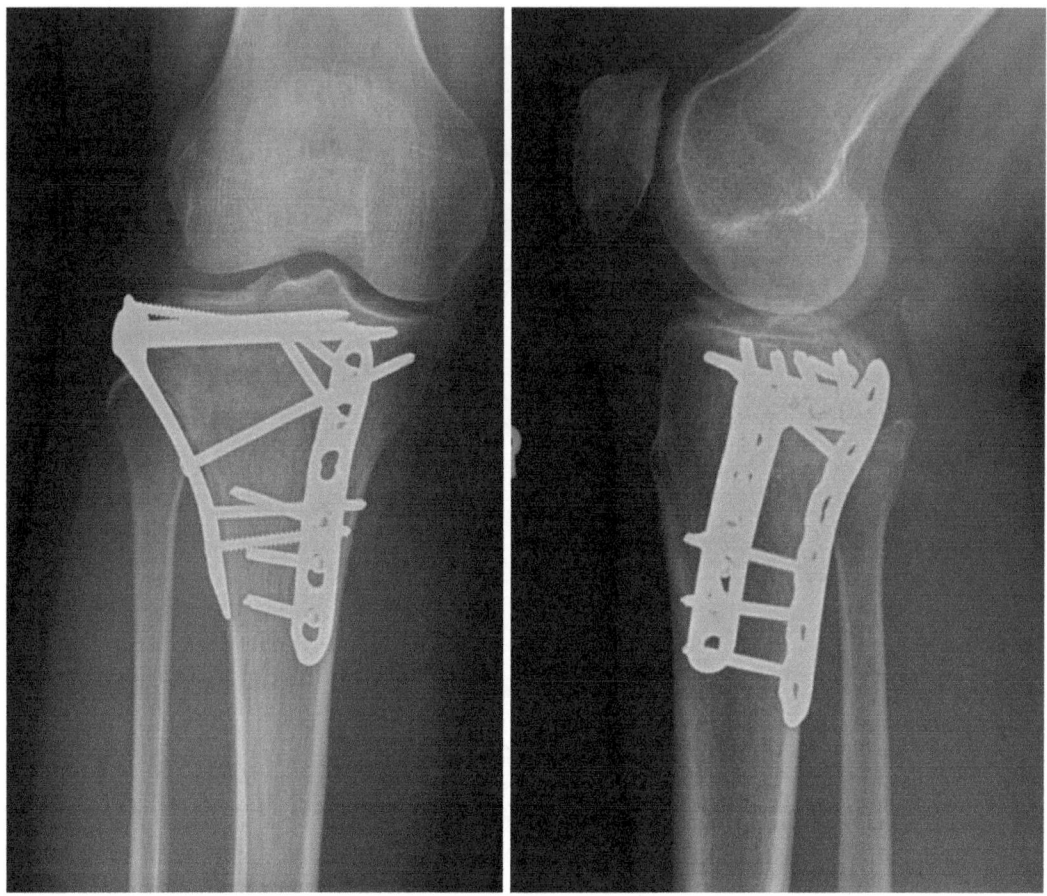

Fig. 11.6 (continued)

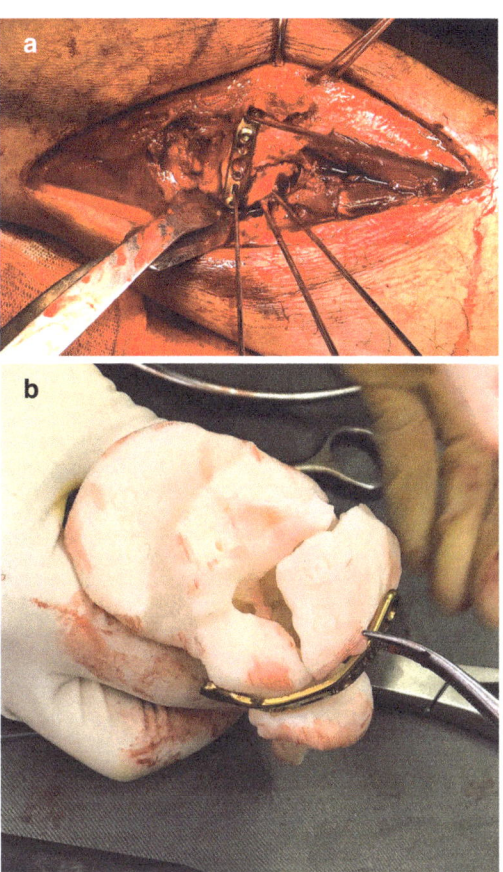

Fig. 11.7 (**a**) Direct lateral approach to the tibial plateau. The posterolateral rim is visualized. A Hohmann retractor can be placed anterior to the fibula, protecting the LCL and the common peroneal nerve while exposing the posterolateral corner of the plateau. A horizontal 2.7 mm rim plate is placed around the posterolateral corner. (**b**) A 3D printed model us useful to precisely contour the rim plate

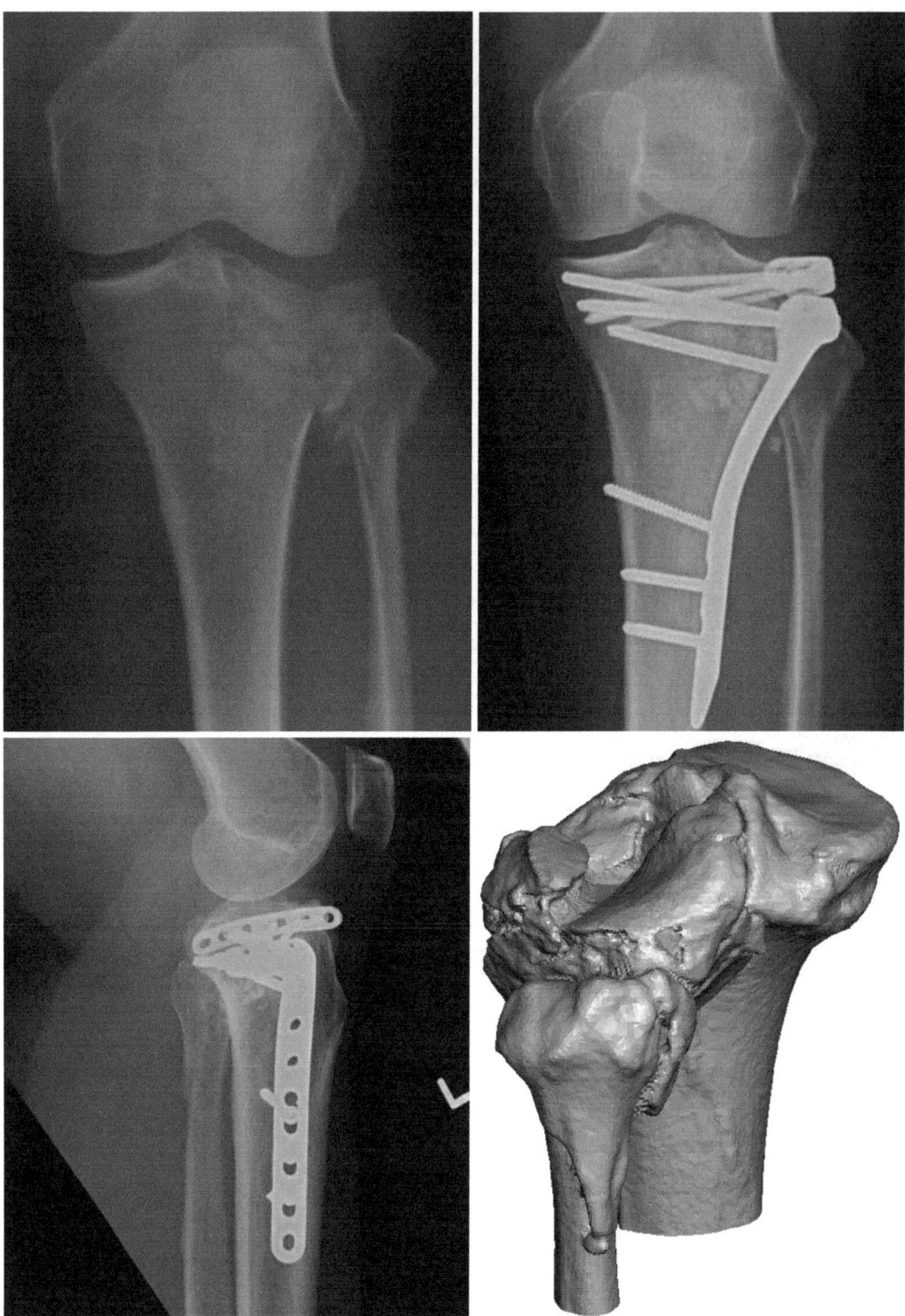

Fig. 11.8 A 68-year-old patient with lateral plateau split depression type injury. There is significant comminution and depression of the posterolateral aspect. Rim plating with an additional 2.7 mm plate deep to the LCL, cranial to the standard 3.5 mm anterolateral plate provides additional buttressing stability around the posterolateral aspect for early mobilization

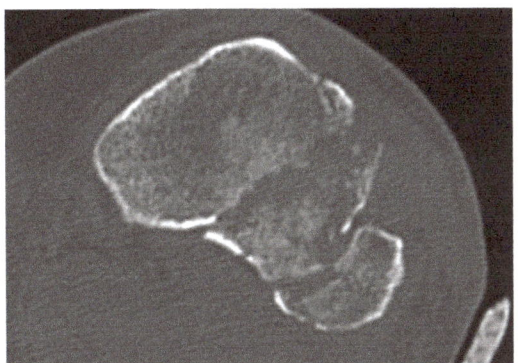

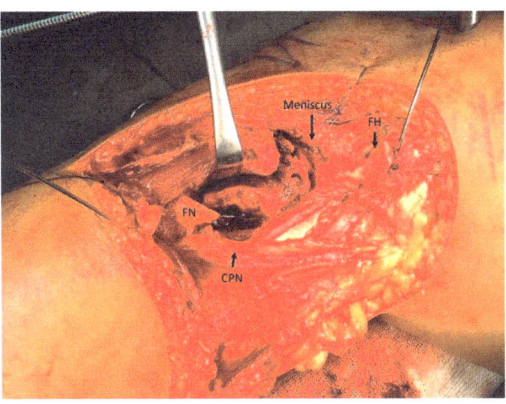

Fig. 11.9 Visualization of the posterolateral tibial plateau via fibula neck (FN) osteotomy. The fibula head (FH) remains attached to the LCL and the biceps femoris and mobilized cranially and temporarily pinned to the lateral femoral epicondyle using a K wire. The common peroneal nerve (CPN) is released and viewed along its course around the fibula neck. A temporary suture is used to elevate the meniscus. This provides excellent view of the posterolateral plateau and metaphysis

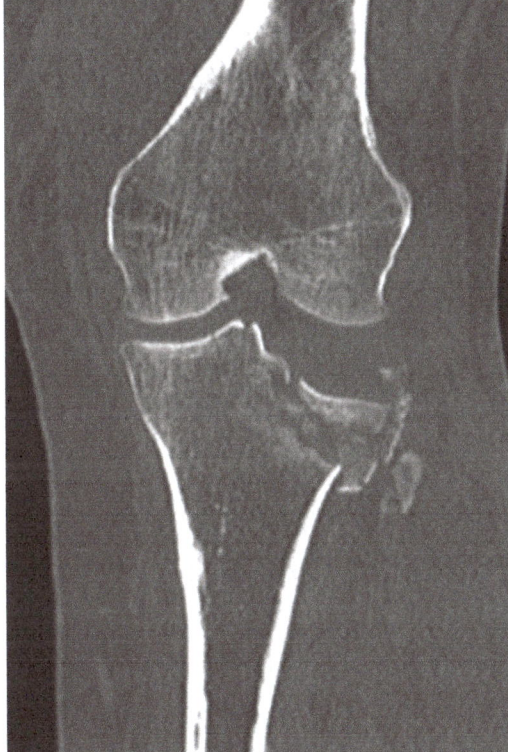

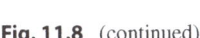

Fig. 11.8 (continued)

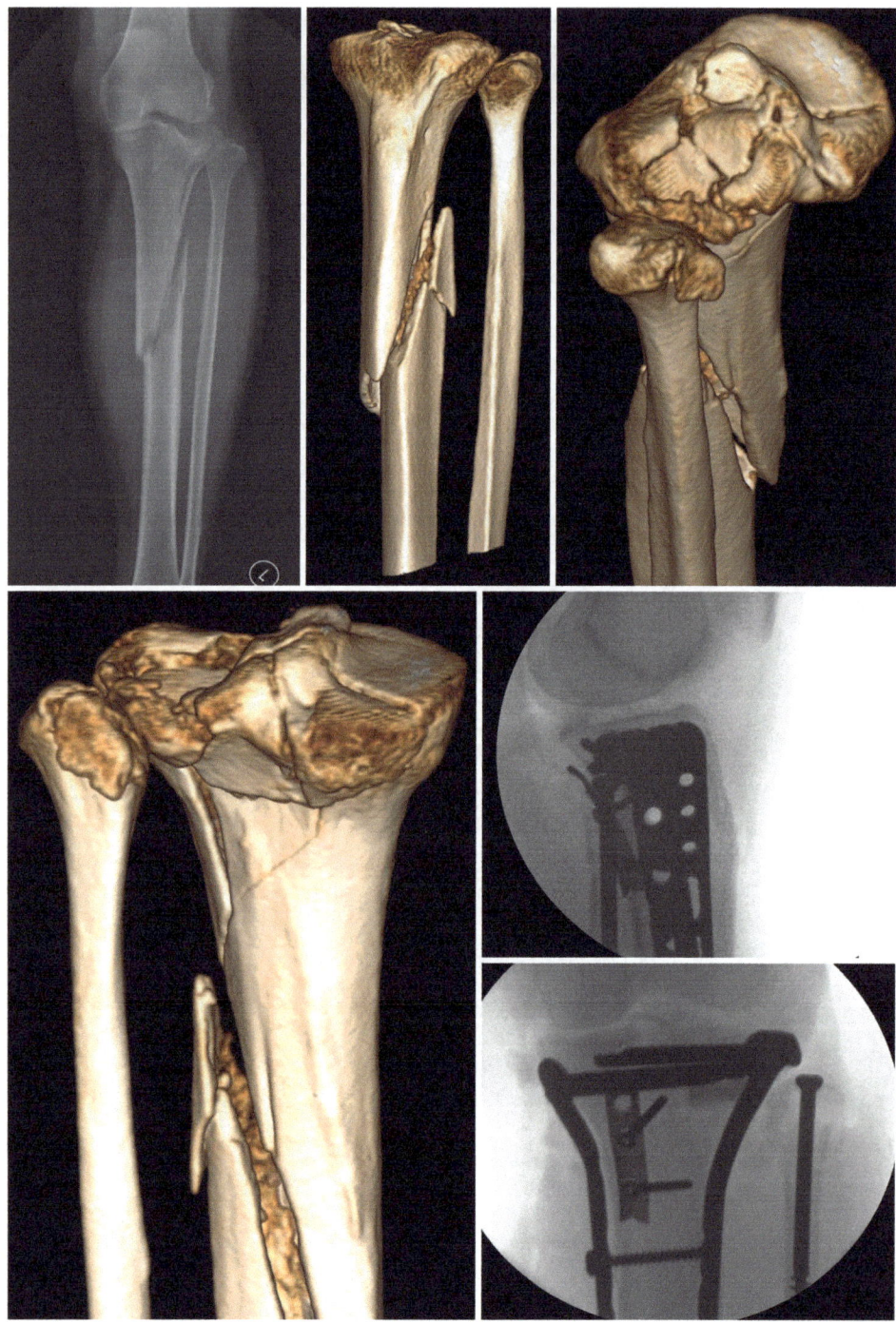

Fig. 11.10 A 65-year-old patient with Schatzker VI fracture, posterolateral and posteromedial plateau involvement with a long metaphyseal fragment. A fibula osteotomy approach is used for the posterolateral plateau reduction. A posteromedial approach with small buttressing reduction plate and a long spanning locking plates extending to the tibial shaft distally. Satisfactory reduction and healing are obtained. Achieving anatomical reduction via such extensive approaches requires attention to the soft tissue status and should be reserved for physically fit elderlies with higher physical demand and good bone quality

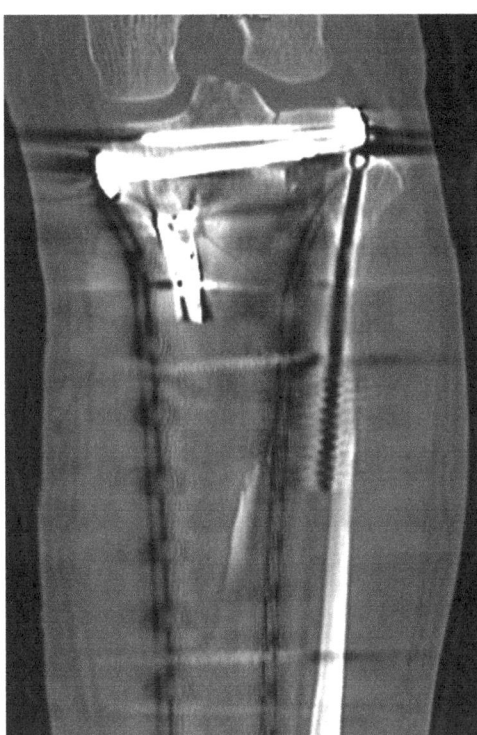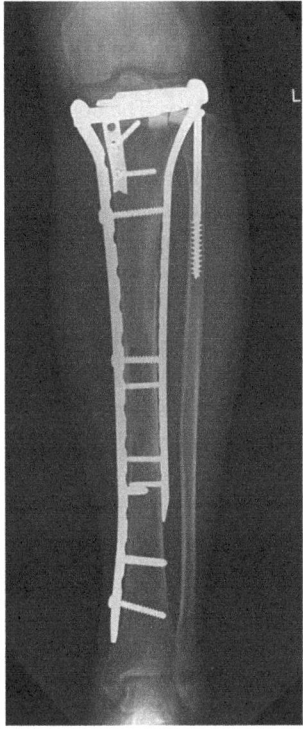

Fig. 11.10 (continued)

11.3 Plate Fixation

The objective of open reduction and internal fixation (ORIF) is to restore articular congruity, correct lower limb mechanical axis and rotation. This is the most common method of treatment for proximal tibial intraarticular fractures. Modern anatomically pre-contoured, angle stable 3.5 mm or 4.5 mm locking plate systems are available. A secure bi-columnar angularly stable fixation can allow patients to mobilize their knee throughout the physiological range of motion immediately following surgery.

The four operative steps are articular reconstruction, bone void filling, articular rim containment, and stabilization of the metaphyseal extension. The first part of surgery is to restore the articular surface. The reduction of the articular surface can be done through the articular fracture itself. The depressed subchondral fragments can be disimpacted by introducing an elevator through the articular splits. If the depression is central without a significant displacement of the rim, a round headed bone grafting punch can be introduced via a cortical window and elevation of the articular fragments can be done en masse. Once the articular surface is restored, large peri-articular clamps can be placed on top of fixation plates. A few subarticular K wires piercing the opposite cortex and skin are inserted to provide sufficient preliminary stability for detailed fluoroscopic assessment before committing to the fixation. Once the reduction is confirmed, subarticular raft screws are placed. Long 3.5 mm cortical screws provide better support as raft screws than 6.5 mm cancellous screws.

Deep positions of the articular surface are not always easily assessed with the sub-meniscus approach and articular depressions and gaps may be missed. Intraoperative use of fluoroscopy remains the best for assessment of articular reduction and the overall mechanical alignment. The lateral plateau is slightly convex and 2–3 mm cranial to the concave medial plateau, therefore constituting to the normal 3° medial sloping in the anteroposterior (AP) view. Residual depression of the lateral plateau is easily overlooked if the above features are not accounted for. The posterior tibial plateau is sloped downwards at around 5°. Therefore, the true anteroposterior view of the plateau is best obtained by slight knee flexion where the X-ray beam is directed parallel to the articular surface. On the lateral view, medial and lateral plateaus surfaces can be individual assessed by slightly shifting the lower limb in adduction or abduction. 3D-Fluroscopy are invaluable for intraoperative assessment of the articular surface. For all proximal tibial fractures, the neutral AP mechanical axis of the lower limb should be obtained with a long metal rod or straight diathermy wire passing though the hip-knee-ankle centreline.

Small articular depressions can be mechanically supported by tricalcium phosphate bone substitute granules filling in subarticular bone defects. They can provide good mechanical strength and support with less malunion and subsidence. The majority of the bone substitutes can be incorporated within 6 months. Autogenous bone graft is not indicated, especially in the face of the osteopenic nature of the graft. Then the metaphyseal splits and depressions are buttressed to contain the articular rim. Finally, the metaphysical and shaft extensions are bridged with

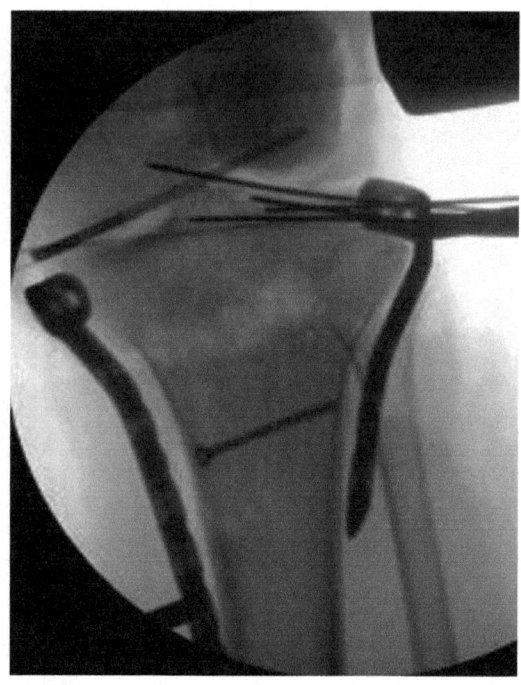

Fig. 11.11 Placement of subchondral K wires to maintain reduced fragments. In some cases, these can be cut short to stay buried inside the subchondral bone

the correct mechanical axis. The general principle of long spanning fixation applies to osteoporotic bone where fixation is commonly extended to the mid-distal tibial shaft (Figs. 11.11, 11.12 and 11.13).

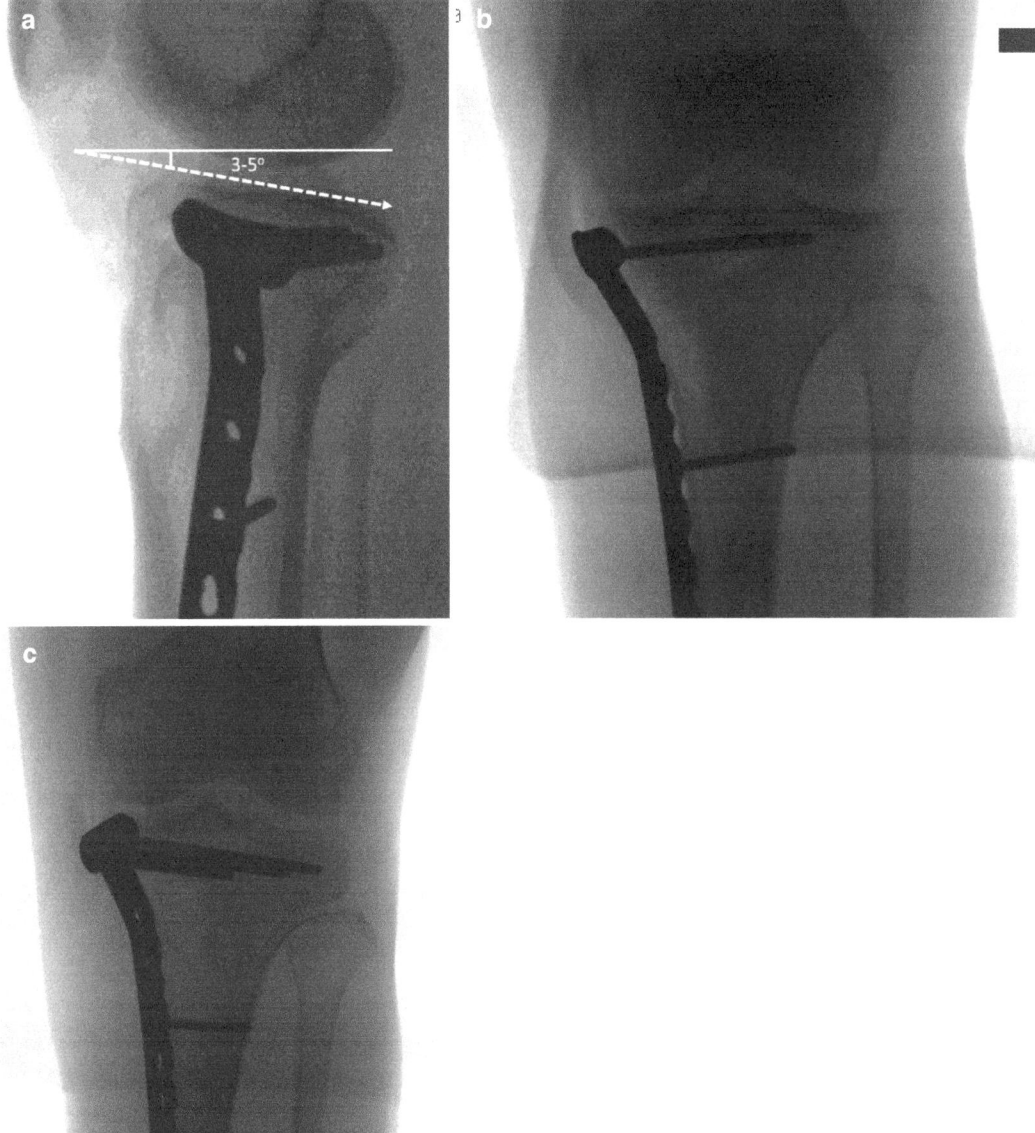

Fig. 11.12 The proximal tibial joint surface has a 3–5° posterior slope (**a**) therefore when screening for the AP fluoroscopy, the X-ray beam should be directed towards this plane by slight flexion of the knee (**b**). The plateau joint surface is obscured with the X-ray beam oriented vertically (**c**)

Fig. 11.13 Patient with Schatzker II fracture and a background of knee osteoarthritis and varus alignment. Full correction of the depression is unnecessary. The depressed lateral plateau is stabilized by minimal invasive osteosynthesis using a locking plate and subarticular raft screws. Immediate full-weight bearing is allowed. Patient is independently ambulatory and pain free with opportunistic correction of the pre-existing varus alignment

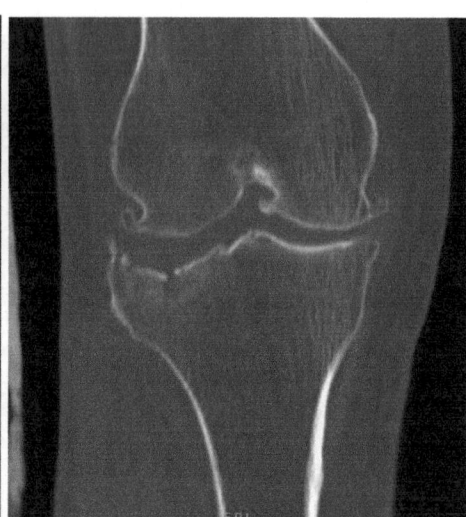

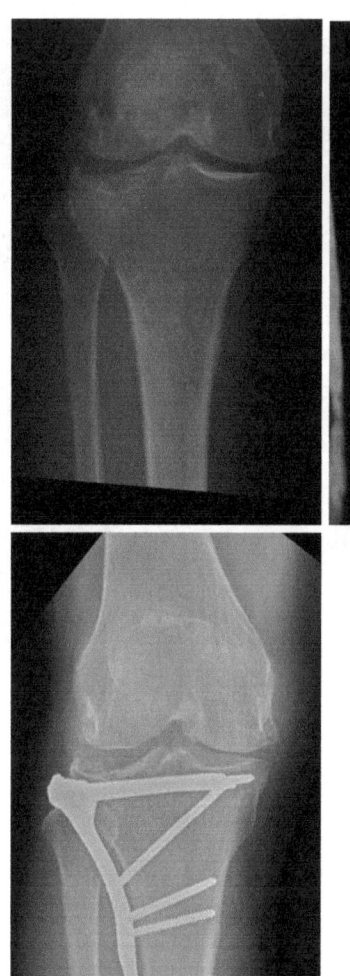

11.4 Intramedullary Nail Fixation

Intramedullary (IM) fixation of the tibia is the standard treatment for mid and distal tibial shaft fractures but less so in proximal tibial fractures. IM nailing is useful for elderly with easily reducible proximal or segmental shaft extension fractures. Because of osteoporosis and inferior mechanical stability, intramedullary nailing is technically demanding of proximal tibia metaphyseal fractures. The use of blocking (Poller) screws is commonly needed, and correct identification of the entry site is critical. Compared to plating, the use of intramedullary nailing is associated with higher risk of valgus and procurvatum deformity but a lower risk of soft tissue and wound complications. While the supra-patellar approach for nailing may facilitate reduction and entry site placement, this is unsuitable for patients with knee osteoarthritis and a tight joint capsule.

11.5 External Fixation

The use of external fixation is generally reserved as a temporary measure for higher energy fractures, open fractures, and those with significant soft tissue compromise. Early loosening is common in osteoporotic bone. Cumbersome equipment, and pin tract infections risks are generally not well tolerated by the elderly.

11.6 Total Knee Arthroplasty (TKA)

Non-reconstructable articular fractures and patients with pre-existing osteoarthritis benefit from immediate TKA with favourable outcomes [10]. Patients are allowed full-weight bearing and a secondary surgery following failed fracture repair is avoided. TKA using a posterior stabilized prosthesis is straightforward when the articular depression is contained without disruption of the metaphyseal cortical rim. This is less so with large metaphyseal fragment when the collateral ligaments are compromised, necessitating the use of stemmed and semi-constrained implants [11]. Adjunctive peri-prosthetic fixation with long spanning plates may be necessary in special situations. It is noteworthy that proximal tibial fracture managed with primary [12] or secondary [13] TKA carries a higher risk of complications such as infection, stiffness and implant loosening than patients receiving primary TKA for osteoarthritis and the functional results are slightly inferior (Fig. 11.14).

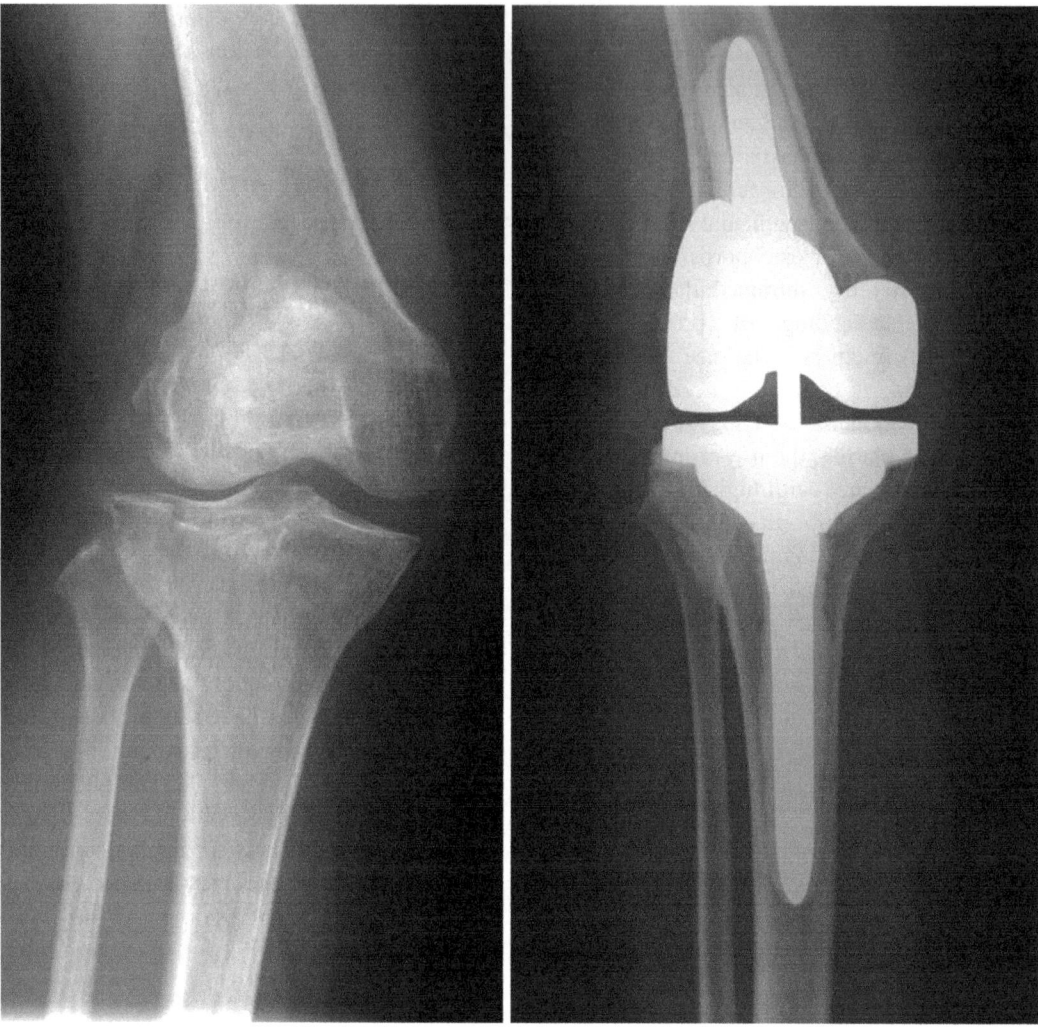

Fig. 11.14 Elderly with delayed presentation of a split depressed lateral plateau fracture. The fracture is already partially united. Fracture repair was deemed too difficult and a stemmed semi-constrained TKA is performed with good outcome

11.7 Rehabilitation

Elderly patients with impaired cognitive function are generally unable to comply with limited weight bearing regimen. Postoperative bracing is of minimal role and immobilization beyond 2 weeks following surgery leads to poor outcomes [14, 15]. Patients are practically either allowed full-weight bearing [16] or no weight bearing at all. This is the reason why surgical fixation should be sufficiently stable for immediate weight bearing. Slight trade-offs regarding maintenance of fracture reduction are favourably offset by the benefits of routine early mobility and ambulation of the elderly. Range of motion exercise should be started immediately. The use of continuous passive mobilization devices is beneficial for early range and stiffness prevention. End range exercise is best prescribed manually because continuous passive mobilization is only effective through the mid-range of motion.

11.8 Outcomes

In general, tibial plateau fractures in the elderly have favourable results. Slight steps or gaps on the lateral articular surface <3 mm are well tolerated provided that the mechanical axis is restored. Complications of proximal tibial fractures are most often related to soft tissue, wound breakdown, and infections. Knee osteoarthritis is common after tibial plateau fractures especially with failed articular reduction, but only a minority of patients would eventually undergo knee arthroplasty. Implant removal is generally avoided for the elderly except for symptomatic implant impingement.

11.9 Summary

Proximal tibial fractures are challenging to manage in the elderly. Non-operative treatment by immobilization of the knee joint is suitable for minority of patients with undisplaced stable fractures. For the majority of patients with displaced and unstable fractures, the objective is to restore the mechanical axis of the lower limb and articular congruity. Stable internal fixation and early mobilization are associated with good outcomes. Pre-existing osteoporosis, osteoarthritis, medical comorbidities and thin, soft tissue envelope are important surgical considerations in preventing complications.

References

1. Schatzker J. Compression in the surgical treatment of fractures of the tibia. Clin Orthop Relat Res. 1974;105:220–39.
2. Chang S-M, et al. A surgical protocol for bicondylar four-quadrant tibial plateau fractures. Int Orthop. 2014;38(12):2559–64.
3. Martínez-Rondanelli A, et al. Reliability of a four-column classification for tibial plateau fractures. Int Orthop. 2017;41(9):1881–6.
4. Kfuri M, Schatzker J. Revisiting the Schatzker classification of tibial plateau fractures. Injury. 2018;49(12):2252–63.
5. Frosch KH, et al. A new posterolateral approach without fibula osteotomy for the treatment of tibial plateau fractures. J Orthop Trauma. 2010;24(8):515–20.
6. Yu B, et al. Fibular head osteotomy: a new approach for the treatment of lateral or posterolateral tibial plateau fractures. Knee. 2010;17(5):313–8.
7. Cho JW, et al. Approaches and fixation of the posterolateral fracture fragment in tibial plateau fractures: a review with an emphasis on rim plating via modified anterolateral approach. Int Orthop. 2017;41(9):1887–97.
8. Weil YA, et al. Posteromedial supine approach for reduction and fixation of medial and bicondylar tibial plateau fractures. J Orthop Trauma. 2008;22(5):357–62.
9. Hartigan DE, et al. Arthroscopic-assisted reduction and percutaneous fixation of tibial plateau fractures. Arthrosc Tech. 2015;4(1):e51–5.
10. Wong MT, et al. Understanding the role of total knee arthroplasty for primary treatment of tibial plateau fracture: a systematic review of the literature. J Orthop Traumatol. 2020;21(1):7.
11. Sabatini L, et al. Primary total knee arthroplasty in tibial plateau fractures: literature review and our institutional experience. Injury. 2023;54 Suppl 1:S15–23.
12. Parratte S, Ollivier M, Argenson JN. Primary total knee arthroplasty for acute fracture around the knee. Orthop Traumatol Surg Res. 2018;104(1s):S71–s80.
13. Aurich M, Koenig V, Hofmann G. Comminuted intraarticular fractures of the tibial plateau lead to posttraumatic osteoarthritis of the knee: current treatment review. Asian J Surg. 2018;41(2):99–105.
14. Gausewitz S, Hohl M. The significance of early motion in the treatment of tibial plateau fractures. Clin Orthop Relat Res. 1986;202:135–8.
15. Polat B, et al. Factors influencing the functional outcomes of tibia plateau fractures after surgical fixation. Niger J Clin Pract. 2019;22(12):1715–21.
16. Williamson M, et al. Immediate weight bearing after plate fixation of fractures of the tibial plateau. Injury. 2018;49(10):1886–90.